P9-DNF-923

AIDS

Ethics
and Public
Policy

AIDS

Ethics and Public Policy

CHRISTINE PIERCE
DONALD VANDEVEER
North Carolina State University

Wadsworth Publishing Company
Belmont, California
A Division of Wadsworth, Inc.

Philosophy Editor: Kenneth M. King
Production Editor: Leland Moss
Interior Designer: Donna Davis
Print Buyer: Barbara Britton
Copy Editors: Bill Reynolds & Leland Moss
Compositor: G&S Typesetters, Inc.
Cover: Adriane Bosworth

Printed in the United States of America

2 3 4 5 6 7 8 9 10—92 91 90 89 88

Library of Congress Cataloging-in-Publication Data

AIDS: ethics and public policy.

 Bibliography: p.
 1. AIDS (Disease)—United States—Prevention—Moral
and ethical aspects. 2. AIDS (Disease)—Government
policy—United States. 3. AIDS (Disease)—Patients—
United States—Social conditions. 4. Homosexuality—
Law and legislation—United States. I. Pierce,
Christine. II. VanDeVeer, Donald.
[DNLM: 1. Acquired Immunodeficiency Syndrome.
2. Ethics, Medical. 3. Public Policy. WD 308 A2881]
RA644.A25A362   1988   362.1'969792'00973   87-10695
ISBN 0-534-08286-6

CONTENTS

Preface

We're running scared. . . . [I can]not imagine a worse health problem in this century. . . . We stand nakedly in front of a very serious pandemic as mortal as any pandemic as there ever has been. I don't know any greater killer than AIDS, not to speak of its psychological, social, and economic maiming.

—Dr. Haldan Mahler, head of the World Health Organization

AIDS (acquired immune deficiency syndrome) was identified in 1981. More widespread medical attention developed somewhat later. Serious exploration of questions about the threat to public health and about the ethics of private and public policy responses must be dated in the mid-1980s. Early views about AIDS have been marked by substantial misinformation, frequent recriminations against persons with AIDS, and calls for radical "solutions," such as banishment to an island, tattooing of carriers, quarantine, and wholesale exclusion (or dismissal) from certain workplace situations.

The aim of this collection is not primarily to recount the history of AIDS, to explore biological and medical research, to tell the stories of conflicts or cooperation among various interested parties, or to describe the psychology of persons coping with AIDS. The collection touches on all these matters, but our overriding concern is: *What should we do about the AIDS problem(s)?* Among other things, of course, we should try to find a cure and a vaccine (to heal and to prevent a harm). Such efforts are vigorously under way, after a slow start. Short of achieving such desirable goals, what should be done about the thousands already dying? What will happen to, and what should be done with respect to, the 1–2 million asymptomatic carriers of the AIDS virus in the United States? Who is at risk? What restrictions on liberty are justifiable with respect to these groups, or the public at large, in order to slow or halt the spread of this potentially lethal virus? According to one pessimistic interpretation, of the 2 million carriers in the United States, 30 percent will develop a full-blown syndrome within five years or so. Hence, over half a million persons could die from AIDS by 1991 or so. A more standard prediction estimates about 180,000 cumulative deaths by 1991. (We note here that the figures cited in this volume quickly go out of date. Hence, readers should attend to the temporal context.)

Proposals to mandate screening, to close gay bathhouses, to criminalize certain sexual activities thought to transmit AIDS, to tattoo, to banish, and to exclude carriers—all involve coercive restrictions on the liberty of competent, typically innocent persons. Thus, a wide range of public responses to persons thought to have AIDS or to carry the virus(es) raises the fundamental moral question of just when it is permissible or obligatory to restrict the liberty of competent persons. A good portion of this volume is therefore devoted to an examination of the ethical and public policy aspects of controversies over AIDS.

The materials have been organized along the following general lines. The General Introduction and Part I attempt to provide a broad overview and to focus especially on factual questions about AIDS (what it is, modes of transmission, and so on). To promote a broader perspective, these sections also sketch a number of the actual and possible ways AIDS may be viewed (societal conceptions of the issues, for example). Part II focuses on an identification and examination of the leading (most influential) moral grounds purporting to justify restrictions on liberty. Part III explores specific public policy or legislative proposals for dealing with various aspects of the AIDS crisis (such as mandatory testing or the use of tests by insurance companies) and the concerns they raise regarding privacy, use of test data, job discrimination, funding for health care for persons with AIDS, and so on.

Part IV examines the consequences of a general, widespread tendency to associate AIDS with sexually immoral behavior. The fact that AIDS is often perceived as a disease of gay white males makes it difficult to separate gay issues from AIDS issues. Hence, even though *in principle* it might be possible to discuss proposed policies with respect to coping with an epidemic without discussing the morality of sexual preference as such, it would be unwise to ignore the reality that the moral conviction of many Americans (condemning even consenting adult homosexuality) affects their views about, and reactions to, public policies regarding AIDS. For example, in its June 1986 ruling in *Bowers* v. *Hardwick,* the Supreme Court invoked, in support of the majority opinion (upholding a Georgia statute criminalizing consensual sodomy among homosexuals), the argument that Judeo-Christian morality condemns homosexual behavior. Thus, the Court, by affirming the conviction that only certain "standard" forms of sex are all right, provided implicit justification for the view that it is all right to restrict coercively those whose behavior is nonconventional.

A problem as serious as AIDS tends to bring out the best and the worst in a society. The main aim of this volume is to explore the questions of what is the best and what is the worst—with an eye to answering the key question: What should we do about AIDS?

We are grateful to a number of people for their suggestions, comments, and other help in our research efforts—in particular, Lina Cofresi, Tracy Reid, Arlene Rogers, Alan Soble, Deborah Merritt, Martin Benjamin, Robert Hambourger, and Barbara Levenbook. The overseeing of our production editor Leland Moss was enormously helpful. We also wish to thank our reviewers, Professors Laurence B. McCullough of Georgetown University and Hans Uffelmann of the University of Missouri.

A special thanks to Lisa VanDeVeer and Beth Timson, and, for their patient secretarial assistance, Adea Allen and Ann Rives.

General
Introduction

What AIDS Is

Terms and Definitions.* AIDS (acquired immune deficiency syndrome) is a break-down of the body's immune system caused by the human immunodeficiency virus (HIV);[1] when this occurs, the body is less able to defend itself against various infections and diseases caused by common bacteria, viruses, and parasites. These infections and diseases are referred to as *opportunistic* because they succeed in impairing the body when the immune system is weakened.

Different investigators have isolated the AIDS virus and given it different names. The American researcher Robert Gallo named the virus *human T-lymphotropic virus* (HTLV-III). What is apparently the same virus was labeled *lymphadenopathy-associated virus* (LAV) by the French researcher Luc Montagnier. Often the AIDS virus is referred to as *HTLV-III/LAV*, in an attempt to give credit to both American and French researchers. Recently, an international committee of scientists proposed calling the cause of AIDS by a new, politically neutral name: *human immunodeficiency virus*, or HIV.

AIDS is fatal. Some say this is so by definition, because the term *AIDS* is reserved for "full-blown" cases that result in death. People with lesser illnesses caused by HIV, which nonetheless range from mild to serious, are said to have *ARC* (AIDS-related complex). Lastly, there are asymptomatic carriers of HIV: those who are infected with HIV and presumably capable of infecting others but who show no clinical symptoms of AIDS; for this condition we coin the acronym *ACH*, for asymptomatic carriers of HIV. In March, 1987 the Centers for Disease Control in Atlanta proposed a revised definition of AIDS which might, if employed, raise the number of cases categorized as AIDS as much as 20 percent.[2]

A Few Statistics. In 1981, when AIDS was first recognized in the United States, there were fewer than 60 cases. As of November 1986, there were 27,000 cases of AIDS and 15,000 deaths from the disease.[3] As of March 1987, there were more than 32,000 cases of AIDS and about 20,000 deaths.[4] Beginning in 1990, according to Dr. Frank Press, president of the National Academy of Sciences, "we will lose as many Americans each year to AIDS as we lost in the entire Vietnam War."[5] About 58,000

---

*For a number of technical terms, see the glossary near the end of this volume.

Americans died in that war. According to federal health officials, 1–1.5 million Americans are now asymptomatic carriers of HIV;[6] the Public Health Service estimates a cumulative total of 270,000 cases and 179,000 deaths in the United States by 1991.[7] As of 1987, no cure had been found.

A Terrible Death. Many people with AIDS develop a rare form of pneumonia (pneumocystis carinii pneumonia, or PCP), and many others suffer from Kaposi's sarcoma (KS), a skin cancer evidenced by purple lesions. People with AIDS are also attacked by other infections, viruses, and fungi, such as herpes; Epstein-Barr virus (the suspected cause of mononucleosis); cryptococcosis, a fungus that may infect the skin, body organs, lungs, or brain; and *Candida*, or thrush, a yeast infection often seen in newborn babies whose immune systems are not fully developed. The case of a 31-year-old man who was hospitalized with thrush is described by Dr. Michael Gottlieb of UCLA's School of Medicine: "The man had been admitted . . . with candidiasis of the esophagus so bad he could hardly breathe. His throat was blocked by the fluffy white growth."[8] Frequent fecal incontinence is not unusual. When the virus crosses the blood-brain barrier, dementia may set in.

Because AIDS was first discovered among gay men in New York, Los Angeles, and San Francisco, society has externalized its anxiety over AIDS by directing it toward an enemy, and that enemy has been homosexuality. Meanwhile, gay men have had to deal with death not only in terms of its physical and psychological terrors, but also within a context of social alienation and invisibility. Michael Bronski describes this experience:

> There is very little—and in many cases *no*—social, legal, or psychological support from outside of the gay community to help deal with these issues. There are no secure legal rights for homosexual lovers, many times no hospital visiting privileges for gay friends. But most of all there is no basic respect for the gay world in which the person with AIDS has lived his life.
>
> It is hard being a gay male today and not think of AIDS all of the time. In Boston, a city that has not been very hard hit by the epidemic, I know of 15 men who have died or been diagnosed. People who live in New York or San Francisco may know as many as 30 or 40 men who have died or who have AIDS.
>
> Because the gay male community is large and loosely knit—made up of groups of friends as well as large socializing networks or bars and baths—it is possible to know a great many people casually or just by sight. It has become commonplace over the last two years to presume that a bar regular may be dying or dead if he is absent for a while. The friendship networks are informal enough that one might not know who to ask about a missing man. Often the news of a friend's diagnosis is simply too hard to talk about in the bars or baths the man used to frequent. Sometimes it feels like living under a fascist regime as people just disappear without a word. . . .
>
> [P]apers like the *Bay Area Reporter* in San Francisco run every week anywhere from 10 to 20 obituaries of regular, everyday gay men who have died of AIDS. This is a chilling sight to see, a regular *memento mori*, especially because many

people first see the paper in bars or other gay establishments where it is given away.

Of course, the straight press is still worse. . . . There is no mention of the 37-year-old underwriter for an insurance company who died after being hospitalized for eight months and leaves no family because they have not spoken to him since he moved from upstate New York eighteen years ago after telling him that he was gay. Nor was AIDS cited in the extensive obituaries of a Boston Latino community leader who died of respiratory complications at the age of 35 this spring. Every time this happens, every time one of these obituaries appears, it is not only AIDS that is rendered invisible, but also the existence of all gay people.[9]

What Causes AIDS

It is now believed that AIDS is caused in important part by a virus that is primarily spread by sexual contact, the sharing of contaminated needles, or the transfusion of infected blood products. Normally, viral and fungal diseases are repelled by certain white blood cells called *T-lymphocytes* or *T-cells*. The AIDS virus attacks the subset of T-cells known as *T-4* or "helper" cells, which defend the body against infections. When the immune system is working properly, it destroys antigens—substances that the system recognizes as foreign. According to Dr. Susanna Cunningham-Rundles of Memorial Sloan-Kettering Hospital in New York, "We've never before encountered a primary immune-regulatory illness—one that doesn't need a specific infection or antigen to cause immune changes. In AIDS any infection will cause a further imbalance of the immune system. It's like a computer that has been programmed so that any input will result in a distorted picture."[10]

Genuine medical controversy exists over whether AIDS is caused by a single virus (such as HIV) alone, or whether cofactors are involved in getting the disease. As of 1986, only 20–30 percent of those infected with HIV were developing full-blown AIDS. Such data suggest that cofactors may account for why some infected people develop the disease and some do not. Life-style, environmental conditions, other viruses (such as those causing African swine fever), and the use of certain drugs (especially "poppers," or amyl and butyl nitrates) are among the factors that challenge the view that HIV is the sole cause of AIDS. Among the least plausible suggestions regarding causes is the conjecture that "AIDS is the result of being bombarded by strobe lights."[11]

Transmission of AIDS

Some modes of transmission are well established and some not. We list the main modes here.

1. *Established modes of transmission*
   a. Anal intercourse
   b. Vaginal intercourse

    c. Intravenous needles and syringes

    d. Blood transfusions

    e. Pregnancy

2. *Possible modes of transmission*

    a. Oral sex

       (1) Swallowing semen

       (2) Oral-anal contact ("rimming")

    b. Kissing—in other words, the exchange of saliva, as in "wet kissing," "French kissing," or "deep kissing"

    c. Sharing household items that may come into contact with blood, such as toothbrushes or razors

    d. Being bitten by infected insects

Dr. Gerald Friedland, a physician who has treated nearly 300 men and women with AIDS, maintains that the sort of proof we now have about the transmission of HIV amounts to little more than "circumstantial evidence." He distinguishes between biological proof and epidemiological proof:

> To obtain biological proof of how the virus is transmitted, as opposed to epidemiological proof—which is essentially circumstantial evidence—we would have to take infected body fluids, inject them into subjects, and wait for infection to occur. Because this is impossible to do in humans, researchers must find an animal that can become infected with the virus and duplicate the disease. Work in this area began only recently. Today, we can only make admittedly circumstantial assumptions about how the virus is transmitted.[12]

Friedland does not raise important questions about the ethics of experimenting on animals,[13] nor does he admit that circumstantial evidence can be compelling. He simply laments that the small amount of work done in this area forces us to rely on epidemiological evidence.

Epidemiology, a discipline concerned with tracking and discovering the cause(s) of an epidemic, uses such techniques as interviews and statistical studies of the behavior patterns of those afflicted with the disease. Like a detective, a researcher must figure out what questions to ask. Harold Jaffe reports: "I found myself hanging around Spanish Harlem looking for drugs to buy, and sitting at card tables in neighborhoods in which homosexuals live, asking impertinent questions and trying to get a fix on what it was they might be doing or coming into contact with that was making them so ill."[14] Over time questions like the following have come to assume importance: (1) How many sexual partners have patients had in an average month? (2) How many patients regularly use poppers? (3) How many health care workers who take care of AIDS patients develop AIDS themselves? Epidemiologically speaking, the frequency of AIDS in people having multiple sex-partners suggests that repeated exposure to the virus may be necessary. The absence of AIDS in those who care for AIDS patients (both health workers and families) suggests that AIDS is not spread by casual contact; the fact that "needle sticks" with contaminated blood are, for the most part, insufficient to give AIDS to health care workers leads us to believe that one must receive a fairly large dose of HIV to get AIDS. In one study of 543 nurses who accidentally cut or stabbed themselves while tending AIDS patients, only two caught the virus.[15] Hence, one probably cannot get AIDS from a mosquito because the amount of infected blood transferred is insignificant.[16]

Although HIV has been found in many body fluids, only blood and semen have been implicated as common sources of infection. Activities in which semen is exchanged (such as when a male ejaculates into his partner's anus) or blood is exchanged (such as the reuse of needles among IV drug users) can almost certainly transmit the AIDS virus. However, because HIV has also been isolated in saliva, tears, and vaginal secretions, it is reasonable to suppose that *any* body fluids that contain lymphocytes, including urine, feces, and cervical secretions, may harbor the virus.

This uncertainty makes safe-sex guidelines difficult to write. Some authors, for instance, include warnings against "fisting" (the insertion of a hand into the anus) and the sharing of anal sex toys in the same category with warnings against anal intercourse. In fact, given all the various possible definitions of the term *sexual intercourse,* any attempt to explain modes of transmission of the AIDS virus must describe explicit sexual practices and not leave meanings to the imagination (or lack thereof) of the reader.

Safe-sex guidelines also need to be explicit as to who is at risk. Some scientists maintain that HIV is more efficiently transmitted through anal sex than vaginal sex, thus implying that heterosexuals who practice only vaginal intercourse are at very low risk. However, the possibility of heterosexual transmission is not in question. The *New England Journal of Medicine* reported an example of sexual transmission of HIV from a man to a woman to a man: A 37-year-old married man engaged in homosexual activity while on business trips in New York. He and his 33-year-old wife had vaginal intercourse accompanied by heavy mouth-kissing about twice a month. After her husband died from pneumocystis carinii pneumonia, the wife had a sexual relationship with a 26-year-old male neighbor. She too then died from PCP. The neighbor, who developed ARC, reported no drug use and no sexual contact except for the above-mentioned relationship, which included only vaginal intercourse and deep kissing.[17]

Comparatively few cases of vaginal transmission (particularly from woman to man) exist today. The "efficiency thesis" attempts to explain this fact: The lining of the anus is thought to be easily torn, thus facilitating the entry of infected semen into the bloodstream. "The rugged vagina," in the words of John Langone, unlike "the vulnerable rectum," is "designed to withstand the trauma of intercourse . . . ."[18] Although it may be true that rectums and vaginas are respectively tender and tough, it has not been demonstrated that a traumatic event is necessary for the transmission of HIV. Artificial insemination is not a traumatic procedure, yet women can get AIDS from undergoing this process if the sperm is contaminated. Moreover, if it turns out that HIV can cross mucous membranes (the possibility of which is as yet unknown), no trauma will be required to transmit AIDS.

Who Gets AIDS

The major groups at risk for AIDS in the United States today are:

Sexually active homosexual and bisexual men

Intravenous (IV) drug users

Regular recipients of blood transfusions (such as hemophiliacs)

People who are sexually intimate with those infected with HIV

Newspapers and magazines repeatedly report that gay and bisexual men make up 73 percent of AIDS cases. Even "Facts About AIDS," a brochure released by the United States Department of Health and Human Services, cites this figure. Statistics, however, can be misleading. Until July 1986, the Centers for Disease Control (CDC) in Atlanta, Georgia (the organization that is the main source of statistical data on AIDS in the United States), automatically classified any gay or bisexual man as a homosexual, even if he also happened to be a hemophiliac or an intravenous drug user. In its July 28, 1986 weekly report, the CDC added "Homosexual Male and IV Drug User" as a new transmission category.[19] However, as Jonathan Lieberson points out, the effect of the CDC's long-standing reporting practice on this matter is that the number of cases contracted through needles has been insufficiently recognized.[20] Biologist Chris Jennings estimates that 12 percent of all gay or bisexual men with AIDS are also IV drug users and may have caught AIDS that way.[21] Thus, even disregarding hemophiliacs (who account for just under 1 percent of AIDS cases), less than 65 percent of all people with AIDS are *simply* gay or bisexual men. Furthermore, Jennings warns, the CDC defines a man as "homosexual" if he has had one homosexual encounter in his lifetime.[22] If we were to use this definition of homosexual in ordinary speech, the number of men in our society counted as gay would rise considerably. In the view of Dr. Robert Redfield, an infectious-disease specialist at the Walter Reed Army Institute of Research in Washington, D.C., there has been considerable "bean-counting epidemiology, where you only recognize patients who fall into categories that epidemiologists have already decided exist. If you were a male who'd had more than one homosexual experience, you were automatically a homosexual. If you were a female prostitute who'd slept with 2,500 men, but you'd shot up heroin twice five years ago, you went into the IV drug-user caseload."[23]

IV drug users are commonly reported as constituting 17 percent of United States AIDS cases. Jennings attaches the 17-percent figure to *heterosexual* IV drug users.[24] If we add 12 percent, as he suggests, to include homosexuals and bisexuals who may have caught AIDS by IV drug use, the problem of drug abuse looms larger than we might otherwise suppose. In certain geographical areas, the drug problem is an enormous one. For example, 34 percent of New York and 53 percent of New Jersey AIDS cases are attributable to IV drug use.[25] Newark, says Wayne Barrett of *The Village Voice*, "with virtually no gay community, now has the fourth largest caseload in the country."[26]

Although at present women make up only about 7 percent of AIDS cases in the

United States, new statistical studies as described in the press are ominous. Dr. James Curran, head of AIDS research at the Centers for Disease Control, has stated that "in certain pockets of the U.S. and among new military recruits, the proportions of infected men and women are approaching equality." [27]

In central Africa and Haiti—where AIDS has reached epidemic proportions—roughly equal numbers of women and men are affected. In the mid-section of Africa, sometimes referred to as "the AIDS belt," an estimated 10,000 cases occur every year, and the total cases of AIDS since 1981 number around 50,000—twice the 1986 United States total. [28] Haitians (both in Haiti and in the United States) have AIDS in such large numbers that in the early days of the AIDS crisis, the CDC classified (United States) Haitians as a risk category: "In Miami, the incidence of AIDS is greater than one per thousand Haitians—almost as great as among gays in New York." [29] As a result, Haitians have suffered discrimination in jobs and housing, and their children often have been ostracized. A Haitian taxi driver in New York reported: "I am black and speak with a French accent. For that, my children are not allowed to play with children in school. Now I say I am from Martinique." [30] Storms of protest from insulted Haitians, who feared a decline in the tourist industry in Haiti, resulted in the elimination of the Haitian category and the reclassification of Haitians as "None of the Above/Other." The ethical argument marshaled against the original classification was similar to the one discussed by Ronald Dworkin in Part II of this collection: To "blame" people for who they involuntarily are, whether black, female, or homosexual, rather than what they do, is irrational. Effective July 28, 1986, United States Haitian AIDS cases have been reclassified by the CDC from the "None of the Above/Other" category to "Heterosexual Cases." [31]

Blacks and Hispanics constitute 40 percent of U.S. AIDS cases [32]—a disproportionately high percentage, given that blacks represent 12 percent of the United States population, while Hispanics account for 6 percent. Black women account for 52 percent of all female cases of AIDS in the U.S., and at least 60 percent of the children with AIDS are black. [33] The study of military recruits mentioned above found that "black men and women are showing evidence of exposure to the disease at a rate four times that of whites." [34]

Although not often included in reports of AIDS cases, lesbians are a statistically significant category in one major respect: As of May 1986, not a single case of lesbian-to-lesbian transmission has been medically documented. [35] Of course, a lesbian could get AIDS: She might be an IV drug user, or she might have had sexual relations with a man. Or she might have gotten HIV from a blood transfusion, an organ transplant, or semen used for artificial insemination.

Even celibates can get AIDS through blood transfusions, organ transplants, contaminated needles, or *in utero*. In New York City alone this year, some 2,000 HIV-infected women will become pregnant. [36] The chance of these women passing the virus to their children is estimated to be between 5 and 56 percent. [37]

Perceptions of
Who Gets AIDS

To date, media attention, public health efforts, and righteous indignation have focused much more on the gay community than on IV drug users. AIDS has often been referred to as the "gay plague." Wayne Barrett complains: "There is, ironically, a greater governmental investment in public health efforts targeted at gays than there is in attacking it among junkies, despite the obvious fact that junkies are much more likely to transmit AIDS to the rest of society."[38] Dr. June E. Osborn, dean of the School of Public Health at the University of Michigan, agrees that IV drug use is the primary way in which AIDS will spread among heterosexuals in the United States; she sees it as "the great gaping hole in the dike as far as AIDS spreading into new and different segments of society."[39]

Although the issue of closing gay bathhouses and other gay establishments has received much public attention, no similar outcry has arisen to close the more than 1,000 shooting galleries in New York City. One may wonder how many Americans know what a "shooting gallery" is. Yet Freddy, a 29-year-old AIDS patient, tells the following story:

> "People come in and out of the galleries like they ride the subway. Twenty-four hours a day," Freddy says. "Inside galleries, there are boxes of needles. You don't know if you're getting a clean one or a used one." According to Freddy, many junkies who have difficulty finding veins pay "hitmen" who work the galleries to shoot them up. Neck, groin, and chest specialists frequently shoot all day with the same needle.[40]

Some IV drug users gather in groups of 40–50 in abandoned buildings to share their drug experiences in a communal way. The same hypodermic needle is handed from user to user in what is described as a "blood-bonding rite."[41] Not all IV users participate in what might be called a "junkie life-style." We must envision as well the youth who, instead of choosing to drink beer, is tempted to try a shooting gallery.

There has been little or no public uproar about drug use (either habitual or recreational) in relation to AIDS. There has been no criticism by feminists to the effect that because AIDS is primarily a disease of males (upwards of 90 percent of AIDS cases are male), men, by and large, are responsible for spreading it. Arye Rubinstein, a professor of microbiology and immunology who directs the AIDS research program at Albert Einstein College of Medicine in New York, said he had found "in his hospital that most pregnant women who were told they were infected with the AIDS virus did not want to abort their fetuses, because they believed they would die and wanted their children to outlive them."[42] Yet there has been no public outrage concerning this intentional risk of harm to fetuses and/or future human beings. No significant ethical or political conclusions have been drawn from the fact that 40 percent of AIDS victims are black or Hispanic. In August 1986, a group of black and white fundamentalist ministers tried to recall the mayor of Durham, North Carolina, for signing a proclamation against discrimination based on sexual preference. In the minds of these ministers, one bad consequence of a tolerant attitude toward gay men and lesbians would be the admission of AIDS patients from other cities and AIDS research at Duke University Hospital.[43] As the controversy raged in the newspapers, no one said, "We don't want AIDS patients here because they are black IV drug users" (despite the fact that infected IV users in New York City are mostly minority men).[44]

The public perceives AIDS as a disease of male homosexuals partly because gay males have rallied as a group in response to the threat of AIDS, whereas blacks and IV drug users have not.[45] New York City's Gay Men's Health Crisis (GMHC), founded in September 1981, has an annual operating budget of $4 million, only 40 percent of which is supplied by the U.S. government. Gay magazines and newspapers repeatedly publish safe-sex guidelines. There is even a collection of short fiction—called *Hot Living: Erotic Stories about Safer Sex*—that attempts to make responsible sex enjoyable and desirable.[46]

AIDS is also perceived as the gay plague for historical reasons. In an article entitled "Heterosexuals: A New Risk Group," Christopher Norwood says:

> While the first man to have contracted AIDS from a woman was diagnosed in 1982, the first homosexual male patient had been diagnosed in 1978. This lag gave Americans four years to convince themselves that HTLV-III was the first virus in the universe to target a sexual orientation. The CDC did not establish "heterosexual contact" cases as a reporting category until June 1984.[47]

Dennis Altman, a noted author on AIDS and the gay community, also points to the influence of certain historical accidents in our conceptualization of AIDS. Altman says, "Had this disease been first recognized in Central Africa, where there appears to be no homosexual link whatsoever involved in its transmission, and had it then, later on, been discovered among those people whom it is known to affect in other parts of the world, it would, I suspect, have been seen by all of us very differently."[48] In addition, Altman mentions another phenomenon—which he calls "first world centeredness"—that clearly plays a role in the way Americans view AIDS. As Altman puts it, one of the ways in which

> the AIDS story, the treatment of AIDS, becomes the same as the gay story and the treatment of homosexuality . . . is the somewhat racist [aspect], and certainly first world centeredness, of our view whereby the many thousands of people who are dying from AIDS in Central Africa have somehow been removed from our vision. We don't think about them, they are not part of this epidemic, yet the reality is . . . the majority of people who are dying of this disease live in third world countries and are not in any sense gay men.[49]

On a worldwide basis, AIDS is primarily a black, heterosexual disease. Facts about Uganda and Zaïre, however, are very unsexy; of much more interest to Americans is the fact that the first 50 gay male AIDS patients studied each had an average of 1,100 sexual partners in their lifetimes. Sexy facts—especially when they concern a group that is hated and feared—are the stuff of which public perceptions are made.

Conjectures About Origins

Some Americans and Europeans have conjectured that AIDS originated in the African green monkey. According to this view, infected Haitians brought the disease from Africa to Haiti. The virus then made its way to New York via gay men who had vacationed in Haiti.

Another theory holds that HIV was developed as part of a government germ warfare program. Some attribute this program to the Soviet Union, while others implicate the CIA. It has even been suggested that the CIA-developed virus was intentionally (but secretly) tested on gay men. Whatever the truth, neither the CIA nor green monkeys have been the victims of widespread blame.

Groups Versus Behavior

Dr. Mathilde Krim, who chairs the AIDS Medical Foundation in New York, has recommended that "[t]he breakdown of reported cases of AIDS into 'risk groups' be abandoned."[50] In her testimony at a government subcommittee hearing, she said that

> since [this practice] highlights the sexual inclinations of one group and does not do so for others, it has contributed significantly to the erroneous interpretation that AIDS was, one, exclusively a "gay disease," and, two, a disease of a world alien to that of most "good Americans." In New York, the public is now astounded to learn suddenly that over 30 percent of AIDS patients are heterosexuals, whether drug abusers or not, and that there may be close to half a million people infected by HTLV-III in this city, many of whom are heterosexuals who certainly are having sexual relations with other heterosexual men and women, and so pass on the infection.[51]

If we abandoned talk about "high-risk groups" in favor of talk about "high-risk behavior," some misleading readings of the data could be clarified, as the following examples show. When two males engage in anal sex, Haitians do not consider the active partner a homosexual. Male homosexuality, then, is defined according to a conception of masculinity, not by the gender of the partner. Hence, the above-mentioned effort on the part of the CDC to reclassify Haitian AIDS cases as "heterosexual" is to some extent suspect. Conversely, some members of the group classified by the CDC as "homosexual" may in fact be primarily heterosexual. To support the view that AIDS in the United States is not spreading to heterosexuals in any alarming way, John Langone states that according to the CDC, about 93 percent of AIDS cases fall into two major high-risk groups: "homosexuals . . . and the estimated 750,000 Americans who inject heroin and other illicit drugs at least once a week."[52] Langone defines "homosexuals" as "some 2.5 million men, ages 16 to 55, who are exclusively homosexual throughout their lives, and some 5 million to 10 million others who have had even one homosexual contact."[53] Surely a significant number of these 5–10 million "homosexuals" who are not exclusively so have also engaged in heterosexual activity. Risk of AIDS, then, is not so much a matter of what group one is in, but rather of what one does—that is, of one's *behavior*.

AIDS and Afraids

In the lyrics of a song about AIDS and the public's reaction to it, songwriter Tom Wilson Weinberg writes, "Now we need a cure for two diseases." The first disease is AIDS; the second—a disease in a metaphorical sense—is the public hysteria surrounding AIDS. Two physicians recently remarked: "Historically, the sudden appearance of any new disease has always elicited some fear; however, the transmissible nature of this fatal disease has escalated fear to phobia, as public dread of AIDS spreads rapidly through the country."[54] Public fear is largely a curious mixture of homophobia (fear of homosexuality) and the fear of catching AIDS through casual contact. Examples follow:

> An AIDS patient arrived at North Carolina Memorial Hospital (from another small hospital) in a body bag normally used to ship a corpse. Nurse Suzi W. Perry reported: "They'd zipped it up." Sticking out the top was a small air tube so that the patient could breathe. When the nurses unzipped the bag, the patient blinked. "He was alert and well oriented."[55]

> Forty-four percent of Americans, according to a Gallup poll, are avoiding places where they expect homosexuals to be as a precaution against contracting AIDS.[56]

> Delta Airlines proposed a rule to forbid carrying AIDS patients. (The proposal was dropped in February 1985.)[57]

> A telephone company attempted to sell disposable telephones for AIDS patients to hospitals in Arkansas. A sales brochure recommended that "patients be told when they are admitted that they must purchase one of the phones as part of the hospital's 'infection control policy.'"[58]

> While Rock Hudson lay in a hospital dying from AIDS, Americans worried about whether Linda Evans (who kissed Hudson on the television series *Dynasty*) might contract the disease.[59]

> Realtors in California were instructed by their association to advise prospective home buyers about whether a house on the market had been owned by an AIDS patient.[60]

> A sculpture of two men standing next to each other and two women sitting together—called "Gay Liberation"—is on loan from New York City to a park in Madison, Wisconsin. The Madison Park Commission voted unanimously to allow the sculpture a temporary home. Critics of the Commission's decision said their reasons to reject the statue were the Bible, motherhood, and AIDS. One woman who objected to the statue said that "one of the men is well endowed and one of the women doesn't wear underwear."[61]

Arkansas Health Department officials publicly stated that "it would be almost impossible for anyone to contract AIDS from using the telephone."[62] Jim Fauntleroy, the reporter of the Madison sculpture story, commented, "[W]e have reason to believe [that AIDS] cannot be transmitted by even the most intimate contact with a life-size bronze statuary group."[63]

Prospects and Projections

In four years, the CDC research staff grew from a few researchers to nearly 100 scientists and other full-time workers. The research endeavor expanded from a $2-million-a-year program to one with an annual budget of $62 million by the fall of 1986.[64]

At least 61 companies are seeking an AIDS vaccine. Scientists, however, disagree as to whether such a thing is possible. Some predict a vaccine might be ready by 1990; others, wary of predicting dates because the AIDS virus mutates so rapidly, warn that researchers, at any point, may be forced back to the drawing board. HIV modifies its genetic structure so frequently that, in the words of Dr. William Haseltine, "trying to develop a vaccine for AIDS is like trying to hit a moving target."[65] As Dr. Mathilde Krim explains, "It's quite possible that an antibody that works against one strain of the virus might be powerless against another strain, which is exactly the difficulty we have in developing a flu vaccine."[66] Many variants of HIV have been found in a single patient.[67] In December 1986, the World Health Organization announced a plan to test vaccines for AIDS on humans, but vaccines are not expected to be generally available for several years. Indeed, it was reported later in that same month that French and Zaïrian researchers in Zaïre had already inoculated asymptomatic human subjects carrying HIV, with the aim of immunizing such subjects from developing AIDS. In March, 1987, one French researcher, Dr. Daniel Zagury, injected himself with an experimental vaccine and the effect was to enhance his immune system's defense against two varieties of the AIDS virus.[68]

If an effective vaccine were available today, it would not help those who already have AIDS or ARC or are ACH. Their only hope is the development of effective drugs. The U.S. government has announced it will provide $100 million to 14 research centers for drug trials.[69] Azidothymidine (AZT), a drug developed by Burroughs Wellcome Company, has significantly prolonged the lives of some AIDS patients. Initial test results show a lower death rate among patients receiving AZT than among patients in a control group who received placebos. Of those receiving AZT, 1 patient out of 145 has died since testing started in February 1986; 16 of the control group, which numbered 137, have died.[70] AZT is a treatment, not a cure. It does not eliminate the virus. Nonetheless, because a treatment for AIDS is so desperately needed, placebo testing of AZT has ended, and the drug has been made available for compassionate use to (at least) victims of PCP. It was federally approved and made commercially available in the spring of 1987 at which time its annual cost was estimated to be anywhere from $7,000 to $10,000.

In the midst of these difficulties, the rising cost of health care poses important policy problems. Some experts predict that by 1991, it may cost the United States health care system as much as $16 billion to treat AIDS patients.[71] Who should pay? In particular, the role of private insurance companies in this matter is a hotly debated issue. In Part III of this collection, Chambers, Mohr, and Bayer address the policy issues surrounding the costs of insurance and health care.

Despite difficult obstacles, the search for an effective vaccine and utilizable drugs will go on. In the meantime, according to Dr. June E. Osborn, the medical profession "must communicate patiently and clearly to a frightened public":[72]

As always happens in times of panic, fringe groups are arising to raise the level of static and make the message hard to hear, and we will have to shout our message of prevention . . . . [P]reventive medicine—in its drab and unattractive garb— turns out to be the solution. I often like to point out that, if you "do" preventive medicine and public health exactly right, exactly nothing happens and things are very dull. Let us all pray for a little boredom.[73]

Conceptual Matters

It seems a mere truism to say that if we want to think clearly about issues, we need to recognize unclarities or confusions that arise because the concepts or terms we use are imprecise or ambiguous, or that the employment of certain terms presupposes claims or viewpoints that themselves may be controversial and in need of scrutiny.

We shall highlight here a few slippery terms whose uncritical use may generate confusion. As noted earlier, casual talk of a person's "having AIDS" often wanders ambiguously between (1) those who are asymptomatic carriers of HIV (ACHs); (2) those with ARC (AIDS-related complex), who show some limited signs of moderate breakdown of the immune system; and (3) those with AIDS—those who, as a result of a more thorough breakdown of the immune system caused by HIV, have serious diseases, such as Kaposi's sarcoma or pneumocystis carinii pneumonia. In the United States it is estimated that in 1986, 1–3 million people "had AIDS" (were carriers of HIV) in the first sense, but closer to 26,000 in the third sense. Clearly, in appraising proposals to quarantine or cure those who have AIDS, no little difference is made whether we are discussing the first, second, or third populations noted.

Is it all right to discriminate against those with AIDS? A quick argument might proceed as follows: "No, because discrimination is wrong." However, whether we should believe that *all* discrimination is wrong depends, in part, on what we mean by *discrimination*. The term, indeed, is often used to mean at least two quite different things: (1) differential or special treatment; and (2) wrongful differential treatment. We may think that it is fine for a person to be "discriminating" about wines, clothes, art, or whom to marry. To favor one person over another (as in marriage or for a business partner) need not be wrong. However, if what someone means by *discrimination* is wrongful treatment of some sort, then referring to an act or policy as "discriminatory" (in this evaluative sense) assumes that the act or policy is wrong. Maybe it is, but a serious moral question arises here that deserves discussion and argument. The use of value-laden expressions to refer to, or identify, an act or policy is liable to blur two tasks that ought to be kept distinct: identifying an act or policy, and morally appraising it. In the spring of 1986, the United States Department of Justice issued an advisory opinion to the effect that employers reliant on federal funds may dismiss people with AIDS when such employers *believe* that infection of others on the job by such people is a likely result of their retention. At the least, House of Representatives Bill 504 (which prohibits discrimination against the handi-capped) does not, according to the Justice Department, preclude such differential treatment. This policy is "discriminatory" at least in the first sense noted above. Whether it is also wrongfully differential treatment is a substantive ethical issue. We leave it an open question here; at least the matter cannot be settled by the "quick argument" noted. A fuller discussion surrounding the issues of AIDS and discrimina-tion against the handicapped including a 1987 Supreme Court judgment which ex-tended the protection of HR 504 to those with contagious diseases can be found in the preview to Part III.

Let us consider another slippery bit of terminology, one often tossed about with little analysis—*promiscuity*. Many people believe that homosexual acts are wrong and appeal to such an assumption as a reason for placing restrictions on such behav-ior. The claims that homosexual acts are wrong and that if an act is wrong it is all right to restrict the liberty of those who engage or intend to engage in it will receive serious discussion later (in the introduction to Part II). Worth noting here is that one complaint made about some or all homosexuals concerns promiscuity. Whether a person is promiscuous depends on what is meant by "promiscuous" (a conceptual question) as well as what sorts of practices that person engages in (the empirical question). Once more, we suggest that conceptual caution is in order. On reflection it seems that several meanings are associated with the term *promiscuous*:

1. Having a large number of sexual partners
2. Failing to be discriminating in choosing sexual partners
3. Having too many sexual partners
4. Having premarital sex

One who has a series of bona fide marriages might be said to be promiscuous in the first sense. A person who is promiscuous in the first sense may or may not be promiscuous in the second sense. The claim that one is promiscuous in the second sense may involve only an accusation of having bad taste (aesthetically). Analogously, we might observe that a person is only concerned with quantity of food and does not discriminate in terms of quality. More evidently, a moral evaluation often is being expressed when someone is judged promiscuous in the third sense. The question arises: On what moral grounds is a certain number of partners *too* many? Those committed to celibacy believe that one is too many (for them at least). A person who is committed to one other person may believe (reasonably) that two is too many. More generally, labeling someone as promiscuous may be an empirical claim (compare the first sense) or an ethical or moral claim (compare the third sense). Both kinds of claims may need defense, but recognizing what is at issue is a necessary first step. Gay men (but not lesbians) are reputed to have, on average, a large number of sexual partners. Thus, they may be promiscuous in the first sense. It does not follow, of course, from that fact alone that a gay male is promiscuous in the second or third sense. Many heterosexuals are also evidently promiscuous in the sense of having a large number of sexual partners; King Solomon, for example, was described as "wiser than all men" (I Kings 4:31), as one who "loved many strange women" (I Kings 11:1), and who "had seven hundred wives, princesses, and three hundred concubines" (I Kings 11:3). Because homosexuals generally cannot legally marry, any sex they have is *inevitably* pre- or extramarital ("promiscuous" in the fourth sense). The choice is between no sex or extramarital sex. Heterosexual women, of course, can wait until marriage (if they wish), but studies indicate that about 80 percent of women in the United States have sexual intercourse prior to marriage.

Another accusation against homosexuals is that homosexual behavior as such is *unnatural*. This matter is explored in Part IV by David Richards and Richard Mohr, but again it is important to ask if we have a clear conception of what is natural and what is unnatural. Some possible meanings of *unnatural* are

1. Wrongful
2. Statistically unusual
3. Not conducive to reproduction of the species
4. Resulting from human artifice or action

Note that *deviant* wanders between (1) and (2). Homosexual sex, arguably, *is* unnatural in sense (2), (3), and (4). Those facts, however, do not seem to provide any compelling reason for concluding that it is unnatural in the first sense—the sense in which *unnatural* functions as a purely evaluative term. After all, pole vaulting, running in a marathon, the use of contraceptives, celibacy, fasting, and sculpting are all, plausibly, unnatural in senses (2), (3), and (4), but they are not, therefore, wrong. An influential viewpoint in the history of ethical thought, the Natural Law tradition, tends to assume that what's right (obligatory or permissible) is whatever is natural (or some variation on this theme). This approach to moral decision making, as it has been applied to questions about sexuality, is explored in Part IV by Susan Nicholson as well as David Richards. As noted, clarity about these matters depends in a crucial way on discerning what is meant by *natural* and considering reasons for accepting or rejecting an alleged connection between what is right and what is natural, or between what is unnatural and what is wrong.

No little confusion often develops about what is meant by the terms *homosexual* and *homosexuality*. Hence, some further conceptual analysis is in order. If we were to define a homosexual as one who has engaged in sexual relations of some sort with a member of his or her own sex, some interesting implications would result. Studies suggest that about one out of every six adult males has had some such sexual experience by age 18. Intuitively, it seems wrongheaded to classify all such males as homosexuals; evidently many function primarily as heterosexuals, become fathers, and so on. A more plausible definition may be "one whose dominant sexual orientation is toward members of his or her own sex." Dispositional, dominant preferences seem to be the central feature of sexuality, not actual experience. How these orientations arise is an interesting and greatly disputed question that we set aside here. On the suggested dispositional analysis of the category "homosexual," some homosexuals are bisexuals, and many are fathers as well. When one sees claims about percentages of homosexuals who have AIDS or do this or that, it is not always clear whether some of those referred to might fall in other categories (such as "bisexual") as well. We have already noted the potential overlap between two risk categories: homosexual males and IV drug users. We note again that references to AIDS as a "homosexual disease" are misleading in part because hardly any lesbians have AIDS; indeed, more male heterosexuals have AIDS than do lesbians.

John Osborne, in an article in the *National Review*, states that "to be gay is to be obsessed with one's homosexuality. That too is what 'gay' *means*."[74] For reasons noted, that is not what "gay" *means*. Are some gay people obsessed with their sexuality? Undoubtedly, but that is also true of many heterosexuals, notoriously those who are young and male. When society severely stigmatizes people for their sexual orientation and in some subcultures regards "queer bashing" as a sport, those so victimized have special reasons to think a lot about their own sexual preference. Only a few decades ago some men committed suicide when their homosexuality was made public—so great was the social stigma and associated (internalized) shame. One way to recruit spies was to be able (effectively) to threaten to make public that the potential recruit was a homosexual. If heterosexual sex were illegal in many states and if widespread social disdain resulted when, say, a male and a female held hands in public, heterosexuals no doubt would be a bit "obsessive" about their sexual identity. Further, it is important to distinguish between (1) a person's *being* a homosexual and (2) the sexual acts in which a person engages. A homosexual, as we have defined the term, may never engage in "homosexual acts," just as a heterosexual (dispositionally defined) may never engage in heterosexual acts, for reasons ranging from lack of opportunity to castration (young boys used to be castrated in Italy to preserve their soprano voices) to being struck by lightning to moral conviction (as in the case of priests and nuns).

But what is a "homosexual act," and what is a "heterosexual act"? The questions seem deceptively easy to answer. Clear cases abound where only a male-female pair can perform a given sexual act; call such acts "heterosexual," then. But other sexual acts are performable by male-male, by female-female, or by male-female pairs.

In Part IV, a selection is included from the United States Supreme Court decision *Bowers* v. *Hardwick*, which upheld the constitutionality of the Georgia law prohibiting sodomy. *Sodomy* is sometimes defined as oral or anal intercourse. According to one interpretation of "oral intercourse"—fellatio—at least one male is required; so, possible pairings are limited. On the broader analysis sometimes used (as in North Carolina)—contact between the mouth of one person and the sexual organ(s) of another—any pair can conceivably engage in oral intercourse. Indeed, if the skin is a sexual organ (as some say), kissing so counts! *Sodomy* is sometimes defined as anal intercourse involving penetration of one person's anus by another person's penis.

On this analysis, two females ostensibly cannot commit sodomy, but any other pair can. The evidence strongly suggests that HIV can be transmitted through anal intercourse, through vaginal (heterosexual) intercourse, and possibly through oral intercourse (fellatio). These facts are relevant to identifying ways to avoid transmission of the AIDS virus. They also suggest a frequent lack of clarity when people speak generally of homosexual or heterosexual "acts." Anal intercourse, as defined above, or buggery, is a practice of both heterosexuals and male homosexuals (usually thought more common among the latter). As such, it is neither homosexual nor heterosexual. Thus, one sexual means of the spread of the AIDS virus cannot, without serious reservation, be described as "homosexual." Correlatively, the *main* sexual thing to be avoided, to prevent the spread of the AIDS virus, is not homosexuality as such, nor male homosexuality as such, but unprotected intercourse (coitus), traditional or otherwise. In this regard, note that in central Africa the sexual spread of AIDS is said to occur almost solely among heterosexuals.

For centuries, sodomy often has been referred to in U.S. state laws as "the unspeakable crime against nature" (a term that has referred to other acts as well—but *never pollution!*). Being unspeakable, the expressions used to designate certain acts have not been discussed very much; hence, little explicit attention has been paid to them. No wonder, then, that a lack of conceptual clarity often exists about terms people have been reluctant to use—even in the law, where normally it is crucial to specify clearly which acts are criminal so that citizens can voluntarily avoid their performance, if they choose. Numerous arguments are presented in the discussions that follow, close scrutiny of which requires a keen eye and an active search for those terms or expressions that serve more to mystify and obscure than to clarify. Very important policy matters have been and will be decided on the basis of what we believe and how we (or legislators or the courts) are moved by the arguments. Hence, we recommend an active, probing look at other key terms surrounding discussions of AIDS, such as *public health, society, responsible for, cause, liberty, morality, a right, medical issue, moral issue, risk, privacy, decent,* and *autonomy.*

Ethical Matters

Ethical and Empirical Claims. Here we review some basic distinctions in contemporary ethical theory as a step toward sorting and appraising different proposals about what to do concerning AIDS. Earlier we characterized an empirical claim as (roughly) any claim about what is, was, or will be the case and whose truth or falsity is not solely a byproduct of the structure of the sentence or the meanings of the terms. So, "duty is duty" and "bachelors are unmarried" are not empirical claims. Whether true or false, the following are empirical claims:

1. AIDS is caused by a virus.
2. AIDS does not exist in Greenland.
3. Originally, green monkeys had AIDS.
4. AIDS is punishment sent from God.

5. Among males and females, straight and gay, the group at lowest risk for AIDS is gay females.
6. A vaccine for AIDS will be created by 1995.
7. The Reverend Pat Robertson can heal hemorrhoids by faith.

In contrast, a useful, albeit rough, characterization of an ethical or moral claim is: any claim about what rational agents ought or ought not to do (or what is permissible), all relevant things being taken into account—or, relatedly, any claim about what are good or bad traits of character. This characterization is a broad one; in this view ethical claims, contrary to a certain popular inclination to think otherwise, need not be about sex. The following are all ethical claims (reasonable or not):

1. The United States ought unilaterally to reduce its nuclear stockpile.
2. The Soviet Union ought to allow less freedom of speech.
3. Experimentation on animals is all right.
4. Sex in the missionary position is perverse.
5. Dowry murders in India are unjust.

Claims *about* moral beliefs or practices may be empirical claims; for example:

1. Many Nazis thought it permissible to kill Jews.
2. Many Americans prior to the Civil War thought it a duty to return escaped slaves to their masters.
3. The New Testament suggests that wives should be subordinate to their husbands.
4. John Calvin believed that adulterers should be burned to death.

Law and Morality.   Frequently we believe that we should settle questions about what we ought to do by reference to what prevailing law permits or requires. Note, however, that we may believe that what the law requires and what a rational ethical position requires are, in principle, distinct considerations. For example, United States law prior to the Civil War required that one seek to help return escaped slaves to their masters. To the contrary, one may believe, as do we, that slavery is unjust and indeed, that one has a duty *not* to obey such a law. One might hold a similar moral view about Nazi law, which required Jews to identify themselves by wearing yellow stars of David on their clothes. Whether one, by law, must drive less than 55 miles per hour is a legal question. Whether one ought to obey that law or any other law is a moral question. Whether legislatures ought to *change* the laws with respect to abortion, sodomy, euthanasia, or immigration are moral questions that cannot be settled by consulting *existing* law. Of course we often believe that what morality requires (rape is wrong) coincides with the stance of the law (rape is legally prohibited).

A common view is that we have a prima facie moral duty to obey laws duly enacted by a legitimate government. A duty is called "prima facie" (sometimes "conditional") to suggest that sometimes one may be justified in disobeying it. Just when, if at all, disobedience is morally defensible is a substantive question. If duties exist that we must never disobey (or "override"), they might be called "absolute" duties (*absolute* is one of those slippery terms one should scrutinize).

Kinds of Duties. Duties toward others are often divided into those that are positive and those that are negative. A *negative duty* is one whose fulfillment requires us to omit or refrain from treating others (those owed the duty) in a certain manner. A duty not to kill or rape requires one to refrain from performing such acts. A *positive duty* is a duty whose fulfillment requires performance of an act. Duties to return a book, repay a debt, fix a car, host a party, or give blood would all be positive duties.

We may also distinguish between *natural* and *acquired* (or *positive*, in an archaic use of the term) duties. Some duties (the acquired ones) we have only because of some *prior act*, such as a contract or a promise. For example, Michelle has a duty to drive Philip all over Paris, but only because Philip and she have so contracted for Michelle to be a driver and guide. In contrast, Michelle also has a duty not to kill Philip, but not because of some prior agreement. Normally, we have an *unacquired* or *natural* duty not to kill other people (the duty must be prima facie if some killings are all right, such as in self-defense). Such a duty is, it seems, prima facie, negative, and natural, whereas Michelle's duty to be Philip's driver seems to be a prima facie, positive, acquired duty.

We are beginning to develop some ways of sorting out, and hence assessing, certain claims of duty. It is widely held that we have certain natural, negative, and quite stringent duties toward other people, as for example not to kill, maim, or torture them. It is also widely held that we do not have so many or so stringent positive, natural duties to others. Hence, to claim that we have a natural duty to donate organs to strangers, to pay their medical bills, or to claim that a country should place no restrictions on immigration is controversial. The question of the nature and extent of our positive (or "Samaritan") duties is not unrelated to the issue of what sort of health care (or what level of care) should be provided for those ravaged by injury or disease, such as AIDS.

Before leaving our brief discussion of duties, we feel some "duty questions" regarding AIDS are worth noting.

1. What duties do those with AIDS (who know they have it) have toward others? Not to donate blood? Not to share needles? A (positive) duty to warn sexual partners of their condition? A (positive) duty to cooperate with a William Buckley–type proposal to tattoo AIDS carriers (to protect others)?
2. Must insurance companies insure those carrying the AIDS virus? Must they ignore such information if available? Must drug companies with a possible cure for AIDS provide the drug (outside of a controlled trial) for those willing to take the risk? If those with AIDS pay the cost? If they do not?
3. Should the government more aggressively fund research on AIDS, educate the public, or set up hospice programs for those dying from AIDS? Should legislators prohibit those with AIDS from performing certain jobs? Should legislators sup-

port quarantine legislation? Should legislators close down shooting galleries or gay bathhouses? Should children with AIDS be prohibited from attending public schools?

Consider for a moment the relationship between the concept of what is *permissible* and what is a *duty*. To say that one has a duty to perform a certain act is to imply, or presuppose, that it is permissible to so act. If Jane has a duty not to punch Dick in the nose, it is permissible for Jane not to do so. However, many acts are permissible without (normally) being duties—to go to a movie, to donate an organ, or to volunteer to be a subject in an experiment to test an AIDS vaccine, for example. In brief, a more basic moral question than that of duty is often whether or not a certain act or policy is morally permissible:

1. Is it permissible to quarantine, given the risks associated with AIDS?
2. Is it permissible to offend a considerable number of citizens in order to disseminate specific information about safe sex?
3. Is it permissible to infect chimpanzees with AIDS to find a cure or vaccine for AIDS?
4. Is it permissible to require blood testing in order to slow the spread of AIDS?
5. Is it all right to inform those tested of a positive result? If they do not wish to know? Or if the test is not completely reliable? Or even if it is?

Questions of duty to perform an act arise, then, only if the act is permissible; so the permissibility question often is a more natural, initial focal point.

Questions of Rights.   Surprisingly, we have not yet in this section couched any moral issue in terms of rights. Indeed, some philosophers believe that for a person to have a certain right is simply to mean that other agents have certain duties toward this person, and that is all. Such a view is controversial. In the United States especially—a nation much influenced by the writings of theorists of natural rights (such as John Locke, Jean Jacques Rousseau, and Thomas Paine), one that has an important Bill of Rights and has been influenced by a Civil Rights, a women's rights, and recently an animal rights movement—conceiving ethical questions as often being questions about rights is a familiar step. To put one point a bit enigmatically, and without exploration, believers in rights generally think that many, if not all, duties are dependent on the existence of certain natural rights—and not the other way around. In discussions about AIDS, references to a right to equal treatment, a right of autonomy, liberty, or privacy, a right to health care, rights of majorities and minorities, and a societal right to protect itself or to maintain a "decent society" are all mentioned. Hence, we should initially sort out certain questions about rights.

Although it is impossible to do so thoroughly, we will note certain fundamental questions, and, as we proceed through this volume, their ties to specific questions concerning AIDS will become increasingly apparent.

Not all assertions of rights are reasonable (for example, the editors of this volume have a right to all your worldly goods) any more than are all assertions of duties (for example, we ought to eliminate everyone with genetic defects). One important question concerns the ground or basis for possession of a certain right. Natural rights theorists usually assume that human beings have certain rights just because they are human (or sentient or rational, as the case may be). In this view rights are not merely conventional or the result of a prior act. Some rights, however, are conventional and may be possessed, in contrast, because one is a French citizen or because one is a member of the Wimbledon Tennis Club. The question of the grounds for possessing rights often has important implications for personal action and public policy. For example, if, to have any rights at all, one must be a human (a member of the species Homo sapiens), then no nonhuman animal has rights, and no experiments on such animals violate "their" rights (for, in this view, they have none).[75]

A Right to Liberty. More important for many questions related to AIDS is the matter of which rights people have. Many people believe in the right to liberty (or autonomy). A crucial question is: What is the *content* of such a right (or, alternatively, what is the right a right *to* or *from*)?

We offer no full analysis here, but a few observations are in order. It is unreasonable to believe that people have a right to be free to do whatever they may choose. Otherwise, Harold would have a right to burn down Harvey's house, perhaps because Harold just likes to see things burn. Harold's right to be free presumably does not entail the right to violate Harvey's rights—and vice versa. Perhaps one has a right to do whatever violates the rights of no one else, and conversely. Still, the view that all people possess equal and reciprocal moral rights does not tell us which rights people have. For example, do people have a right to life, to health care, to self-defense, to be told the truth, to privacy, and so on?

Liberty, Privacy, and Restraint. Because the right to liberty is important in policies dealing with AIDS, it may be helpful to think about what is involved in being free. To be free to choose with respect to doing some act, X, or free to do X, would seem to involve the *presence* of certain things (for instance, money for the plane ticket to London) or the *absence* of something (such as an electrified fence, a straitjacket, or the threat that one will be jailed for 10 years if one does X). All of the criminal law, then, can be thought of as placing constraints on a person's liberty of choice. Citizens of the United States think of themselves as living in a "free country," but the expression cannot mean a country with no institutionalized constraints on liberty.

Indeed, if we believe murder, rape, child abuse, kidnapping, theft, and maiming the elderly to be serious wrongs, we will most likely approve of the use of the coercive powers of the law to prevent or reduce the performance of such acts. If so, we are committed to the permissibility (and perhaps the obligatory nature) of some restrictions on the liberty of individuals by coercive means. The more important moral question is, then: Just when is it permissible to restrict the liberty of persons (our focus here generally is on competent adults), and on what grounds? A considerable portion of this volume can be thought of as an attempt to explore this issue by attending to this central and specific question: What restrictions on the liberty of people are permissible—especially in light of (1) the (noncontroversial) goal of reducing and eliminating the suffering and premature deaths involved in the spread of AIDS, and (2) the (controversial) widespread assumption that certain of the activities that facilitate the spread of AIDS are seriously wrong (and wrong, it is often held, independently of the fact that they facilitate the spread of AIDS)?

What sorts of laws or policy proposals with respect to the AIDS problem would result in important constraints on the liberty of people? We note a few here. Mandatory screening of blood to detect antibodies to the AIDS virus involves an obvious constraint. If not all people are required to undergo testing, but rather only "high-risk" groups, the possibility of arbitrary discrimination is no remote worry. As noted earlier, why not high-risk behavior? Further, how is the term *high-risk group* to be defined? Also related to voluntary or involuntary testing is a worry about respect for privacy or retention of confidentiality. For example, according to Thomas B. Stoddard of the Lambda Legal Defense and Education Fund, six states (Colorado, Idaho, Minnesota, Montana, South Carolina, and Wisconsin) require physicians to report the name and address of anyone whose blood registers positive on the test for antibodies to HIV.[76]

It might be argued that the right to privacy is not so much a right to do things when one is in a private area, or a right to a private area, but rather a right to exercise some control over what others can observe of one's behavior or what they know of one's attitudes, habits, or interests. Arguably, failure to grant and respect another's privacy is one mode of invasive interference with that person's choices and actions; it is an interference with another's liberty. Not all interferences with liberty, however, seem to be invasions of privacy. If we constrain by force a gang of subway muggers, we restrict their liberty but do not invade their privacy.

Other proposals—the proposal to close gay bathhouses or to prohibit gay males from being blood donors, health care workers, or restaurant employees—also restrict choices. Note that many of the proposed restrictions are often couched in terms of a response to the "gay plague," even though it is now quite obvious that the AIDS virus is present in heterosexuals and homosexuals, children and adults. Further, the high rate of the incidence of AIDS is not found in all gay people but rather in gay males, especially urban gay males. Finally, although AIDS is rampant among IV drug users, the burdens on constrained choice implicit in many policy proposals seems to fall on gay populations. Again, this fact tends to support the view that the American public finds it difficult to respond to the AIDS crisis on the basis of considerations that are independent of their commonly negative moral views about homosexual behavior, views deeply entrenched in the Judeo-Christian tradition.

Indeed, such negative views are not only implicit in the expressions—such as "queer bashing" or "faggots"—used by (among others) heterosexual male gangs who intimidate or beat up gay males. Some such view, arguably, was the basis, or partial basis, for the majority Supreme Court decision, in *Bowers* v. *Hardwick* in June 1986—a decision deeming constitutionally permissible a state's criminalization of homosexual sodomy. These matters receive further attention in Part II and, especially, Part IV of this volume.

It might be argued that, on the face of things, all people have an equal right to be free. Further, a liberty important to all is the liberty to form intimate and sexual associations with other like-minded people. For reasons not so obscure, this liberty seems to be a very important one, one in the absence of which a primary good of life is unobtainable—in contrast to certain other liberties (such as the liberty to take books from the library for a six-month period). However, it may be argued that just as one should not have the liberty to rape (because rape is wrong), so gay people should not have the liberty to engage in homosexual acts (because such acts are wrong). This latter claim, one variation of which is called *legal moralism*, will be discussed in Parts II and IV.

Emergency Situations and the Public Health.   Consider, in contrast, a line of argument in favor of liberty-restricting policies that does *not* suppose that homosexual acts are inherently wrong (wrong independently of any bad consequences that may result). Certain acts more effectively spread AIDS than others, such as blood donation by carriers, anal intercourse with at least one carrier, and the use of nonsterile needles for intravenous injections. Further, the spread of AIDS threatens to decimate large numbers of people, a total of almost 180,000 in the United States by 1991, cutting them down quickly (often in months to a couple of years) and often in their prime. In short, there is an epidemic, an increasingly devastating one, and hence a major public health problem—indeed, not just a problem for the public of one nation, but a problem soon to be seen (barring an effective vaccine or cure) as the global health issue that it is. In such a situation, it may be argued, rights must give way. By way of analogy, if the only way to save a dying person is to take your neighbor's car (without her consent) and drive the victim to the hospital, that justifies the infringement of your neighbor's property right. It may be claimed that cases abound in which to infringe rights is justified—roughly, those cases in which a great good can thereby be obtained or (more relevantly) thereby a great harm can be avoided. Similarly, by the legal right of eminent domain your property may be taken against your will, so that a hospital, for example, may be built (and you may be compensated for its market value). Another related case concerns the "law of necessity," a rather well-established principle of Anglo-American law, which holds that, although one cannot normally dock one's boat in a private port, one may use another's port even without the owner's consent if a storm constitutes a serious threat to one's safety. These three cases are a few of many one might consider in reflecting on the question of the legal and moral permissibility of infringing on others' rights to prevent a serious harm or to promote an important good.

In some cases (such as the hospital example) it may be claimed that it is in the public interest or for the public good to do that which is presumptively wrong (such as to restrict a person's liberty) and, hence, morally justifiable to so act. A well-established precedent in legal cases exists in the United States that the sta⁷ rather extraordinary (for example, coercive) measures in order to pro⁷ health against serious threats. As Larry Gostin has noted, some cour⁷ States have taken the view that "quarantine does not frustrate c⁷

because there is no liberty to harm others."[77] Whether this sort of appeal is acceptable and to what extent, if at all, it provides a justification for placing possibly severe
restrictions on the lives of citizens pose serious moral questions. These matters are
frequently implicit, if not explicit, issues in much of the discussion in Parts II and III
of this volume.

Review.   To summarize a few points, many of the moral questions raised by proposed policies to cope with AIDS concern the justification for restricting the liberties
of competent adults. We have sketched here one line of argument for restrictions
that appeals to legal moralism. We have also sketched a nonmoralistic "appeal to the
public interest" or "appeal to public health" line of argument for restrictions. Our
purpose here is largely to identify basic issues that are more closely examined elsewhere in this volume. We also noted an issue that does not focus on coercive restriction on the liberties of others; namely, what duties carriers of AIDS have. What re-
straints, if any, should they voluntarily place on themselves? These matters do not
exhaust the moral questions surrounding AIDS. There are questions of justice:
Would a just society or a just system of health care spend more (or less) funds on
AIDS research? Would it provide hospice care for AIDS victims? If so, is this a matter
of compensation for societal discrimination? In any or all cases? There are, of course,
additional questions about the government's legitimate role in educating the public
about AIDS. For the same reason some people oppose sex education in the schools
(because disseminating such information is said to encourage promiscuity), some
object to forthright public education regarding AIDS. Consider also research and experimentation: Should the Food and Drug Administration disallow AIDS victims (facing imminent death) from trying anti-AIDS drugs not yet proven to be "safe and
effective"? Further, can we justify experimenting on nonvolunteer humans if that is
the only likely way to discover an adequate vaccine? May we kill or torture thousands
of other mammals if that is the only way? Finally, in a random clinical trial in which
one group of subjects is receiving a placebo and another group an experimental
drug for AIDS, at what point during the trial must one halt the trial and allow placebo
recipients to have the drug being tested, if the testing indicates that the drug may be
an effective cure of AIDS? Indeed, was the halting of just such a trial by Burroughs-
Wellcome in the fall of 1986 defensible?

We have elaborated some of the prime scientific challenges with respect to dealing with AIDS in order to find an effective, inexpensive means of preventing and
curing the disease. As we have gone some length to suggest, powerful moral questions remain to be answered as well—questions concerning what we morally may
do or what we morally must do as we try to prevent, cure, or ameliorate the burden
of the AIDS epidemic. The essays that follow seek to advance publicly the intelligent
answering of these questions.

Notes

1. Strictly speaking, scientists agree that there are several viruses that can cause AIDS and that more may be discovered. The one believed to be the cause of AIDS in the overwhelming majority of cases is designated variously as HIV, HTLV-III, or LAV. See *The News and Observer,* Raleigh, N.C., November 20, 1986 (from the New York Times News Service).
2. *USA Today* (March 18, 1987).
3. Tom Morganthau and Mary Hager, "AIDS: Grim Prospects," *Newsweek* (November 10, 1986), p. 20.
4. *The New York Times* (March 16, 1987).
5. *The New York Times* (October 30, 1986).
6. *The New York Times* (June 13, 1986).
7. *The New York Times* (June 13, 1986); see also *Discover* (August 1986), p. 85.
8. Ann Guidici Fettner, *The Truth about AIDS: Evolution of an Epidemic* (New York: Holt, Rinehart and Winston, 1984), pp. 11–12.
9. Michael Bronski, "Death and the Erotic Imagination," *Gay Community News* (September 7–13, 1986), pp. 8–9. Used by permission.
10. Fettner, *op. cit.*, p. 45.
11. David Black, *The Plague Years: A Chronicle of AIDS, the Epidemic of Our Times* (New York: Simon and Schuster, 1986), p. 217.
12. Gerald Friedland, "AIDS: What Is to Be Done?" *Harper's* (October 1985), pp. 43–44.
13. Researchers have successfully infected chimpanzees with HIV. They have even engaged in what David Black calls "bunny bondage": In an effort to test the thesis that depositing semen from one male into the rectum of another might cause the receiver to produce antibodies to foreign semen and in turn suppress the immune system, researchers "took rabbits and gave them rabbit semen rectally once a week. . . . Healthy males were restrained and 1 ml of fresh semen . . . was deposited . . . to a depth of 5 cm . . . with a No. 7 French rubber catheter." Black, *op. cit.*, p. 97.
14. Fettner, *op. cit.*, p. 65.
15. *The News and Observer* (Raleigh, N.C.: September 7, 1986).
16. In Paris, tests to date have disclosed no insects containing HIV. However, in Zaïre, mosquitoes, ticks, and even cockroaches have been found to possess AIDS-like genetic material. Some researchers conjecture that mosquitoes and ticks can get AIDS from humans but cannot give it back. However, since cockroaches are not blood-sucking insects, how they could get or transmit HIV remains a mystery. *Ibid.*
17. From a letter written by L. H. Calabrese and K. V. Gopalakrishna, in *The New England Journal of Medicine* (1986), Vol. 314, No. 15, p. 987.
18. John Langone, "AIDS," *Discover* (December 1985), pp. 40–41.
19. Marcos Bisticas-Cocoves, "CDC Revises AIDS Risk Hierarchy (a Little)," *Gay Community News* (August 24–30, 1986), p. 3.
20. Jonathan Lieberson, "The Reality of AIDS," *The New York Review of Books* (January 15, 1986), p. 44.
21. Chris Jennings, *Understanding and Preventing AIDS* (Cambridge, Mass.: Health Alert Press, 1985), p. 29. See also *Gay Community News* (May 24, 1986), p. 1, where a breakdown by patient group of people with AIDS reveals that 64.4 percent are gay and bisexual men who are not IV drug users. (At the time of this study, the total number of U.S. AIDS cases had passed the 20,000 mark.)
22. Jennings, *op. cit.*, pp. 28–29.
23. Robert Redfield, M.D., quoted in "Heterosexuals: A New Risk Group," *The Village Voice* (May 27, 1986), p. 20.
24. Jennings, *op. cit.*, p. 29.
25. Wayne Barrett, "Straight Shooters," *The Village Voice* (October 29, 1985), p. 16.
26. *Ibid.*
27. James Curran, M.D., quoted in "Spread of AIDS among Women Poses Widening Challenge to Medical Field," *The Wall Street Journal* (June 26, 1986), p. 5.

28. John Langone, "AIDS Update: Still No Reason for Hysteria," *Discover* (September 1986), p. 32.
29. Fettner, *op. cit.*, p. 115.
30. *Ibid.*, p. 113.
31. Bisticas-Cocoves, *op. cit.*, p. 3.
32. Lieberson, *op. cit.*, p. 44; see also *The New York Times* (June 13, 1986).
33. "Blacks Face Far Greater AIDS Risk, Army Says," *Louisville Courier-Journal* (July 22, 1986); see also *Gay Community News* (July 13–19, 1986).
34. *Ibid.*
35. Barbara Herbert, M.D., quoted in "Lesbian/Gay Health Conference," *Off Our Backs* (May 1986), p. 3. Herbert was also quoted as saying: "Only nuns have less incidence of Sexually Transmitted Diseases (STDs) than lesbians. . . . [W]here you see an STD there's been a penis in the picture."
36. Arye Rubinstein, M.D., quoted in "Pediatricians Warn of Increase in Cases of Children with AIDS," *The Chronicle of Higher Education* (May 28, 1986).
37. Keith Krasinski, M.D., quoted in "Pediatricians Warn of Increase in Cases of Children with AIDS," *The Chronicle of Higher Education* (May 28, 1986).
38. Barrett, *op. cit.*, p. 15.
39. June E. Osborn, quoted in "Women and AIDS," *Newsweek* (July 14, 1986), p. 61.
40. Barrett, *op. cit.*, p. 16.
41. *Ibid.*, p. 14.
42. Rubinstein, *op. cit.*
43. See, for example, "Effort to Recall Durham Mayor Fails as Petition Drive Comes Up Short," *The News and Observer* (Raleigh, N.C.: August 9, 1986).
44. Barrett, *op. cit.*, p. 15.
45. This may change; for example, a national conference on AIDS in the black community was held in Washington, D.C., on July 18, 1986.
46. John Preston, ed., *Hot Living: Erotic Stories about Safer Sex* (Boston: Alyson Publications, Inc., 1985).
47. Christopher Norwood, "Heterosexuals: A New Risk Group," *The Village Voice* (May 27, 1986), p. 19.
48. Dennis Altman, "Dilemma of the Homosexual Connection," a paper read at the "AIDS: Ethics, Law and Social Policy" conference organized by the Center for Human Bioethics (Monash University: April 7, 1986), p. 1. Used by permission.
49. *Ibid.*, p. 2.
50. Mathilde Krim, *Federal and Local Government's Response to the AIDS Epidemic*, a paper read at hearings before a subcommittee of the Committee on Government Operations of the House of Representatives, 99th Cong., 1st sess., on July 3, September 13, and December 2, 1985 (Washington, D.C.: Government Printing Office, 1986), p. 329.
51. Krim, *op. cit.*, pp. 329–330.
52. Langone, *op. cit.*, p. 34.
53. *Ibid.*
54. Paul Volberding, M.D., and Donald Abrams, M.D., "Clinical Care and Research in AIDS," *Hastings Center Report* (August 1985), p. 16.
55. *The News and Observer* (Raleigh, N.C.: June 15, 1986).
56. *Bay Windows* 3 (July 24, 1986).
57. William Check, "Public Education on AIDS: Not Only the Media's Responsibility," *Hastings Center Report* (August 1985), p. 31.
58. *The Advocate* (August 5, 1986).
59. "The Rock Hudson Story," Part II, *People* (June 16, 1986), pp. 95–96.
60. *The New York Times* (June 26, 1985).
61. *Gay Community News* (July 20–26, 1986).
62. *The Advocate* (August 5, 1986).
63. Jim Fauntleroy, *Gay Community News* (July 20–26, 1986).
64. *The News and Observer* (Raleigh, N.C.: September 7, 1986).
65. Quoted in Allan M. Brandt, *No Magic Bullet*, 2nd ed. (Oxford: Oxford University Press, 1987), p. 185.

66. Krim, *op. cit.*, p. 45.
67. *The Citizen* (Auburn, N.Y.: June 13, 1986).
68. *The News and Observer* (Raleigh, N.C.: March 19, 1987).
69. *The New York Times* (July 1, 1986).
70. *The Durham Morning Herald* (September 20, 1986).
71. David Holzman, "New AIDS Victim: Hospital Budgets," *Insight* (August 25, 1986), p. 54.
72. June E. Osborn, M.D., "The AIDS Epidemic: Multidisciplinary Trouble," *The New England Journal of Medicine* (March 20, 1986), p. 782. Used by permission.
73. *Ibid.*
74. John Osborne, "The Politics of AIDS," *National Review* (May 23, 1986), p. 26.
75. A discussion of the moral status of animals can be found in *People, Penguins, and Plastic Trees: Basic Issues in Environmental Ethics*, Donald VanDeVeer and Christine Pierce, eds. (Belmont, Calif.: Wadsworth Publishing Company, 1986). For an essay critical of human experiments on animals, see Tom Regan, "Ill-Gotten Gains," in *Health Care Ethics*, Donald VanDeVeer and Tom Regan, eds. (Philadelphia: Temple University Press, 1987). This volume also contains essays on the ethics of informed consent and the use of random clinical trials. See also, for a contrary view and an extensive bibliography, Michael Allen Fox, *The Case for Animal Experimentation* (Berkeley: University of California Press, 1986).
76. Tom Stoddard, "Patients Must Have Laws Providing Privacy," *USA Today* (August 1, 1986), editorial page.
77. Larry Gostin, "Public Fears Versus Private Rights in AIDS Patients: The Use of Traditional Infection Control Strategies" (unpublished manuscript), p. 12. Gostin is on the faculty of the Harvard School of Public Health.

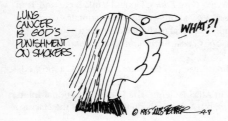

LUNG CANCER IS GOD'S — PUNISHMENT ON SMOKERS.

WHAT?!

© 1985 JULES FEIFFER 9-8

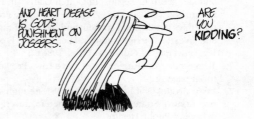

AND HEART DISEASE IS GOD'S PUNISHMENT ON JOGGERS. —

ARE YOU KIDDING?

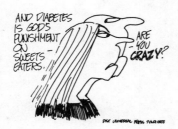

AND DIABETES IS GOD'S PUNISHMENT ON SWEETS— EATERS.

— ARE YOU CRAZY?

DIST. UNIVERSAL PRESS SYNDICATE

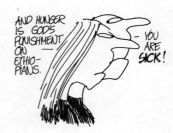

AND HUNGER IS GOD'S PUNISHMENT ON — ETHIO— PIANS.

— YOU ARE SICK!

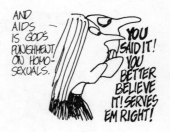

AND AIDS — IS GOD'S PUNISHMENT ON HOMO— SEXUALS.

YOU SAID IT! YOU BETTER BELIEVE IT! SERVES EM RIGHT!

□ □ □ ■

Part I

Perspectives

AIDS in Historical Perspective

ALLAN M. BRANDT

Despite George Santayana's famous injunction that those who do not remember the past are condemned to repeat it, history holds no simple truths. Nevertheless, there are a number of significant historical questions relating to the AIDS epidemic. What does the history of medicine and public health have to tell us about contemporary approaches to the very difficult dilemmas raised by AIDS? Is AIDS something totally new or are there instances in the past which are usefully comparable? Are there some lessons in the way science and society have responded to epidemic disease in the past that could inform our understanding of and response to the current health crisis? There are obviously no simple answers to such questions. History is not a fable with the moral spelled out at the end. Even if we could agree on a particular construction of past events, it would not necessarily lead to consensus on what is to be done. And yet, history provides us with one means of approaching the present. In this regard, the history of responses to particular diseases can inform and deepen our understanding of the AIDS crisis and the medical, social, and public health interventions available.

The way a society responds to problems of disease will reveal its deepest cultural, social, and moral values. These core values—patterns of judgment about what is good or bad—shape and guide human perception and action. This, we know, has most certainly been the case with AIDS; the epidemic has not only been shaped by powerful biological forces, but by behavioral, social, and cultural factors as well. This essay briefly analyzes the process by which social and cultural forces shape our understanding of disease and examines several analogues to the current health crisis.

One model has already been proposed in Susan Sontag's brilliant polemic *Illness As Metaphor*. In this work, Sontag assessed the important ways in which tuberculosis

Reprinted by permission of the author.

and cancer have been used as metaphors. Using techniques of literary analysis she demonstrated prevailing cultural views of these diseases and their victims.[1] But disease is more than a metaphor. These "social constructions" have very real sociopolitical implications.

An examination of the first decades of the twentieth century, a moment of intense concern and interest in sexually transmitted diseases not unlike those today, may demonstrate how this process has worked. Indeed, the first two decades of the twentieth century witnessed a general hysteria about venereal infections. The historical analogues are striking; they relate to public health, science, and especially social and cultural values.

This period, often referred to as the Progressive Era, combined two powerful strains in American social thought: the search for new technical, scientific answers to social problems as well as the search for a set of unified moral ideals. The problem of sexually transmitted diseases appealed to both sets of interests. The campaign against these infections—the "social hygiene" movement—was predicated on a series of major scientific breakthroughs. The identification of the specific organism which causes gonorrhea, the gonococcus, and the causative agent for syphilis, the spirochete, [had been] achieved. By the end of the first decade of the twentieth century diagnostic exams had been established.[2] In 1911, the first major chemotherapeutic agent effective against the spirochete—Salvarsan—was discovered on the 606th attempt by German Nobel Laureate Paul Ehrlich. Science had the effect of reframing the way in which these diseases were seen. The enormous social, cultural, and economic costs of venereal disease were finally revealed.

Doctors came to define what they called *venereal insontium*, or venereal disease of the innocent. The tragic familial repercussions of syphilis within the family were traced by Victorian physicians. Perhaps the best known example of venereal insontium was ophthalmia neonatorum, gonorrheal blindness of the newborn. As late as 1910, as many as 25 percent of all the blind in the United States had lost their sight in this way despite the earlier discovery that silver nitrate solution could prevent infection. Soon many states began to require the use of the prophylactic treatment by law.[3]

But doctors stressed the impact on women even more than children. In 1906, the AMA held a symposium on the Duty of the Profession to Womanhood. As one physician at the conference explained:

These vipers of venery which are called clap and pox, lurking as they often do, under the floral tributes of the honeymoon, may so inhibit conception or blight its products that motherhood becomes either an utter impossibility or a veritable curse. The ban placed by venereal disease on fetal life outrivals the criminal interference with the products of conception as a cause of race suicide.[4]

The train of family tragedy was a frequent cultural theme in these years. In 1913, a hit Broadway play by French playwright Eugene Brieux, *Damaged Goods*, told the story of young George Dupont, who, though warned by his physician not to marry because he has syphilis, disregards this advice only to spread the infection to his wife and, later, to their child. This story was told and retold and it revealed deep cultural values about science, social responsibility, and the limits of medicine to cure the moral ailments of humankind.[5]

But physicians expressed concerns which went beyond the confines of the family; they also examined the wider social repercussions of sexually transmitted diseases. The last years of the nineteenth century and the first of the twentieth were the most intensive periods of immigration to the United States in its entire history; more than 650,000 immigrants came to these shores each year between 1885 and 1910. Many doctors and social critics suggested that these individuals were bringing venereal disease into the country. As Howard Kelly, a leading gynecologist at Johns Hopkins, explained, "The tide [of venereal disease] has been raising [sic] owing to the inpouring of a large foreign population with lower ideals." Kelly elaborated, warning, "Think of these countless currents flowing daily from the houses of the poorest into those of the richest, and forming a sort of civic circulatory system expressive of the body politic, a circulation which continually tends to equalize the distribution of morality and disease."[6]

Although examinations at the ports of entry failed to reveal a high incidence of disease, nevertheless, nativists called for the restriction of immigration. How were these immigrants spreading sexually transmitted diseases to native, middle-class, Anglo-Saxon Americans? First, it was suggested that immigrants constituted the great bulk of prostitutes who inhabited American cities; virtually every major American metropolis of the early twentieth century had defined red-light districts where prostitution flourished. These women, it was suggested, were typically foreign born.[7]

But even more importantly, physicians now asserted that syphilis and gonorrhea could be transmitted in any number of ways. The various modes of transmission were catalogued by doctors: pens, pencils, toothbrushes, towels and bedding, and medical procedures were all identified as potential means of communication.[8] As one woman explained in an anonymous essay in 1912:

> At first it was unbelievable. I knew of the disease only through newspaper advertisements [for patent medicines]. I had understood that it was the result of sin and that it originated and was contracted only in the underworld of the city. I felt sure that my friend was mistaken in diagnosis when he exclaimed, "Another tragedy of the common drinking cup!" I eagerly met his remark with the assurance that I did not use public drinking cups, that I had used my own cup for years. He led me to review my summer. After recalling a number of times when my thirst had forced me to go to the public fountain, I came at last to realize that what he had told me was true.[9]

The doctor, of course, had diagnosed syphilis. One indication of how seriously these casual modes of transmission were taken is the fact that the Navy removed doorknobs off its battleships during the First World War, claiming that [they] had been a source of infection for many of its sailors (a remarkable act of denial). We now know, of course, that syphilis and gonorrhea cannot be contracted in these ways. This poses a difficult historical problem: Why did physicians believe that they could be?

Theories of casual transmission reflected deep cultural fears about disease and

sexuality in the early twentieth century. In these approaches to venereal disease concerns about hygiene, contamination, and contagion were expressed, anxieties that
reflected a great deal about the contemporary society and culture. Venereal disease
was viewed as a threat to the entire late Victorian social and sexual system, which
placed great value on discipline, restraint, and homogeneity. The sexual code of this
era held that only sex-in-marriage should receive social sanction. But the concerns
about venereal disease also reflected a pervasive fear of the urban masses, the
growth of the cities, and the changing nature of familial relationships. Finally, the
distinction between venereal disease and venereal insontium had the effect of dividing victims; some deserved attention, sympathy, and medical support, others did not.
This, of course, depended on how the infection was obtained. Victims were separated into the innocent and the guilty.

In short, venereal disease became a metaphor for the anxieties of this time, reflecting deep social and cultural values about sexuality, contagion, and social organization. But these metaphors are not simply innocuous linguistic constructions; they
have powerful socio-political implications, many of which have been remarkably
persistent during the twentieth century.

These concerns about sexually transmitted diseases led to a major public health
campaign to stop their spread. Many of the public health approaches which we today
apply to communicable infections were developed in the early years of the twentieth
century. Educational programs formed a major component of the campaign. But to
speak of "education" is far too vague. The question, of course, is the precise content
of the education offered. During the first decades of the twentieth century, when
schools first instituted sex education programs, their basic goal was to inculcate fear
of sex to encourage premarital continence. Indeed, it would be accurate to call these
programs antisexual education.

In addition to education, the ability to diagnose syphilis and gonorrhea led to the
development of a series of important public health interventions. American cities
began to require the reporting of venereal diseases around 1915. Some states used
reports to follow contacts and bring individuals in for treatment. By the 1930s many
states had come to require premarital and prenatal screening; some municipalities
mandated compulsory screening of food handlers and barbers, even though it was
by then understood that syphilis and gonorrhea could not be spread in these ways;
the rationale offered was that these individuals were at risk for infection anyway and
that screening might reveal new cases for treatment.

Perhaps the most dramatic public health intervention devised to combat sexually
transmitted diseases was the campaign to close red-light districts. In the first two decades of the twentieth century, vice commissions in almost all American cities had
identified the risk which the prostitute posed for American health and morals, and
decided the time had come to remove the sources of infection. Comparing the red-
light districts to swamps which produced malaria, they attempted to "drain" these
swamps. During the First World War more than 100 red-light districts were closed.
The attack on the prostitute constituted the most concerted attack on civil liberties in
the name of public health in American history. Not surprisingly, in the atmosphere of
crisis that the war engendered, public health officials employed radical techniques in
their battle against venereal disease. State laws held that anyone "reasonably sus-

pected" of harboring a venereal infection could be tested on a compulsory basis. Quarantine, detention, and internment became new themes in the attack on sexually transmitted diseases, centering on the figure of the prostitute.[10] As Attorney General T. W. Gregory explained:

> The constitutional right of the community, in the interest of the public health, to ascertain the existence of infections and communicable diseases in its midst and to isolate and quarantine such cases or take steps necessary to prevent the spread of disease is clear.[11]

In July 1918, Congress allocated more than $1 million for the detention and isolation of venereal carriers. During the war more than 30,000 prostitutes were incarcerated in institutions supported by the federal government. As one federal official noted:

> Conditions required the immediate isolation of as many venereally infected persons acting as spreaders of disease as could be quickly apprehended and quarantined. It was not a measure instituted for the punishment of prostitutes on account of infraction of the civil or moral law, but was strictly a public health measure to prevent the spread of dangerous, communicable diseases.[12]

Fear of venereal disease during the war had led to substantial inroads against traditional civil liberties. Although many of these interventions were challenged in the courts, most were upheld; the police powers of the state were deemed sufficient to override any constitutional concerns. The program of detention and isolation, it should be noted, had no impact on rates of venereal disease, which increased dramatically during the war. Although this story is not well known, it was not unlike the internment of Japanese Americans during World War II.

THE ANALOGUES THAT AIDS poses to this brief history are striking: the pervasive fear of contagion; concerns about casual transmission; the stigmatization of victims; the conflicts between protecting public health and assuring civil liberties. How these issues will be resolved as the AIDS epidemic continues to unfold in the years ahead is far from certain, and we know that history is not a predictive science. AIDS is not syphilis, and 1986 is not 1918. But one thing is certain: The response to AIDS, as already can be seen, will not be determined strictly by its biological character; rather, it will be deeply influenced by our social and cultural understanding of disease and its victims. It is an understanding of this process which gives the historical record relevance and meaning. How will the response to AIDS be shaped by prevailing social and cultural values? Recognizing this process provides us with an opportunity to guide and influence the response to AIDS in ways which may be more constructive, effective, and humane. Moreover, it may shape our views of the important legal issues that the epidemic has already posed.

As was the case in the early twentieth century, public health measures which require dramatic infringements of civil liberties are again being proposed. All too often these measures have had no positive impact on the public health. For example, rates of venereal disease climbed rapidly during the First World War, despite the government's efforts. This is not to suggest a purely pragmatic notion that if it works it is right, but rather that if it does not produce results, and yet it is supported by officials and the public, one must look for secondary reasons to support these activities.

The issue thus becomes not the desire to protect the public from hazard—an idea so basic to modern governments that few would question it in principle. Indeed, our notion of social welfare is based upon it. Rather, these activities indicate a transformation from protection to punishment, a clear signal that the disease and those who get it are socially disvalued. These punishments, of course, do not fall randomly across society.

The question is how will social and cultural values concerning AIDS influence the public policy response to the disease now and in the years ahead? A series of difficult dilemmas are just offstage. How can the impact of this disease be mitigated? Can we protect the rights of victims of the disease while avoiding the victimization of the public? What types of policies should be employed? And how will these policies reflect our cultural notions of the disease?

In the months and years ahead the problems of constructing cost-benefit ratios for various policies will be confronted. Who will bear the burdens of any particular intervention? What will the motives be? How will information be used? Ideally? In practice? What are the potential unintended consequences of any particular policy? Already there has been a tendency to invoke traditional public health policies: screening, testing, reporting, contact tracing, isolation, and quarantine. Will these measures be effective in the case of AIDS, which is complicated by the large number of healthy carriers perhaps infectious for life? Does the fact that no effective treatment for the disease currently exists change the nature of potential public health interventions? In short, how do you construct a just, humane, and effective policy? How do we protect civil liberties while protecting the public good? All these issues will be resolved in the context of our legal system.

But the answers to these difficult questions will be shaped by our scientific, social, and cultural understanding of the disease. This, of course, has been further complicated by the substantial fear surrounding the epidemic. While there is much that we know about AIDS, there is much that lies outside current scientific understanding. While scientists and physicians have experience tolerating such ambiguities, this level of uncertainty is often hidden from or denied by the larger society. Policies relating to AIDS will, of course, be created in this atmosphere of uncertainty. Moreover, the decline of the authority of experts—from Three Mile Island, to Love Canal, to the space shuttle, to Chernobyl—has had the effect of creating significant distrust among the public. The fact that as a society we have been fortunate not to have to address any major infectious disease on an epidemic level since polio reflects our relative lack of social and political experience in dealing with such problems. And, indeed, we would probably have to go back to the influenza pandemic of 1918 to identify a pathogen as dangerous as the AIDS virus. In this light, we have few models for dealing with public health issues of this magnitude and complexity.

Second, the notion of relative risk is generally undefined in our culture. How is the danger of AIDS considered vis-à-vis other risks? How will the courts, for example, make determinations about the relative risk posed by individuals who carry the AIDS virus? We need to develop better measures for making more sophisticated assessments of the risks we face.

Third, our notions of cost-benefit analysis and social policy are characterized by a belief in policies without costs. All social policies carry certain costs, but in our political culture, we tend to reject policies when the costs become explicit, even if they promise significant potential benefits. This has recently been seen in two proposals to slow the spread of the infection. As in the early twentieth century, education has been put forward as one of the few positive activities which might slow the further spread of the disease. But such discussions must assess the meaning and content of such education. Explicit sexual education has been rejected because it is viewed as encouraging homosexuality; the costs are thus evaluated as being too high. Another recent proposal has met a similar fate—the idea of providing sterile needles to intravenous drug abusers to prevent the rapid spread of the disease, which has already occurred in that community. This idea has been rejected because it is seen as contributing to the drug problem.

In the context of fear that surrounds AIDS, there is a clear potential for policies which, despite having little or no potential for slowing the epidemic, could have considerable legal, social, and cultural appeal. What can be done to separate realistic concerns from irrational fears? How can victim-blaming and stigmatization of high-risk groups, already socially disvalued, be avoided? In many respects the process of dividing victims between the blameless and blameful—analogous to early twentieth-century notions of venereal insontium—has been activated once again. This can be seen, for example, in assessments such as the following, offered by a journalist in *The New York Times Magazine*:

> The groups most recently found to be at risk for AIDS present a particularly poignant problem. Innocent bystanders caught in the path of a new disease, they can make no behavioral decisions to minimize their risk: hemophiliacs cannot stop taking bloodclotting medication; surgery patients cannot stop getting transfusions; women cannot control the drug habits of their mates; babies cannot choose their mothers.[13]

In some quarters the misapprehension persists: AIDS is caused by homosexuality rather than a retrovirus. In this confused logic, the answer to the problem is simple: Repress these behaviors. Implicit in this approach to the problem are powerful notions of culpability and guilt.

AIDS' high mortality could become the justification for drastic measures. "Better safe than sorry" could well become a catch phrase to justify dramatic abuses of basic human rights in the context of an uncertain science. Moreover, the social construction of this disease, its close association in much of the public's eye with violations of the moral code, could contribute to spiralling hysteria and anger, which has already led to further victimization of victims, the double jeopardy of lethal disease, and social and legal oppression.

The social costs of ineffective draconian public health measures would only augment the crisis we know as AIDS. But such measures may only be avoided if we are sophisticated both in our medical and [in our] cultural understanding of this disease;

if we are sophisticated in our ability to create an atmosphere of social tolerance. For we need to perform a difficult task, that of separating deeply irrational fears from scientific understanding. Only when we recognize the ways in which social and cultural values shape this disease will we be able to begin to deal effectively and humanely with a problem so serious and complex as AIDS.

Notes

1. Susan Sontag, *Illness As Metaphor* (New York: Farrar, Straus & Giroux, 1978).

2. The following discussion is abbreviated from my book, *No Magic Bullet: A Social History of Venereal Disease in the United States Since 1880* (New York: Oxford University Press, 1985; rev. ed., 1987).

3. On the problem of ophthalmia neonatorum, see Abraham L. Wolbarst, "On the Occurrence of Syphilis and Gonorrhea in Children by Direct Infection," *American Medicine*, n.s. 7 (September 1912): 494; Carolyn Von Blarcum, "The Harm Done in Ascribing All Babies' Sore Eyes to Gonorrhea," *American Journal of Public Health* 6 (September 1916): 926–31; and J. W. Kerr, "Ophthalmia Neonatorum: An Analysis of the Laws and Regulations in Relation thereto in Force in the United States," *Public Health Service Bulletin* 49 (Washington, D.C., 1914).

4. Albert H. Burr, "The Guarantee of Safety in the Marriage Contract," *Journal of the American Medical Association* 47 (December 8, 1906): 1887–88.

5. See Eugene Brieux, *Damaged Goods*, trans. John Pollack (New York: Brentano, 1913). On the critical reception of the play, see "Demoralizing Plays," *Outlook* 150 (September 20, 1913): 110; John D. Rockefeller, "The Awakening of a New Social Conscience," *Medical Reviews of Reviews* 19 (February 1913): 281; "Damaged Goods," *Hearst's Magazine* 23 (May 1913): 806; "Brieux's New Sociological Sermon in Three Acts," *Current Opinion* 54 (April 1913): 296–97.
See also Barbara Gutmann Rosenkrantz, "Damaged Goods: Dilemmas of Responsibility for Risk," *Health and Society* 57 (1979): 1–37.

6. Howard Kelly, "Social Diseases and Their Prevention," *Social Diseases* 1 (July 1910): 17; Kelly, "The Protection of the Innocent," *American Journal of Obstetrics* (April 1907): 477–81.

7. On prostitution in progressive America, see Paul S. Boyer, *Urban Masses and Moral Order* (Cambridge: Harvard University Press, 1978); Ruth Rosen, *The Lost Sisterhood: Prostitution in America, 1900–1918* (Baltimore: Johns Hopkins, 1982); and Mark Thomas Connelly, *The Response to Prostitution in the Progressive Era* (Chapel Hill, N.C.: University of North Carolina Press, 1980).

8. On nonvenereal transmission, see especially L. Duncan Bulkey, *Syphilis of the Innocent* (New York: Bailey and Fairchild, 1894).

9. "What One Woman Has Had to Bear," *Forum* 68 (October 1912): 451–54. See also "New Laws About Drinking Cups," *Life* 58 (December 21, 1911): 1152.

10. The wartime policy for the attack on the red-light districts and the testing and incarceration of prostitutes is described in greater detail in Brandt, *No Magic Bullet*, pp. 80–95.

11. T. W. Gregory, "Memorandum on Legal Aspects of the Proposed System of Medical Examination of Women Convicted Under Section 13, Selective Service Act," National Archives, Record Group 90, Box 223. See also Mary Macey Dietzler, *Detention Houses and Reformatories as Protective Social Agencies in the Campaign of the United States Government Against Venereal Diseases*, United States Interdepartmental Social Hygiene Board (Washington, 1922).

12. C. C. Pierce, "The Value of Detention as a Reconstruction Measure," *American Journal of Obstetrics* 80 (December 1919): 629.

13. Robin Marantz Henig, "AIDS: A New Disease's Deadly Odyssey," *New York Times Magazine* (February 6, 1983): 36.

Ethics and the Language of AIDS

JUDITH WILSON ROSS

If names are not correct, language is not in accordance with the truth of things. If language is not in accordance with the truth of things, affairs cannot be carried on to success.
—Confucian Analects, Book XIII

Introduction

AIDS has proven a difficult phenomenon medically, but it is equally problematic from a linguistic perspective. As many writers have commented, the problems that AIDS presents appear new to us because very few remember the great influenza epidemic of 1918–19 and not many have more than dim memories of the pre-1944 fear of tuberculosis or the relatively small polio epidemic of the 1930s and 1940s. For the most part, we have spent our lives in a culture in which infectious disease does not represent a significant threat and thus we had consigned living in fear of life-threatening contagious disease to the pages of history books. New phenomena, however, whether they are new in cultural or in personal history, demand explanations. We need to place them in some context so that we can account for them in our world view. The language that we choose to describe new phenomena displays both the context and the meaning we give to them. In particular, the metaphors we use convey much of the deeper meaning that we attribute to these new events.

Public policy, ethical judgments, and personal choices can all be deeply influenced by the metaphors we have chosen or have grown accustomed to using and

Judith W. Ross, "Ethics and the Language of AIDS," in *AIDS and the Medical Humanities*, Eric T. Juengst and Barbara Koenig, eds. (forthcoming from Praeger Publishers, a division of Greenwood Press, New York, New York). Copyright © by Eric T. Juengst and Barbara Koenig. Reprinted by permission.

hearing others use throughout the last few years. We may talk of facts and objective judgments, but facts can be arranged in many ways to prove many things. They are not as immutable as the scientists would have us believe. Scientific facts past mathematics cannot long exist as independent entities: They are quickly integrated into the linguistic patterns of everyday use where decision making takes place. Everyday language—the jars, as it were, into which these facts are poured—is itself shaped by our perceptual patterns. The metaphors of AIDS—death, sin, crime, war, and civic division—are the shaping perceptions that make the language of AIDS so dangerous.

The Death Metaphor

AIDS is perhaps first of all a metaphor of personified death. The personal account literature is full of references to people who "lost" lovers or friends to AIDS. "AIDS took three people on this street," an acquaintance told me. A young man with AIDS says, "Why did it get me?" In *Life* magazine, "AIDS struck the Burk family"; it "laid their bodies open to lethal infections."[1] Here, AIDS becomes powerful and independent. It goes about choosing its victims, a grim reaper hiding behind ordinary sexual relationships. In *Rolling Stone*, Edmund White uses this metaphor quite specifically: "Gay sex has become equated with death. Behind the friendly smiling face, bronzed and mustachioed, is a skull. . . ."[2] The ubiquitous use of the word *victim* is part of the *AIDS as death* metaphor. Death in our culture is not a kindly God looking to bring his people back into his presence. It is a skeletal figure, stealing people and taking them into the realm of darkness. AIDS is death, out looking for victims.

This image of AIDS as death is reinforced throughout the popular and quasi-academic literature by the unrelenting joining of the word AIDS with the phrase "inevitably/invariably fatal." It is as if one expected a diagnosis of AIDS to lead to instant death. Yet, many people with AIDS live for months and even years and live for the most part outside the hospital. The metaphor of AIDS as death permits us to forget those who have the syndrome: They are dead to us, making it easier to withhold aggressive treatment or financial assistance.

Here, scientific information could help to straighten out our metaphor. From a medical perspective, AIDS is considered to be "invariably fatal" only because it has, historically, been defined that way.[3] When the CDC provided its definition for surveillance purposes, little was known about the natural history of the disease. Now, four years later, it is obvious that AIDS is not an isolated disease or even disease syndrome. The CDC maintains its definition for the limited purposes of epidemiological surveillance, although it is not accurate for other purposes.[4] The disease is obviously a spectrum disease caused by infection with HTLV-III/LAV. Its effects range from a brief and transient illness, through to generalized lymphadenopathy, to what is called AIDS-Related Complex (ARC), and on to frank or full-blown AIDS. Dr. Robert Gallo, as well as other scientists, has argued for change in this nomenclature.[5] Yet, we cling to AIDS as death, to AIDS as an invariably fatal disease, perhaps because it better fits the drama that we have constructed about the coming of and the meaning of AIDS.

The Punishment Metaphor

The metaphor of AIDS as death leads directly to the metaphor of AIDS as punishment for sin. If Death is about, looking for new victims, then the victim inevitably asks, "Why me? Why was I chosen?" Those who feel threatened also look to find reasons why they may be protected: They ask, "Why not me?" To answer these questions, [people characterize] the disease as the result of something over which [they] have some control, most particularly their own behavior.

Historically, new and threatening events have frequently (some would say invariably) been explained by reference to God's punishment. In the Bible, God repeatedly punishes with disease and with plagues. In Defoe's semifictional account of the 1665 plague, *A Journal of the Plague Year*, he describes the ways in which, at the beginning of the plague, the people looked first to astrologers to explain the plague as a result of astral doings, then to dream interpreters, and finally to preachers who explained it in terms of God's judgment, the "dreadful judgment which hung over their heads."[6]

Fundamentalist ministers have been the most reliable exponents of this version of AIDS as punishment for sin. Thus, the Moral Majority's Jerry Falwell is reputed to have claimed that "AIDS is the wrath of God upon homosexuals."[7] Other fundamentalist ministers have been as forthright in their claims.[8] More ecumenically, the Anglican Dean of Sydney, Australia, is quoted as saying that "gays have blood on their hands."[9] In a secular vein, President Reagan's Pat Buchanan, an ultraconservative, has written that "the poor homosexuals have declared war on nature and now nature is exacting an awful retribution."[10] Although cleansed of religious implications, this is the same view of AIDS as punishment for sin, but here sin is seen as a violation of the natural law rather than as a violation of God's law. A variation of this metaphor appears in the account of the young man with AIDS who promises his doctor that, if he recovers, he will get a girlfriend.[11] This is sin followed by penance.

It is easy to dismiss this kind of talk as merely the babblings of exceedingly smallminded souls or minds overstressed by illness, and yet the metaphor of AIDS as punishment for sin flourishes as well in academic and liberal forums. AIDS is transmitted sexually and through the blood. Two behaviors statistically account for 90 percent of these transmissions in the U.S.: homosexual intercourse and illegal IV drug use. Both these behaviors are regarded as sinful by many and perhaps most people; gay sex is still illegal in half of the United States, and IV drug use without a prescription is illegal in all states. Because behavior that is regarded as sinful has resulted in exposure to disease, it is easy for the disease to become the punishment for the sin.

Thus, Dr. James L. Fletcher, in an editorial in the *Southern Medical Journal*, cautioned that "a logical conclusion is that AIDS is a self-inflicted disorder for the majority of those who suffer from it. . . . Perhaps, then, homosexuality is not 'alternative' behavior at all, but, as the ancient wisdom of the Bible states, most certainly pathologic." He concludes by suggesting that physicians would do well to seek "reversal treatment" for their gay patients.[12] Similarly, UCLA Medicine Professor Joseph Perloff denies that there is any scapegoating going on with AIDS because "it is not correct to say that nobody is to blame. . . . Ninety percent of all AIDS cases are contracted by either specific sexual acts or specific IV drug abuse. The remaining 10 percent—recipients of blood transfusions, children of female AIDS patients, hemophiliacs—may well be regarded as mere 'victims.'"[13]

The overflow of this metaphor is seen in the insistence on "promiscuity" as the source of AIDS contact. Matt Herron, writing in *The Whole Earth Review* in an article that is clearly not intended to be punitive toward gays, nevertheless comments that when "AIDS arrived, . . . the doors of the candy store started to close." Gays, in his account, had been feasting on forbidden fruits and AIDS was a predictable result of this excess. AIDS was not just a disease in this account, nor even *merely* personal punishment for sin. According to Herron, "the teaching of AIDS" is that "[if you] mess around on a grand enough scale, you will begin to disturb human biology itself."[14]

In the general medical literature, writers frequently refer to promiscuity as the source of AIDS, easily confusing a statistical phenomenon with a judgmental one. Even if they were genuinely trying only to indicate that an increased number of sexual partners heightens the risk of having a partner who carries the virus, the choice of the word *promiscuity* is suspect. *Promiscuous* carries with it a moral judgment: It does not simply mean multiple sexual partners. *Promiscuous*, in America's sexual nervousness, very probably means more sexual partners than the speaker currently has, [that is], an inappropriate or morally reprehensible number.[15] Incorporating this word into serious general or medical writing is probably far more effective than Falwell and Buchanan could ever hope to be in driving home the message that AIDS is punishment for sin.

The gay press, too, has writers in this vein. Ned Rorem, writing in the national gay journal *The Advocate*, wonders whether (with respect to AIDS) "some chastisement is at work."[16] Writers who are encouraging reduced numbers of sexual relationships for gay men are now beginning to make a virtue of this reduction, so that monogamy is seen as a morally correct gay life-style. Although monogamy will statistically reduce one's chances of coming in contact with HTLV-III, that in itself is certainly no endorsement of the moral splendor of monogamy or even of its safety, if one's single partner happens to be carrying the virus. Yet, the metaphor of AIDS as punishment for sin makes the virtue of gay monogamy seem a correct analysis.[17]

A final way in which AIDS as punishment for sin is foisted upon us is in the idea of "innocent victims." *Innocence* belongs to the vocabulary of sin. Gay people who never heard of AIDS until they were diagnosed with it are never referred to as *innocent*; nor are IV drug users who met up with HTLV-III entirely to their surprise. *Innocent* victims of AIDS are babies, elderly women, and nuns, all of whom are presumed to have led, for a variety of reasons, blameless lives. This language of "innocent" and, by indirection, "guilty" victims is translated into action in hospitals, in public agencies, and in the news media, where gay men or drug users with AIDS are treated with less sympathy than "innocent" AIDS patients—that is, those who have not sinned on their way to illness, those for whom disease does not represent just deserts.

The Crime and
Criminal Metaphor

The AIDS *victim* (guilty *or* innocent) also belongs to the metaphor of AIDS as crime. It is almost impossible to find an article in the popular press about people with AIDS that does not use the word *victim* several times. When Los Angeles's Archbishop Mahoney announced that the diocese intended to open a hospice for those with AIDS, he could scarcely get through a sentence without talking about "victims." In an interchange that particularly demonstrated the strained use of language, he finally declared, when asked if the hospice would be open only to Catholics, that it would indeed be open to "victims of any faith or belief." [18]

When the person with AIDS is portrayed as a victim, it is because he has had something unexpected done to him [or her], something that is somehow against the law, if only the scientific law as we imaginatively perceive it. Thus, AIDS becomes a supercriminal able to get away with violating the law. It is seen as amazing, Lex Luthor-like, someone who sweeps across the world, striking terror in hearts. *Newsweek* describes AIDS [as] "embark[ing] on an intercontinental killing spree." It becomes a serial killer that "strikes men and women" and "makes deep incursions on heterosexuals." [19] It goes on "a deadly odyssey." [20]

For the *Los Angeles Times*, AIDS becomes a "pathological personality." [21] This language presents a disease that is bigger than life. Its power is awesome and we can only be terrified by it. This kind of image can be used to encourage increased spending (it's so big that you need to spend a lot of money to control it), but it also encourages drastic steps, steps that go outside the ordinary bounds of good sense, good law, and good ethics. Discussions about quarantine usually bring this metaphor into focus. As well, the battle about closing the bathhouses may have been affected by this aspect of the crime/criminal metaphor, because although many acknowledged it to be a drastic action, the action could be justified by the enormity of the "criminal" that was being tracked.

In addition to appearing as a master criminal, AIDS also appears as a new kind of crime. New diseases are easily seen in a crime metaphor exactly because we do not understand them. They then present themselves as puzzles or as mysteries. "An unidentified disease mysteriously focuses on one group." [22] This metaphor feeds directly into our rather trivial fantasies about detective stories and turns physician/scientists into detectives scrambling about, using their superior intellectual abilities to unravel the mystery. It makes "unraveling the secrets of the shifty AIDS virus" the important aspect—not the care of those with the disease. In a recent *New York Times Magazine*, there is a colorful account of the work of four Boston physicians and researchers who are presented as a crackerjack, coordinated and collaborative detective team, out to solve the mystery. [23] The detective story metaphor is widely apparent in the popular press: The *Philadelphia Daily News* warns of a "gay plague baffling medical detectives." [24] "Clues" turn up everywhere. *Medical World News* advises that "mounting evidence suggests that . . . heterosexuals may find themselves tangled in the AIDS web." [25]

The primary problem with this metaphor is that it tends to collapse the *disease* as crime and criminal with the *person who has the disease* as crime and criminal. Thus, whereas *Newsweek* describes *AIDS* as terrorizing the world, *Life* magazine asserts that "the AIDS *minorities* are beginning to infect the heterosexual, drug-free majority,"[26] and *Weekly World News* moves one step further to have "AIDS *victims* terrorizing everybody" (ital. added).[27]

The War Metaphor

The metaphor of medicine as war is so common that we can perhaps scarcely imagine any other way of talking about how physicians deal with diseases and patients. The physician's job is, after all, to fight disease [using] batteries of tests and . . . an armamentarium of drugs[, giving] orders [to] troops, of course, [who] owe . . . obedience and loyalty. This metaphor developed first in the late 19th century with the discovery of bacteria, which were seen as invaders.[28] HTLV-III infection, as a disease that affects the immune system (with its killer cells that fight off foreign invaders), is particularly surrounded with a scientific vocabulary based on war metaphors. For example, one writer explains that "when the battle against the invading microorganisms is done, . . . T-suppressor cells send out signals to call off the troops." When the AIDS virus appears, it "must first invade a host cell and commandeer some of that cell's DNA material." Eventually, "the body is completely at the mercy of the most commonplace of infectious invaders."[29]

AIDS as a war ("The AIDS Conflict," according to *Newsweek*[30]) is reported much as any other war is. Intrepid *Cosmopolitan* reporter Ralph Gardner, Jr., advises his readers that "if this is a battle that pits man against nature, then nature is pushing back our forces. The news from the front is not good."[31] A dedicated troop rallier, Detroit physician John F. Fennessey does not take such news lying down. He issues a clarion call that "AIDS must be confronted, attacked, and bested by the full, coordinated resources and armamentarium of the medical scientific community. . . . AIDS must and will be confronted and controlled."[32]

Although much of this sounds like no more than bad writing, it is important to remember that the primary element of the war metaphor is the existence of an enemy. AIDS or HTLV-III is, presumably, that enemy. As the crime metaphor permits the person who has the disease to become the criminal, so also does the war metaphor encourage transforming the person housing the enemy into the enemy. Thus, *Medical World News* reports that "an infected person could harbor the virus for 14.2 years."[33] *Life* refers to the 1.3 million Americans who "may be harboring—and passing on—the virus without having symptoms."[34]

Outside of ship anchorage, *harbor* is probably most closely associated with spies and criminals (as in harboring criminals or spies). Harboring suggests that the virus is being hidden knowingly, willingly, and with bad intentions. It does not leave the "infected person" a neutral object. In a war, those who "harbor" the virus are like spies in our midst. Demands for quarantine and isolation of those with AIDS or for labeling and tracking asymptomatic people who are antibody positive are calls to locate the enemy. They are reminiscent of World War II internment policies that we now look back upon with great discomfort. No one believed that *all* Japanese residents were a threat to the country but, because the dangerous ones could not be identified, it seemed appropriate to incarcerate all of them. This decision was supported by the public and, ultimately, by the U.S. Supreme Court, because it occurred in the context of a great war. To the extent that the war metaphor dominates our perceptions of AIDS, we will be more likely to sacrifice people and their rights in the name of protecting society. Edmund White, writing in *Rolling Stone*, argues that "gays are quickly losing basic civil liberties. A real state of siege has been declared."[35] Clearly the war has been declared not on the virus but upon those who carry it.

The war metaphor also gives rise to other elaborations. Susan Sontag has commented that writing about cancer is so dominated by war metaphors that the only thing missing was the body count.[36] Newspaper articles on AIDS now routinely include that body count. The last paragraph of news stories almost invariably gives the absolutely up-to-date numbers of cases and deaths. A scientist calls asymptomatic, antibody-positive individuals "time bomb[s]," because doctors are unsure of when they will "go off," [or] develop [the] disease.[37] AIDS itself is a "time bomb," according to the [Los Angeles] *Times*, because of its financial implications.[38] Bombs loom increasingly large. Several writers, including John Brennan (a *Los Angeles Times* medical columnist), have called for a "Manhattan Project" to fight the "war against AIDS."[39] Brennan even goes so far as to say that creating an AIDS Manhattan Project will produce in a short time the necessary weapons ([that is, the] drugs and vaccines) to win the war, just as the Manhattan Project, in only three years, created the atomic bomb, thus "marking the beginning of the use and abuse of nuclear power." The hope of controlling AIDS with something even metaphorically like the atomic bomb is scarcely an encouraging prospect, especially if we must think of it in terms of the abuse of nuclear power. Brennan's statement shows how easily the war metaphor draws one to otherwise unacceptable ideas.

The Metaphor of Otherness: The Divided Community

The most difficult metaphor to illustrate in the language of AIDS may be the most pervasive one. That is the language of otherness, of the divided community. It is heard easily in conversation. Ask half a dozen people what is to be done about the problem of asymptomatic but infectious seropositives and they reliably respond in terms of what "we" must do about "them." The image of AIDS has been carefully sustained as a problem for "them," whoever they may be. Margaret Heckler publicly illustrated this when she announced the availability of the HTLV-III antibody blood test, saying that "we must conquer [AIDS] as well before it . . . threatens the health of our general population."[40] There was considerable distress expressed about this statement, especially from the gay community who thought they were a part of the general public. Nevertheless, the phrase continues to be used when discussing whether AIDS risk groups will change.[41] The speakers seem to believe that they can move the threat of disease further away by casting the high-risk groups out, as if a linguistic distance might provide physical safety.

The persistent recurrence of *leper* and *leprosy* in AIDS discussions and writings is also part of this metaphor. The leper is cast out; he is no longer an integral part of the community. Omnipresent analogies between AIDS and leprosy make it seem acceptable to respond to the newer "plague" in the same way that was acceptable for the older one.

The metaphor of AIDS as otherness permits people to accept lesser treatment for those who belong to that other group than they would demand for themselves. Gardner, for example, points out that "if there was any good news . . . it was only that the great majority of cases (94 percent) remain confined to the four high-risk groups."[42] The idea of otherness is possible only as long as "we" are able to isolate ourselves from linguistic connection with people who have the disease or who are at risk for it. By referring in print to AIDS as a "gay disease" or a "gay plague," those in the straight community are encouraged to think of AIDS as something happening beyond their borders, outside the "general population"—as something happening to people for whom they have no human responsibility. The metaphor of otherness provides comfort to those who use it because it implies that they will be spared harm and responsibility.

Conclusion

In *The Plague*, Camus's penetrating novel of the way in which the residents of the town of Oran, quarantined with bubonic plague, come to grips with their fate, Tarrou tells Dr. Rieux what he thinks must be done. Through the months, he says, "I'd come to realize that all our troubles spring from our failure to use plain, clean-cut language. So I resolved always to speak—and to act—quite clearly, as this was the only way of setting myself on the right track."[43] Susan Sontag, in a much different context, echoes this statement, when she argues that "the most truthful way of regarding illness—and the healthiest way of being ill—is one most purified of, most resistant to, metaphoric thinking."[44]

In Camus's tale, the plague creates community where there had been none: "No longer were there individual destinies; only a collective destiny, made of plague and the emotions shared by all." The metaphors of AIDS, however, work in direct opposition to this sense of community. Crime, sin, war, and the divided polity are all metaphors that oppose a sense of community. They are inherently divisive metaphors that suggest we are not all in this together. But surely we are. There is no question but that ethically one ought not to harm innocent people. But in this situation we are all innocent. Those who are carriers of the HTLV-III virus need to care about and to protect those who are not. Those who have not been exposed also need to care for and to protect those who have. It is not that some of "us" need protection and some of "them" need to sacrifice their rights; that some belong to death, while others embrace life; that some are righteous and others are sinners; that some are criminals and others their victims; that some are enemies and others loyal and deserving citizens; that some may be cast out, while others are kept securely within. Surely those who have been exposed to AIDS have enough to suffer without being victimized by metaphorical myths.

Disease, especially disease that may lead to death, takes on a dramatic quality in this culture. Drama encourages elevated language. A brief stroll through the *Readers' Guide* listings under AIDS will demonstrate the drama that AIDS has provided for readers in the past few years.[45] It is time, however, to speak plainly. There is too much at stake to permit rhetorical flourish to drive our pens. Again quoting Sontag, "nothing is more punitive than to give a disease a meaning—that meaning being invariably a moral one."[46] AIDS has been permitted and encouraged to carry a moral meaning, but that morality is in our minds, not in the disease. If our ethical judgments are not to be based on punitiveness and further divisiveness, it is time for us to confront the inner meanings our language betrays and then to rid not only our speaking and writing but also our thinking of these metaphors.

Notes

1. July 1985, p. 12.
2. Edmund White, "The Story of the Year," *Rolling Stone* 463–64, Dec. 19, 1985/Jan. 2, 1986.
3. Dennis Altman also makes this point: "Although people suffering from ARC can be very sick, relatively few go on to develop the full syndrome and die; one wonders whether the media reaction and resulting hysteria would have been noticeably less had the range of less serious illnesses been included in the conceptualization of AIDS itself from the beginning." *AIDS in the Mind of America*, New York: Anchor Press/Doubleday, 1986, p. 36.
4. See also "The Walter Reed Staging Classification for HTLV-III/LAC Infection," *New England Journal of Medicine* 314(2), 1985, pp. 131–32, in which Redfield et al. create a scale/nomenclature for HTLV-III infection: "The clinical presentation of patients with HTLV-III infections can range from asymptomatic (with viremia or antibody or both), through chronic generalized lymphadenopathy, to subclinical and clinical T-cell deficiency."
5. *American Medical News*, Jan. 10, 1986, p. 36. See also David Dassey, "AIDS and Testing for AIDS," *Journal of the American Medical Association* 255(6), 1986, p. 743.
6. *Journal of the Plague Year*, New Meridien Classic, 1984, p. 36.
7. Falwell has denied this, although several newspaper reporters have insisted that they heard him say it. Altman, op. cit., p. 67.
8. See, for example, Rev. Charles Stanley, president of the Southern Baptist Convention, who has said that "AIDS is God indicating his displeasure toward a sinful life-style." As quoted in *Los Angeles Times*, Jan. 24, 1986, Section 2, p. 5.
9. Altman, op. cit., p. 25.
10. As quoted in *Newsweek*, Aug. 12, 1985, from *New York Post*, May 24 and 25, 1983.
11. See Altman, op. cit., p. 17.
12. *Southern Medical Journal* 77(2), 1984, p. 150.
13. *Los Angeles Times*, Mar. 14, 1986, Section 2, p. 4.
14. Matt Herron, "Living with AIDS," *Whole Earth Review* 48, 1985, p. 52.
15. A recent "Dear Abby" included a letter from a woman who "accepted as due punishment" contracting herpes during a period of "promiscuity." She asks, "What are the facts regarding formerly promiscuous women and AIDS? How many years must I fear retribution for that phase of my life? And how would you define promiscuous?" Abby's reply is that disease isn't punishment

but that anyone "who has a sexual relationship with more than one person at a time is promiscuous." *Los Angeles Times*, Mar. 9, 1986, Section 6.

16. *The Advocate*, Sept. 19, 1983.
17. Another variation of AIDS as punishment for sin is expressed by Joan McKenna, a "renegade scientist," who tells gays that "you can't *catch* the deficiencies of an impaired immune system. You have to create them." McKenna teaches "thermobaric therapy," which involves cooling the body's "core temperature." *East/West Journal* 16 (1), Jan. 1986, p. 44.
18. *Los Angeles Times*, Feb. 3, 1986, Section 2, p. 1.
19. *Newsweek*, Aug. 12, 1985.
20. *New York Times Magazine*, Feb. 6, 1986, p. 28.
21. *Los Angeles Times*, Nov. 25, 1985, Section 1, p. 2.
22. Herron, op. cit., p. 35.
23. *New York Times Magazine*, Mar. 2, 1986. See also "Disease Detectives Tracking the Killers: The AIDS Hysteria," *Time*, July 1985.
24. Aug. 9, 1982.
25. *Medical World News*, May 13, 1985, p. 11.
26. *Life*, July 1985, p. 12.
27. Nov. 26, 1985, p. 35.
28. Susan Sontag, *Illness as Metaphor*, New York: Vintage Books, 1979, pp. 64–65.
29. Herron, op. cit., p. 46.
30. *Newsweek*, Sept. 23, 1985.
31. Ralph Gardner, Jr., *Cosmopolitan*, Nov. 1984, pp. 150, 155–56.
32. "AIDS Hysteria Counterproductive," reprinted in *American Medical News*, Jan. 17, 1986, p. 4.
33. *Medical World News*, May 13, 1985, p. 11.
34. *Life*, July 1985.
35. White, op. cit., p. 124.
36. Sontag, op. cit., p. 64.
37. *American Medical News*, Nov. 22–29, 1985, p. 28.
38. *Los Angeles Times*, Jan. 12, 1986.
39. *Los Angeles Times*, Oct. 15, 1985, View Section, pp. 1, 3. An Assistant Secretary of Health told President Reagan that AIDS research was the "health equivalent of the Manhattan Project" (*Los Angeles Times*, Dec. 20, 1985, Section 1, p. 2).
40. As quoted in *Journal of the American Medical Association* 253(23), 1985, p. 3377.
41. "IV drug users are most responsible for introducing AIDS into the general population." (Herron, op. cit., p. 47.) "So far, the epidemiological evidence suggests that the disease hasn't yet spread widely in the general population." (C. Marwick, "AIDS Associated Virus Yields Data to Intensifying Scientific Scrutiny," *Journal of the American Medical Association* 254 (20), 1985, p. 2867.) A Washington, D.C., lobbyist is quoted by *American Medical News* as saying "the federal government recognizes that AIDS is a public health crisis that has the potential for infecting the general population." (Jan. 10, 1986, p. 9.)
42. Gardner, op. cit., p. 150.
43. Albert Camus, *The Plague*, Random House, Vintage Books, 1972, p. 236.
44. Sontag, op. cit., pp. 5–6.
45. "Fatal, Incurable, and Spreading," "Battling AIDS," "The Plague Years," "AIDS Neglect," "AIDS Panic," "Public Enemy #1," "Death after Sex," "Homosexual Plague Strikes New Victims," and so forth.
46. Sontag, op. cit., p. 57.

The Punishment Concept of Disease

LORETTA KOPELMAN

There is an ancient, powerful, and universal view of disease as punishment. It is found in the plays of Sophocles, criticized in the Book of Job, and used in every epidemic throughout history to account for why some get sick and some do not. Noncontagious as well as contagious, and mental as well as physical, diseases have been explained by means of it.[1]

The punishment concept of disease is here understood as the view that being bad or doing bad things can directly cause disease, and that when it does, blame should be placed on those who get sick or those having special relations to the sick. For example, parents may believe their child's genetic disease is punishment for their sins, or, to escape self-reproach, may blame others. Versions of the punishment concept of disease echo through preventive, wellness, and holistic health programs,[2] but thunder through current debates about the rights and needs of those with acquired immunodeficiency syndrome (AIDS). Some argue that AIDS is a punishment because they disapprove of the life-style of those at greatest risk for getting it (prostitutes, those with multiple sexual partners, homosexuals, and intravenous drug users). I will argue that this is an untenable but influential view of disease. Moreover, it should be identified in its various versions and resisted because it can thwart fair and compassionate responses to people. There are important, potentially conflicting values in setting health policy that are especially evident during the AIDS epidemic—how to allocate funds, provide empathetic care, honor civil liberties, and protect public health and safety. These issues are complex enough without the untoward influence of what I argue is a potent misconception about disease. In what follows, I identify and criticize several versions of it.

Religious versions of the punishment view of disease allege that God (or supernatural forces or gods) deliberately inflicts punishment on an offender in retribution for an offense. It may be a warning or deterrent to others to change their ways lest they too be singled out; or an incentive to be virtuous; or a warning that the bad perish and the good thrive; or a sign that a cosmic order or purpose requires that the sin be negated by punishment; or a chance for the sinner to learn and be rehabilitated by God's paternalistic intervention.[3] Consider:

> Little did the world recognize the three plagues which originated in the mind of the Eternal Father. These plagues were called The Legionnaires' Disease, Herpes, and AIDS. . . . However, these diseases that came upon mankind originated through the merciful heart of the Eternal Father. Sufferings were brought upon those who must cleanse their souls to avoid Hell.[4]

This same publication predicts that God will not permit science to find a cure for AIDS because homosexuality "shall not be accepted nor condoned by the Eternal Father even if He has to send another plague upon you." Charles Stanley (when president of the Southern Baptist Convention, the largest Protestant group in the United States) claimed AIDS was sent by God to show God's displeasure that homosexuality was gaining acceptance in America.[5]

Where disease is seen as punishment, preventive medicine may take the form of good behavior, and therapy includes seeking forgiveness. In the Bible, Job's friends use what I have called a religious version of the punishment concept of disease. When Job loses his family, fortune, and health, they ask him what he did to deserve such terrible punishment from a just God. They implore him to beg God's forgiveness for his sins. Job insists that he has done nothing wrong, that he deserves no blame, and that evil can come from natural sources. In the end God, speaking from the whirlwind, agrees [with Job] and condemns his friends' judgments.

This view expressed by Job's friends is common in prescientific and unscientific medicine. Taboos, rituals, and sacrifice were and are used to promote health, ward off disease or plague, or to seek forgiveness. Duffy writes that throughout history, "pestilences and other catastrophes were widely held to be punishments sent by God; and, without exception, every major epidemic resulted in the proclamation of days of fasting, humiliation, and prayer."[6] Sickness was seen as the result of even minor infractions of God's moral law. But even in our own science-dominated culture, the association of loss and blame is strong.[7] It is not my purpose to question the power of beliefs in supernatural forces to make people feel sick or scare them to death; this power is illustrated by Voodoo practice. My interest is whether it is a rational or plausible view in itself.

There are at least three very serious problems with this religious version of the punishment concept of disease. First, if we look at who thrives and who perishes in the world, it does not seem reasonable to conclude that the wicked perish and the good thrive in accordance with any just system of reward and punishment. Sometimes the good die young from disease and the wicked lead long, healthy lives. Thus, this view fails as a general account of why people get sick. It cannot explain why the innocent get diseases. Infants who get AIDS are not being punished for anything they have done. In response, defenders sometimes claim innocent babies are suffering for the sins of their parents. Infants have AIDS, they point out, because of things done by the parents. Innocent people often suffer for the sins of the others. Once defenders of the religious version of the punishment concept of disease admit some disease is not punishment for what the person did wrong, however, then they must also agree they have modified their view. It is no longer a general account of why people get sick. For in responding in this way they must admit there are two sorts of diseases, those that are due to punishment for one's own action, and those that are not, but no way has been given to distinguish them.

A second problem is that the obscure (why do people get sick?) is explained by the more obscure (because of what a supernatural being intends). For example, if God uses disease to warn or punish us for a bad life, then a just God ought to be consistent in setting similar punishments for similar behavior. Some church figures have claimed AIDS is a plague sent from God to indicate displeasure about social acceptance of homosexuality.[8] If that is true, one might expect a consistent and just God to punish male and female homosexuals equally. But lesbians, unlike male homosexuals, are in a low-risk group for getting AIDS. Essential to our notion of justice is that similarly situated people ought to be similarly treated. Defenders may respond that God does not have to follow our notions of justice. Still, we have no others to use; hence, the explanation is more obscure than what we seek to explain. The problem is that appeals to God's will and intentions have been used in disputes over homosexuality, school curricula, euthanasia, abortion, war, and other issues. Because we cannot agree what God's will or intentions may be, our personal views cannot rationally be used as a final appeal in settling controversies. Such appeals lack substance we can discuss critically and undermine both compassion and recognition of the need for rational inquiry.

Third, even if . . . we knew who got sick from God's punishment, it is not clear what would follow about how we should treat or view others. As we have seen, some defenders believe that these religious views allow us to draw certain conclusions. But this does not seem obvious. If it is wrong to make others suffer intentionally and without cause, and if someone has already been justly punished by God's more perfect means, then arguably it would be wrong for humans to inflict additional punishment. Thus, even granting the truth of the religious version of the punishment concept of disease, one could not obviously use it to justify different treatment of sick people. If sinners have been justly warned or punished by God, then that should be sufficient. Arguably, too, if an individual has been singled out on earth for God's justice, perhaps we should agree that that person is blessed.

Thus, the religious versions of the punishment concept of disease seem neither cogent nor useful. They give no general account of why some people suffer diseases and others do not, and no grounds for why it would be acceptable to treat or view people with diseases in any way differently as a result of viewing disease as punishment from a supernatural being.

There is a second, and very different, nonreligious, secular version of the punishment concept of disease. Unlike the religious versions, there is no supposition that a supernatural being judges us for wrongdoing and inflicts punishment in the form of disease. Rather, it is assumed that we get diseases from living badly. Nonreligious versions employ a different understanding of *punishment* from that used in the religious forms of the punishment concept of disease. *Punishment* in a religious version was taken to be the act of a judge who inflicts a penalty on a wrongdoer for an offense out of retribution, requital, or as an inspiration for deterrence or reform. But there is another understanding of *punishment*.[9] In the moral versions *punishment* is used as it is in sports, meaning the infliction of a heavy blow. When we say boxers or football teams "took a punishment," we mean that they got hurt. A nonreligious version of the punishment concept of disease does not say God punishes us for wrongdoing and irresponsibility, but that we suffer punishing blows in life in the form of diseases if we live badly, act irresponsibly, or fail to attend to our moral or spiritual well-being. Diseases are, in these views, consequences of people's bad attitudes, habits, or actions.

Nonreligious versions of the punishment concept of disease are popular. They are suggested in cereal advertisements and magazine articles that tell us we can avoid the "punishment" of diseases such as cancer for ourselves and our loved ones if we eat high-fiber cereals, or exercise, or have the right kind of thoughts and images. These views are sometimes encouraged by enthusiasts of preventive medicine [or] holistic and wellness programs [who suggest] that illness can be avoided and aging delayed with "good living." The wellness, preventive, and holistic health-care movements emphasize individual responsibility for health.[10] Diseases from smoking, obesity, alcohol, drug abuse, and anxiety are often targeted as being subject to control. Bad attitudes, habits, or actions are credited with causing diseases, and to the degree we are responsible for our bad "life-styles" we are responsible for our diseases. Most advocates of the holistic, wellness, or preventive health programs, I believe, neither want to make people who get sick feel like moral or spiritual failures, nor encourage special treatment of people because a disease is supposed to be "their own fault." But some explicitly conclude that people are responsible for their "wellness" if they live well and to blame for their illnesses if they do not.[11]

Nonreligious versions of the punishment concept of disease avoid some of the problems of the religious versions. For one thing, we do not have to find some way to reconcile the interventionist role of a just and all-powerful supernatural being with the fortunes of good and evil people. For another, we need not claim to explain the obscure (who gets sick) with the more obscure (what supernatural beings intend).

There are, however, some serious problems with this view. One difficulty is similar to the one raised with the religious version: It fails as a general account of why people get diseases. Clearly some sick people are not in any way responsible for their condition, such as infants born with Trisomy-18 or AIDS. Accordingly, advocates may hold to a modified version that states people are directly responsible for some, but not all of, their diseases. Infants are of course not responsible for their diseases. But people who pass around dirty needles, or who have multiple sexual partners, ought to know they are at greater risk for contracting infectious or venereal diseases, even if they do not know about AIDS. So, too, those who smoke or drink heavily ought to know they are more likely to get diseases.

According to the modified, secular punishment view, people directly cause some

but not all disease by their actions, habits, or thoughts; and people who act irresponsibly about their health should be viewed or treated as blameworthy either before or
once the disease strikes. This view may seem initially plausible because most of us
do believe we are to some degree responsible for our health and illness. But can we
reliably assess responsibility for health and illness well enough to justly or usefully
blame or praise, set health policy, or treat and view people differently? And even if
we could, should we?

Suppose we can distinguish responsible and irresponsible health behavior in
some rough way, how should this affect, for example, educational programs, allocation of funds, or health policy when people get sick after knowingly engaging in risky
behavior? Of course, it is useful to educate people about risks, especially those in
high-risk groups. This allows them more informed choices about how to live their
lives. For example, blacks have a higher incidence of high blood pressure than other
groups, and they can learn how to lessen their risks. Education has been very effective in stemming the AIDS epidemic among homosexuals, because they have altered
their behavior. Education has also been useful to reduce some of the alarm and discrimination people who have AIDS or ARC have encountered in schools, at work, or
in obtaining housing.

But education about choice does not settle how people ought to act or whether
they deserve blame for not acting as education programs advocate. First, while
health is a good, it is not the only good. Some risks with one's health may not be
irrational or uninformed when judged in terms of other duties or goods. For example, certain religious groups, such as Jehovah's Witnesses, make unusual medical
choices, such as rejecting blood transfusions or organ transplantation, because of
what they see to be higher goods. Another example is the praiseworthy work of the
physicians and nurses who provided care for AIDS patients even before there was
evidence AIDS was not contracted from casual contact. They knowingly took risks
with their health and well-being for what they regarded to be higher goods or duties.
Those working with blood still take risks.

Second, some education programs have been criticized in themselves for creating unrealistic expectations: Some simplify associations of risky behavior and disease; some fail to communicate that the conditions leading to disease may be very
complex, or that the data used may be rather sketchy. These factors create difficulties
because people who become sick may be unfairly blamed by themselves or others
for getting sick.

Third, educational programs presuppose that people can alter their behavior and
act responsibly to avoid disease and promote well-being. It is difficult, however, to
determine responsibility. The clearest case of ascription of responsibility is where
people could have done otherwise, intended the act done, and foresaw and intended
the salient consequences. But ignorance, temptation, compulsion, ambivalence, or
irrational views can make responsibility hard to determine. Socioeconomic or cultural factors may also predispose people to act in certain ways. These considerations
can be so complex that we should doubt if we could know enough to determine
accurately the relationship between responsibility and disease in order to view or
treat sick people in significantly different ways.[12] In addition to dangers of unjust

blame from others there are also problems of unjust self-blame. For there is a well-established association of loss and self-blame.[13] People who get sick or suffer a major loss may initially feel responsible. They ask what they did to deserve this, or how they might have acted to avoid their loss. Thus, some educational programs may unwittingly promote a punishment view of disease, and when illness occurs fuel self-blame and increase rather than decrease suffering.

Perhaps, however, we should view or treat people as blameworthy *after* a sickness occurs. I will discuss three difficulties with this view. The first is that it presupposes we can reliably mark out diseases that are people's fault with the kind of accuracy fairness requires for health policy. We have seen that there are serious difficulties with this assumption.

The second problem with viewing or treating people as blameworthy once there is sickness is that if we do this we are likely to blame some unjustly. Unjust blame harms others by increasing their suffering, but also harms those who unjustly blame. By encouraging people to take responsibility for what they cannot control, we add to their suffering by encouraging them to bear a sense of failure, guilt, and moral blame. And if we inflict harm on others unjustly, then we also harm ourselves by acting unjustly and by increasing needlessly others' suffering.

A third problem with viewing or treating people as blameworthy once they get sick is that even if we could reliably distinguish between those sicknesses that could have been avoided by living better, we ought not to do so, because it would thwart the kind of [care from] community and health professionals we should want to foster. Special treatment is sometimes made on the basis of an argument for fairness, that it is just or useful to treat people who bring on their own illness differently. But this may be too narrow a view. For we all profit from a system of health care that fosters compassionate care. If we begin to distinguish between those sufferers who are deserving of care and those who are not, then arguably we risk surrendering a compassionate response to people just because they suffer. Encouraging health care professionals to adopt or use a policy restricting care because they judge a disease as the person's own fault could threaten the general relations between professional and patients. Health practice is distinguished by its commitment to care for those who suffer simply because they are in need. Thus, allocation of care on the basis of blame for illness is unreliable and endangers concern and feeling for people who need help.

To conclude, the difficulty with denying people care or penalizing them because disease is "their own fault" centers on our inability to determine responsibility with the kind of accuracy needed to be just. Even if we could, such judgments endanger important values encouraging a caring and compassionate response to people. Blaming people for disease burdens them with the charge of moral weakness and distorts the response of caring for those in need.

The punishment concept of disease may be enduring and universal because it is related to how we employ defense mechanisms. It may help us make a chaotic world fit with our idiosyncratic notions of control or justice. (I am good, I am safe.) Sometimes it seems a ready excuse to ignore or abandon people in need. (We don't have to help, it's their fault and their trial.) Or, it may be, as Nietzsche observed, that we do not want to believe that our suffering has no important purpose.[14] (Why me? I must have done something to deserve this. There must be a reason for it.) I have not addressed why this view is powerful, but why it is untenable.

Notes

1. J. Duffy, *The Healers: A History of American Medicine* (Urbana: University of Illinois Press, 1979), pp. 189–190. H. E. Sigerist, *A History of Medicine* (New York: Oxford University Press, 1955), Vol. I, pp. 180ff, 442ff; and Vol. II, pp. 298ff.
2. See, for example: D. L. Fink, "Holistic Health: Implications for Health Planning," *American Journal of Health Planning* (1976), p. 27. Criticisms of this aspect of the holistic health movement may be found in: L. Kopelman and J. Moskop, "The Holistic Health Movement: A Survey and Critique," *Journal of Medicine and Philosophy* 6 (1981), pp. 209–35; and in L. E. Goodman and M. J. Goodman, "Prevention: How Misuse of a Concept Undercuts Its Worth," *The Hastings Center Report* 16 (1986), pp. 26–38.
3. S. I. Benn, "Punishment," in *Encyclopedia of Philosophy*, Vol. 7, ed. P. Edwards (New York: Macmillan Publishing Company, Free Press, 1967), pp. 29–36.
4. *Roses*, "Our Lady of the Roses" (Flushing Meadow Park, Bayside, New York, August 21, 1985).
5. Charles Stanley, as quoted in *New York Native* (Feb. 10–16, 1986), p. 7.
6. Duffy, *op. cit.*, pp. 189–90.
7. S. Freud, "Mourning and Melancholia," in *Collected Papers*, Vol. 4, tr. under supervision of J. Reviere (New York: Basic Books, 1917, 1959), pp. 152–70. E. Lindemann, "Symptomatology and Management of Acute Grief," *American Journal of Psychiatry* 101 (1944), pp. 141–48.
8. Stanley, *op. cit.*
9. Benn, *op. cit.*, p. 29.
10. Fink, *op. cit.*, pp. 25–29. R. B. Miles, "Humanistic Medicine and Holistic Health Care," *Holistic Health Care Handbook* (Berkeley, Cal.: And/Or Press, 1978), pp. 20–21; H. Bloomfield and R. Kory, *The Holistic Way to Health and Happiness* (New York: Simon and Schuster, 1978), pp. 47–55. O. C. Simonton and S. Matthews Simonton, "Belief Systems and Management of the Emotional Aspects of Malignancy," in *Holistic Health Handbook* (Berkeley, Cal.: And/Or Press, 1978), pp. 212–20.
11. Fink, *op. cit.*, pp. 25–29. Miles, *op. cit.*, pp. 20–21.
12. R. N. Veatch, "Voluntary Risks to Health: The Ethical Issues," *Journal of American Medical Association* 243 (1980), pp. 50–55.
13. Freud, *op. cit.* Lindemann, *op. cit.*
14. F. Nietzsche, *The Genealogy of Morals* (1887), Second Essay, Section 7.

Life After Death

SEYMOUR KLEINBERG

The effort to assess the meaning of one's sexuality—anyone's sexuality—has rarely been characterized by clear thinking or frank self-examination. Arguments and accusations about moral responsibility certainly don't help matters. Such confrontations are, rather, an invitation to defiance, rationalization, and rhetoric. Yet the time for such an assessment is upon gays, literally as a matter of life and death.

Some gay men have been changing, in both unexpected and predictable ways. Former activists are now middle-aged and more prosperous than ever before in their lives. They have steady partners and more settled domestic lives. Even the majority who are single have found that the ageism of gay culture has altered their sexual lives as much as AIDS has. Surprisingly, I find those for whom the caloric value of every mouthful of food was instantly tabulated, who were tanned all year round at the playgrounds of the Caribbean or Long Island, who never missed a day at the gym—they are the men who are putting on weight, and spending time on fundraising, or working at the Gay Men's Health Clinic or elsewhere. One does not have to be political, or even to read with any regularity, to be civic-minded.

SOME HAVE REFUSED to change; they search for safe places to practice old pleasures. Latin America and the Caribbean have long accommodated homosexual men with their informal bordellos, their "muchachos" who are partners to passive men but who do not think of themselves as homosexual. It is only a question of time before these gay men spread AIDS to other islands near Haiti, from which they probably first brought it to the mainland. It is hard to gauge the state of mind of such men. They may be filled with rage and seeking revenge. They may fatalistically believe that their behavior doesn't matter. They don't feel they are doing anything wrong, or they don't care. They have no moral sense, or they are immoral. It's bad enough to live in dread of dying an awful premature death. Yet to be filled with desire for revenge, or to be without desires at all, even for ordinary dignity, is a terrible way to live or die. I

From *The New Republic* (August 11 & 18, 1986), pp. 30–33. Reprinted by permission.

assume that such men act less from conscious indecency than from pure evasion. To emphasize sexual desire and desirability is a very effective way to mask anxiety. The habit of promiscuity doesn't allow much room for introspection.

Promiscuity is a broad term. For some men, it means serial affairs or brief erotic relationships. For others, there are no relationships at all; sexual encounters begin and end with momentary arousal. And for some men, promiscuity is all of these—having a lover, and having someone else, and having anyone else. Promiscuity is time-consuming and repetitious. Still, it also has another history and meaning for gay men; and it is that history, and that meaning, with which gay men in the shadow of AIDS must grapple.

In the last 15 years or so, until AIDS appeared, promiscuity had been a rich if not invaluable experience for gay men, uniting a sense of liberation with a politics of resentment, a feeling of living at the modern edge with an outlet for aggressions created by long-held grievances. Such a combination is explosive, of course, and anti-intellectual. But gay men did not invent sexual liberation. They merely stamped it with their hallmark of aggressive display. Casual sex, freed from commercialism, seemed a glamorous portent of a society free from sexism. After "Stonewall," the riot at a New York bar in which gay men successfully resisted police arrest and inadvertently inaugurated gay liberation, gay activists felt they were going to redefine the old terms, junk the guilt and the remorse. They were already discarding with contempt the shrinks and the moralists, paying some of them back for the years of misery they had helped to create, the self-dislike they had urged gays to internalize for the sake of what now seemed merely propriety. Out the window went "sick" and "bad." Many could hardly believe they were jettisoning that dismal baggage.

THOSE YEARS OF sexual opportunism were a time of indifference to psychological inquiry. Description was a higher priority. After so much silence, the need to explain, and the desire to shock, were first on the agenda of gay writers and intellectuals, while the majority of gay men were exploring an exhilarating sense of relief in discos, bars with back rooms, and the baths. The politics of that eroticism had as much to do with ego as with eros: Gay men said that sexuality did not diminish social status, to say nothing of intellectual or professional stature—no matter how vividly it was practiced.

In the early '70s, when movement politics was at the zenith of its popularity, the values it promoted were very seductive. It said the old romantic pieties were a slavish imitation of straight society, where they were already undergoing vigorous scrutiny from feminists. If women and blacks could use politics to demand that society acknowledge they had been unjustly treated, why not gay men? If the acknowledgment of that injustice took the form of striking down old laws and replacing them with better ones, then that, obviously, was the agenda. But for the most part, neither the victories nor the defeats changed the daily lives of gay men and women very much. With or without sodomy laws, most lived without concern for legality. It was understood that the principal struggle was psychological, a demand first for recognition, then for acceptance; the bold terms in which that demand was couched guaranteed the right to pursue a sexual life-style of their own choosing. After Stonewall, gays chose to be very visible.

BEFORE STONEWALL, PROMISCUOUS SEX was illegal, but it was no particular threat to health. If the heart and heat of gay politics have been to ensure the right to fuck whom, when, and where one pleases, then the consequences now for the movement have a rough poetic justice. The more that sex dominated the style of life, from discos to parades, with rights secured or not, the less need most men felt they had for politics—and the less others, such as lesbians, feminists, and minorities, felt the gay movement offered them. For gay men sexual politics became something oddly literal. Both before and after the movement, promiscuity was honored as the sign of an individual's aggressiveness (no matter how passive he was in bed). To fuck was to defy, as bad girls of the past did, dismantling some of society's dearest notions about virtue. But most homosexuals want to be conventional. They are no more imaginative, courageous, or innovative than their neighbors. They want a good life on the easiest terms they can get. Many regard as uninteresting the activism that a handful of men and women are devoted to.

By the late '70s, movement politics displaced flamboyant effeminacy. The piece of trade (a man who is fellated by another but pretends to be heterosexual), whose very stance of masculinity ensured his contempt for his homosexual partner, had been replaced by that formerly groveling queen himself, now looking more virile than his proletarian idol. The dominant image of rebellion was no longer the defiant queens with their merciless ironies but powerful, strong bodies modeled on working-class youth. This new image exposed the erotic ideal of gay male life more clearly and responsively than anything since classical Greece. It was a vast improvement. Liberation freed gays from a lot of burdens, and one of the biggest was to end the search for masculinity among the enemy.

But paralleling the rise of the macho body has been the decline of the health of the male community—a nasty coincidence, if you believe in coincidence. The deeper truth, however, is that the very values that motivated us to look strong rather than be strong are the same values that elevated promiscuity as the foundation of a social identity. AIDS is mobilizing many to work in agencies caring for the ill, allowing them opportunities for sympathy and generosity—but that, too, is not the basis of an identity. What is killing you is not likely to give you a sense of self.

Even if AIDS were cured tomorrow, the style and identity of gay life in the '70s and '80s will be as dated as the sexual mores of closeted homosexual life are now. Many men may rush back to the baths, but it can no longer be the liberating experience it was. AIDS has nullified promiscuity as politically or even psychologically useful.

AIDS has replaced one set of meanings with another. It has now become mythic as the dark side of sexuality, Thanatos to Eros. The life force that is the sexual drive has always had its counterpart, and AIDS is the most dramatic juxtaposition of the need for another and the fear of the other, of pain and pleasure, of life and death, in modern medical history. From the ancient Greeks on down, without a moment's interruption, the lesson has been the same: unfettered sexuality means death, whether through dishonor, the wrath of the gods, or nature itself. We are the heirs of those legends. AIDS, like a blotter, has absorbed those old meanings.

THERE IS MUCH, then, that gay men must give up. The loss of sexual life, nearly as much as grief and fear, compounds deprivations, and no amount of civic work or marching to banners of Gay Pride compensates for it. The most dramatic changes have occurred among those large numbers of men who have become abstinent, assuming a sense of responsibility to themselves if not to others. Not only must gay men refrain from what alone gave them a powerful enough identity to make a mark on the consciousness of society, a behavior that replaced society's contempt with the much more respectable fear and anger, but they must cease to think of themselves as unloved children. And they must do both before they have evidence that society accepts them or that their own behavior has meaning for each other more nurturing than it has been. It is very hard to give up a sense of deprivation when little that created it has disappeared, and worse, when one is beset with fear.

One thing, however, is clear: Gay men are not acting in concert. If gay men sensed they belonged to a recognized community, instead of struggling still to assert their legitimacy, the task would be simpler. If they felt the larger society was no longer so adamantly adversarial, they could give up the sense of injustice that makes talk of social responsibility seem hypocritical. And if their own experience with each other had provided them with bonds deeper than momentary pleasure, they could trust themselves to act as a group in which members assumed responsibility for each other.

As long as the larger society continues to prefer the old homosexual invisibility, the nice couple next door to whom anyone can condescend, as long as that society fails to articulate its responsibilities to gay men, the harder it will be for gay men to give up their seductive sense of grievance. Those men who act irresponsibly in the midst of this crisis betray their isolation, their failure to feel they belong either to a gay community or to a larger one. They perceive the demand for accountability as a demand from strangers. Society has not acted as the surrogate family in which we all develop our loyalties and moral sense. In fact, too often it acts just like the families of gay men: filled with contempt or indifference.

MANY GAYS ARE now relieved that sex is no longer a banner issue. It is not even so important that we all stand up to be counted; enough of us have stood up to satisfy the curious. Instead, much as other groups in American society have done, the gay community has had to reassess more profoundly its relationship to the larger society. Customarily, that relationship has been adversarial. Now, for the first time in my memory, the gay community expects help. It hopes for sympathy from heterosexual society. It expects that those who are ordinarily silent will be uncomfortable with such neutrality when orthodox religious leaders proclaim AIDS the scourge of God upon homosexuals, or when politicians exploit and promote fear.

AIDS has made it necessary for gay men to begin questioning themselves. For too long we have lived as if we were driven, too impelled to know what we were doing and what, consequently, was happening to us. It takes perhaps half a lifetime before one is capable of the introspection (not self-absorption) necessary to make sense of the past and thus act as a morally free adult. The same is true of groups. There are moments in history when groups, too, must tell the truth about themselves.

□□■■

Part II

Grounds for Restricting Liberty

Preview

The liberty to choose and act is a valuable thing. Admittedly, some liberties are more valuable than others. In general, however, it seems presumptively wrong to interfere invasively with the choices and acts of another competent individual. Such interferences stand in need of moral justification. Shortly, we shall survey some of the leading or most influential proposals for determining when it is morally permissible to restrict the liberty of competent people. Indeed, that is the main purpose of this preview; the further goal, of course, is to assess the acceptability of proposals to cope with AIDS that, if carried out, would limit the liberty of certain people.

Let us consider some ways of trying to influence the behavior of other people. The main ways are:

1. Persuasion
2. Enticement
3. Coercion
4. Raw force
5. Deception

To simplify a bit: Fair attempts to *persuade* seem morally unproblematic, because no invasive interference with individual liberty is involved. Similarly, *enticement*—which offers a benefit for compliance ("Eat your spinach and you can stay up an extra hour") without making noncompliers worse off—seems in itself morally unproblematic (ignoring a few worries about bribing, "making offers one can't refuse," or hiring assassins).

In contrast, *coercion, raw force*, and *deception* are presumptively wrong ways to influence the behavior of competent people. Coercion (roughly) can be thought of as a threat to make another person worse off unless he or she complies with a given directive; thus, a mugger issues a coercive threat by saying, "Your money or your life." Similarly, the criminal law, by prohibiting sodomy, prostitution, rape, child abuse, theft, or use of certain drugs, in effect says, "Comply or you go to jail" (or pay a fine or be killed). Thus, such laws are an indication of our collective support for institutionalized coercion. We may make a distinction between coercion and the use of direct force (putting Rasputin in a straitjacket); however, popular usage of the term *coercion* tends to refer to force as such, as well as to coercive threats. Often deception is an equally, or more, effective way to alter behavior. Someone may get your money, not by coercion or brute force, but by selling you stock in a nonexistent company. Generally one is aware of having been forced to do something or coerced into it, but one may be duped and not know it. Thus, one may continue to look with favor on the deceiver. Hence, deception holds out a special attraction for sellers in the marketplace who wish to influence consumer choices.

Coercion, force, and deception are all examples of "invasive" interferences that undermine the capacity of competent people to direct their own lives; thus, they are morally problematic. When is it all right (if ever) to employ such measures? When, in other words, is it all right to interfere invasively with the choices or acts of others? Shortly, we will review some proposed answers to this fundamental ethical question.

It is worth noting that a number of policy proposals with regard to AIDS involve some coercion and are thus morally controversial. Consider again the following proposals or practices:

1. Mandatory blood screening
2. Prohibiting AIDS carriers from being health-care workers
3. Prohibiting AIDS carriers from being restaurant employees
4. Prohibiting AIDS carriers from donating blood
5. Prohibiting gay bathhouses
6. Prohibiting homosexual sodomy
7. Quarantining AIDS carriers
8. Socially stigmatizing those who are AIDS carriers
9. Dismissing from federal jobs those suspected of being able to spread AIDS
10. Refusal to care for or provide shelter for AIDS victims

This list is not, of course, exhaustive of the measures that have been proposed or implemented to control AIDS by restricting liberty. Because quarantine is one of the more radical proposed restrictions on liberty, it is not without interest that in a poll of over 2,400 people taken by the *Los Angeles Times* in July 1986, some form of quarantine for people with AIDS was favored by close to half of all respondents, and by more than half of the respondents who resided in Los Angeles (a city that is not normally considered one of the more tradition-minded or conservative locations in the United States). Of course, ignorance of the difficulties that quarantine would entail is widespread.

Let us move on now from specific proposals to a more theoretical level for a succinct consideration of the more influential proposals regarding legitimate grounds for (invasively) restricting the liberty of competent adults. Here (in overly simplified form) are some of the leading principles:

1. *The Offense Principle (OP)*: It is permissible to interfere invasively to prevent a person (P) from performing an act (X) if P's doing X:

a. seriously offends another (Q); and

b. Q cannot readily avoid the occasion for offense; and

c. the taking of offense is not a result of Q's having absurd beliefs; and

d. an act of the offending type could be done by P in some nonoffensive manner without great loss to P.

2. *The Harm Principle (HP)*: It is permissible to interfere invasively to prevent P from performing X if P's doing X wrongfully harms others.

3. *The Principle of Legal Moralism (LM)*: It is permissible to interfere invasively to prevent P from performing X if P's doing X is intrinsically wrong.

4. *The Paternalistic Principle (PP)*: It is permissible to interfere invasively to prevent P from performing X if P's doing X will result in serious harm to P.

5. *The Principle of Utility (PU)*: It is permissible (indeed, a duty) to interfere invasively to prevent P from performing X if by doing so one can maximize total net expected utility.

It is worth observing that there is extensive philosophical literature covering most of these principles (or similar variants).[1] Hence, our discussion can only allude to the nuances or complexities that are involved.

The Offense Principle

The offense principle (OP) is a reasonably complex principle and is far more plausible than a simple sort of offense principle that might suggest the acceptability of interference whenever someone is offended. Some of the evidently bizarre or counterintuitive implications of the latter principle are not associated with the more plausible OP. Still, such a principle is more likely to be relevant to questions of restricting *public* performance of certain acts, such as going to class nude, a heterosexual couple copulating on the bed in the furniture section of Sears, displaying certain hygienic devices on television, or marching with Nazi flags through a Jewish neighborhood. For our current purposes, the other principles are likely to be of greater interest (although recall the offensiveness to some of disseminating information about "safe sex" or how AIDS may be spread sexually).

The Harm Principle

When considering the harm principle (HP), the question about how to define *harm* becomes very important and not so straightforward. If to offend someone need not harm them, then there is indeed a need for a distinct offense principle, as our list implies. Whether offending someone should be thought of as a kind of harm is a question we set aside here. Intuitively, to harm another is to make that person worse off. And we normally worsen the lives of others by killing or causing pain to them, or by subverting other interests that they may have. Hard cases do exist: Do we harm someone if we damage her reputation but she never learns of it? Is killing always harming? May not someone be, as we sometimes say, "better off dead"? And is not heightening risks for others a kind of harm?

HP is, it would seem, plausibly characterized in terms of "wrongfully harming others." First, we normally do not believe it all right to interfere with a person's liberty whenever his or her acts do very minor harm to others: Thus, we should not fine Max $50 because he forgot to return his coworker's greeting. Second, it is reasonable to think that it is sometimes all right deliberately to perform acts that will foreseeably result in harm to others. Thus, if you choose to live with person A rather than person B, you may hurt (and, hence, harm) B; yet we usually think it is all right for you to make such a choice. Similarly, if Apple Computer, Inc., hurts IBM's business by producing a more popular product (or vice versa), we usually think that kind of damage is morally permissible—and, thus, not a legitimate ground for restricting Apple's liberty to compete. So, it seems more reasonable to believe that it is only in the case of some *subset* of harmful acts (call them "wrongful harms") that we may legitimately restrict the liberty of the harming agent.

Further complexities abound. Some harms are direct, and some are indirect. Some acts are harmful when considered alone, while some are harmful only in conjunction with the acts of other people (throwing one's garbage in the lake, for example). Some harms are certain and immediate (A stabs B); others are not (A appoints an incompetent person to be a federal judge). Some harmful results may be thought of as ones to which the affected parties consent (as in a business or athletic competition). But more important for our purposes is the virtually universal agreement that something like our harm principle states an acceptable ground for restricting liberty. We assume that serious and unconsented-to harm to others, of some sort, is a legitimate basis for restricting liberty. This assumption, surely, justifies much of the criminal law—the laws forbidding rape, theft, murder, child abuse, fraud, and so on.

How does the harm principle affect decisions about policies with respect to AIDS? We will only sketch some possibilities here. HP supposes that we each have a duty not to impose certain harms on others, and that, if we fail to fulfill that duty, our liberty may be legitimately restricted by others. In one bizarre case, some prison inmates in Florida conspired to introduce blood serum from a person with AIDS (in a vial) into the coffee of another person. Had this act been carried out, the coffee drinker probably would not have been infected. Arguably, however, he would have been placed at greater risk of infection. The common view seems to be that the moral prohibitions on harming others also require not significantly and deliberately increasing the risk of harm to which others are subject. Thus, one ought not to drive quickly near a schoolyard at certain times.

Do AIDS carriers heighten the risks for others? To answer affirmatively is tempting. However, two points deserve reflection. First, many conditions or acts heighten risk for others—selling and driving cars or motorcycles, having the flu, selling liquor, and so on. Second, we should distinguish (1) carrying the AIDS virus from (2) carrying the virus and acting in a manner that significantly increases risks to (or harms) others. We note that a number of social commentators have viewed AIDS as divine punishment for wickedness; according to this view, if you carry the AIDS virus you are blameworthy. For example, as an editorial in the *Southern Medical Journal* put it, "Might we be witnessing, in fact, in the form of a modern communicable disorder, a fulfillment of St. Paul's pronouncement: 'The due penalty of their error.'"[2] Of course, if this is the right view, then children who acquired HIV while in a prenatal state, as well as carriers who received the virus during a blood transfusion, are getting their just deserts. More plausibly, merely *having* AIDS is not something deserving of blame, in spite of the stigma society has managed to attach to the condition. A venerable, ancient tradition, of course, blames the sick and conflates the categories of the immoral and the unhealthy. Recall that in Samuel Butler's fictional world of Erewhon, those who became ill were punished as criminals.

Normally we praise or blame people for what they (more or less) knowingly and voluntarily do. Hence, we may have moral questions about what one did to get or avoid AIDS, or what one does to spread or avoid spreading AIDS. Thus, if a carrier, acting deliberately and voluntarily, significantly increases the risk that others may get AIDS, we may regard such acts as a violation of duty. Must, therefore, an AIDS carrier warn others (especially a potential sexual or marital partner) of his or her condition? Should an AIDS carrier readily agree to wear a Buckley-endorsed warning tattoo? Should an AIDS carrier refrain from risky sex? From virtually all sex? From the standpoint of third parties, or the government, may one intervene to guarantee such behaviors? Would such intervention be required by (and be justifiable by) the harm principle? These important matters deserve further exploration.

Before we set aside the harm principle, we should emphasize that it is often invoked to justify restricting the liberty of those *wrongfully* harming (including causing increased risk to) others, such as the mugger, the killer, or the kidnapper. We normally think that we have a right to defend ourselves or innocent bystanders against wrongful harm (or noninnocent threats). May we use (for example) coercion to restrict the liberty of those who are innocent threats to us? Note that if being blameworthy (or noninnocent) requires a capacity to choose rationally, then a dog, a three-year-old child, or a psychotic (at least during certain episodes) could not be considered noninnocent or blameworthy; yet they could each be threats (the child or the psychotic about to shoot a gun, for instance, or the rabid dog intent on getting his pound of flesh). They are innocent threats. We have no room to explore the matter here, but consider these questions: May we coerce innocent threats? May we use serious, indeed lethal, force to thwart such threats? The standard case of self-defense generally involves a response to a noninnocent threat (the malicious mugger or rapist), and most people believe that it is all right to use force against such a threat (perhaps a tacit acceptance of the harm principle). But may we shoot the innocent child before he shoots us (if that is the *only* way to turn away the threat)?

In brief, what is permissible in the case of innocent threats is not obvious and is a matter of some dispute. Observe, then, that a parallel exists here with the case of AIDS carriers. Some, perhaps, are no threat at all; others may be blameworthy threats. Some, however, may be innocent threats to others. If so, are restrictions on the liberty of such people permissible? As a society we are reluctant to restrict the liberty of those not morally responsible for some (seriously) wrongful act. In such cases we cannot claim that the individual has forfeited a right to be free by having performed some blameworthy act. For such reasons quarantine seems morally suspect.

In focusing here on quarantine, we do not wish to suggest that all restrictions on liberty are so extreme. Lesser restrictions, in principle, may be less difficult to justify.

Legal Moralism

The expression *legal moralism* is not always used invariantly, but it commonly refers to the conjunctive view that (1) some acts are intrinsically wrong, and (2) it is legally permissible to prohibit such acts (typically by the criminal law).

Many acts are thought wrong, as we have observed, because they are thought to harm others in some fashion—typically by directly or indirectly causing pain, frustration of desires, death, or deprivation of some sort (killing, stealing, defrauding, and so on). Some actions that are legally prohibited in various countries do not, it is often claimed, cause (unconsented to) harm to others; examples include blasphemy (or cursing the gods), adult prostitution, consenting adult homosexuality, sodomy among married heterosexuals, certain seditious acts, "mishandling" the flag, selling certain forms of pornography, consenting adult incest, sales of certain goods on Sunday, and the sale or use of certain drugs. Many people label most or all such acts "victimless crimes" and frequently argue for the decriminalization (that is, legalization) of the acts.

"Victimless crime," however, can be a question-begging label and a source of confusion. First, users of drugs such as cocaine or crack often seriously harm themselves. So the term *victimless* may be misleading; rather, the label is usually employed to suggest that there are no unwilling victims (assuming that those who use drugs do so willingly). The slightest reflection, however, suggests that this claim is also at least debatable, in view of the rather notorious amount of deception, robbery, and violence committed by certain drug users to support their habit. (Many economists argue that such illegal acts result from the high prices that are the consequence of legal prohibition; thus, according to this point of view, the solution is to legalize the drugs.)

However, suppose that it can be plausibly argued (although we do not attempt to do so here) that the act or practice in question is victimless or harmless in the relevant sense. The legal moralist's position, in effect, is that the criminalization of such an act may be justifiable anyway, if the act is a serious *intrinsic wrong*. Some people believe, for example, that blasphemy, consenting heterosexual adult sodomy, consenting heterosexual adult incest, or consenting adult homosexual acts are wrong *in themselves*—or intrinsically wrong—*even if no one is harmed*. In this view, the class of wrongful acts and the class of harmful (to others) acts only overlap. Those who, in contrast, believe that an act is wrong only if it is harmful to others disagree in a fundamental way with the legal moralists (over the question of whether the distinction between right and wrong is based ultimately on considerations of whether an act harms others or not).

Logically, it does not immediately follow from the principle of legal moralism that any particular act should be criminalized; rather, it must be argued that the act in question is intrinsically wrong. If such is agreed to be the case, then, in the absence of harm to others, on what basis should a certain act be judged wrong? Is the matter thought to be self-evident?

Often legal moralism is associated with religious assumptions, such as:

1. There is a God.
2. God commands (prescribes) or forbids certain acts.
3. Whatever God commands is right, and what God forbids is wrong.

Assumptions 1, 2, and 3 are sometimes called the divine command theory of ethics. So if one accepts (for example) the further assumption that Yahweh forbids sodomy, it follows from the divine command theory that sodomy is wrong.[3] This conclusion comes close to being an assertion that the act of sodomy is intrinsically wrong: Even if the act harms no others, it is wrong (because Yahweh forbids it).

Perhaps it is now clear why certain acts can be correctly described as "harmless immoralities" according to the legal moralist view (as well as in the divine command theory, because one is not thought to *harm* God by disobeying him). Under the harm principle (which assumes that an act must at least cause harm in order for it to be wrong), there cannot be any "harmless immoralities." Of course, if one adopts a definition of *harm* that is quite expansive (including, for example, ethereal "harms" such as those that threaten the moral tone of society), the harm principle can be used to support policies that are practically similar (cursing, for instance, may be viewed as wrong because it threatens the moral "tone" or "fabric" of society, as well as because it is frowned on by Yahweh).

Perhaps it is also now evident how, from the perspective of legal moralism embellished by religious assumptions, it is all right to criminalize sodomy (regardless of whether it is harmless). On the other hand, if sodomy as such is harmless, and if it is unreasonable to believe any or all of the assumptions of legal moralism or the divine command theory, such a proposal is left floating, with no evident rational support.[4]

Following this preview is Lord Patrick Devlin's now-famous defense of legal moralism. (His essay also includes an appeal to a Societal Right of Self-Defense.) Devlin's essay, "Morals and the Criminal Law," appeared in response to, and as a critique of, the recommendations (in 1957) of a British committee, chaired by John Wolfenden, to legalize private, consensual adult homosexuality and not to alter existing law under which prostitution was not a crime. The Wolfenden Committee based its view on a moral position much like that stated in philosopher John Stuart Mill's classic treatise *On Liberty* (1859). In the passage reprinted below, Mill in effect acknowledged only one legitimate ground for restricting the liberty of competent adults: to prevent (certain kinds of) harm to others. Other grounds, such as paternalistic or (legal) moralist ones, Mill found unacceptable. Let us look at Mill's own words (though not, of course, at his defense of these words):

> The object of this Essay is to assert one very simple principle, as entitled to govern absolutely the dealings of society with the individual in the way of com-

pulsion and control, whether the means used be physical force in the form of legal penalties, or the moral coercion of public opinion. That principle is, that the sole end for which mankind are warranted, individually or collectively, in interfering with the liberty of action of any of their number, is self-protection. That the only purpose for which power can be rightfully exercised over any member of a civilized community, against his will, is to prevent harm to others. His own good, either physical or moral, is not a sufficient warrant. He cannot rightfully be compelled to do or forbear because it will be better for him to do so, because it will make him happier, because, in the opinions of others, to do so would be wise, or even right . . . .⁵

In short, Mill accepted some version of what we have identified here as the harm principle. Further, he rejected other grounds (such as legal moralism) for restricting the liberty of competent people (children, idiots, and the incompetent are another story).

Devlin's view, in part, is that the state need not restrict itself only to the interventions permitted by the harm principle. Devlin's position and arguments have been the target of much criticism. In "Immorality and Treason," H.L.A. Hart, who was at that time a famous professor of jurisprudence at Oxford University, scrutinized Devlin's argument and (like other critics of Devlin) sided in substantial part with Mill's position as to what constitutes legitimate grounds for invasive intervention in the affairs of competent adults (or, similarly, what constitutes the moral limits on state intervention in the choices and acts of its citizens).

A final point concerning legal moralism: The expression "the legislation of morality" seems to have generated rampant confusion. The claim that "one cannot (or should not) legislate morality" is widely held among those who seem not to think twice. In one rather straightforward sense, the state can (and jolly well ought to) legislate morality. We have characterized moral claims mainly as claims about what people ought or ought not to do. Hence, claims such as "One ought not to kill, rape, or torture children" are moral claims. We enforce such prescriptions by legally prohibiting and punishing such acts (food for thought for those who are uncomfortable with "shoulds"). Hence, we do and should enforce "morality" of a certain sort. Quite possibly, when many people say "We should not enforce morality," what they mean to be defending is a different proposition, namely: "We should not legally prohibit certain harmless acts (which some people believe to be harmless *immoralities*)." This claim is a quite different kettle of fish. Critics of Devlin may well defend this latter claim; however, they are committed to enforcing morality in the former sense.

Paternalistic Principles

Paternalistic principles assume that sometimes it is all right (or perhaps even a duty) to interfere invasively in the lives of other people in order to promote their good. The remark "It was for your own good" is a familiar reminder of a widely invoked (alleged) justification for invasive intervention, ranging from mild intervention (as when a friend, thinking you are drunk, takes your car keys) to severe (such as incarcerating someone we believe to be otherwise dangerous to himself; or forcing someone to undergo an operation we think good for her). Paternalism toward people who possess less than a certain minimal capacity for rational decision-making is widely thought to be permissible (for instance, using force to get a child away from a hot stove). Paternalistic intervention with competent adults, however, is a matter of considerable dispute and recent investigation.

The range of cases in which a paternalistic principle is invoked to defend typically coercive constraints on liberty of choice and action is greater than one might think at first. For example, the following acts or policies are often defended as justifiable paternalism:

1. Prohibitions on dueling
2. Prohibitions on driving without buckling one's seatbelt
3. Prohibitions on riding a motorcycle without a helmet or without headlights
4. Prohibitions on using certain drugs without a prescription
5. Prohibitions on using certain unapproved drugs
6. Prohibitions on obtaining certain products or services without a prescription from a licensed professional
7. Prohibitions on driving without having passed certain tests
8. Prohibitions on building certain structures unless they satisfy certain standards
9. Prohibitions on distributing certain products unless they include certain warning labels

The term *paternalistic* often seems to carry images of Big Brother and undue invasiveness; hence, it is often used evaluatively to mean "wrongful." However, it is worth recalling that paternalistic actions, in simple terms, are merely acts whereby one party interferes with another (typically contrary to the will of that other) in an attempt to promote the good of (or prevent harm to) the other party. If you are about to step into an elevatorless elevator shaft, and a friend, as a last recourse, violently knocks you away, that intervention is paternalistic. We assume that such an act is a permissible (indeed a welcome) instance of paternalistic intrusion. The interesting philosophical and moral question would seem to be not *whether* but rather *when* or *under what conditions* paternalistic intervention toward competent people is morally justifiable (and when it is not).

Different principles provide different criteria as to when paternalistic intervention is all right. The very strong (bold) principle—that such intervention is *obligatory* whenever another's good is thereby promoted—seems counterintuitive: There would be little respect for individual autonomy (the right to direct one's life according to one's own values or vision) in a society that acted on such a principle. Similarly, it can be argued plausibly (though we shall not do it here) that a society that acted on the weaker (less bold) principle—that it is *permissible* to intervene invasively with a subject whenever one thereby can promote his or her own good—

would also be intolerable, as it would place too high a value on individual autonomy (or on a competent person's right to direct his or her life in ways that wrong no others). A plausible compromise is that those forms of paternalistic intervention toward competent people are permissible that succeed in respecting individual autonomy (or the right just mentioned). Although it is beyond the scope of this book to explore the point here, it is clear that certain paternalistic interventions may indeed respect an individual's autonomy; for example, a subject may have previously given voluntary, informed consent to the sort of intervention in question. Thus, in the earlier example, you may have agreed (or indeed requested) that if you were approaching a state of inebriation, your friend should take your car keys (in spite of any protests and resistance you might offer). In the elevator example, even though no prior consent exists, it is normally reasonable to surmise that, given your beliefs, desires, and values, you would consent to coercive intervention to save your life. Hence, a certain form of hypothetical or implied consent (as well as an actual, prior consent) may suffice to morally justify intervention on paternalistic grounds.

We have sketched, in a most succinct way, the outlines for a theory of when paternalistic intervention with competent adults is justifiable. Assuming that this viewpoint is correct, what bearing does all this have regarding AIDS? Here, the issues become more complex.

Although most people with AIDS are competent individuals, it is worth noting that the AIDS virus can cross the "blood-brain barrier." When it does so, significant cognitive disability can result, severe enough in some instances to render the victim incompetent to choose rationally. In such cases it is not unreasonable to conclude that different paternalistic considerations come into play, and that the general presumption in favor of respecting autonomous choice no longer exists, or is at least weakened. Hence, more intrusive forms of paternalistic intervention may be all right.[6] This issue needs, of course, a more extensive investigation than we are able to provide here.

According to the view of permissible paternalism sketched above, when competent adults voluntarily and knowingly choose risky courses of action that involve no chance of harming anyone else, they should normally be left alone, out of respect for their autonomy. In some cases, temporary intervention may be justified in order to ascertain competence or to determine if an act or choice is really voluntary and informed. Further, for reasons discussed above, fair attempts to dissuade or persuade are not considered invasive. Thus, many attempts to educate or inform potential victims of AIDS (in other words, everyone) would be permissible acts of a paternalistic sort. Providing clean syringes to IV drug users would also be a noninvasive type of paternalistic intervention.

In some cases, people who are inclined to engage in acts that involve risk of spreading or acquiring AIDS—such as intercourse without a condom, deep kissing, or sharing needles—may choose to create a "Ulysses contract" with their potential partners. Less abstractly, in the same way you might give prior consent to your friend to take your car keys if you get drunk, a potential recipient or carrier of AIDS may wish to make agreements with others, if possible, to avoid risky behavior. By so doing, that person effectively consents to paternalistic interventions with, or refusals to cooperate with, certain acts or practices. The term *Ulysses contract* is derived from the story in which Ulysses (or Odysseus) and his crew are approaching the isle of the Sirens, alluring females who promise great knowledge to anyone who swims the treacherous shores to reach them. Ulysses commands his crew to bind him to the mast to prevent his giving in to this nearly irresistible temptation as they near the island, and to ignore him even if he demands to be released. Those who are at high risk for AIDS, analogously, may impose constraints on themselves by consenting to (even invasive) paternalistic interventions by others in order to steer clear of harm's way.

Much more about this subject needs exploration here, but we have sketched one viable position with regard to permissible paternalism and noted (however briefly) its possible application to AIDS issues.

The Principle of Utility

We have too little room here to do justice to such an influential ethical theory as utilitarianism. The core of this theory states that there is just one rationally defensible principle of morality: that one ought to do whatever will maximize the balance of good over evil—usually interpreted to mean the balance of satisfaction (happiness, pleasure, or *utility*) over dissatisfaction (unhappiness, pain, or *disutility*). The central idea of this secular theory (derived from the work of the 18th-century Scottish philosopher David Hume, as well as the English philosophers Jeremy Bentham, James Mill, and John Stuart Mill) is that we are to consider the likely *consequences* of performing alternative acts with respect to their utility or disutility for all people or sentient creatures affected by such acts. In other words, we should weigh or estimate the magnitude of the aggregate benefit (utility) or harm (disutility) of each alternative act being considered; once we determine which alternative maximizes expected utility (or the balance of good over evil), we are to do that act—notwithstanding intuitive judgments about what is right, traditional moral practices or rules, talk of rights, the Golden Rule, and so on, to the contrary.

Strictly speaking (to emphasize a point), in the utilitarian view the maximization of utility is the only justifiable principle of morality; thus, traditional moral values (such as respect for privacy and telling the truth) are regarded, at best, as rules of thumb—theoretically dispensable and overridable. Likewise, talk of natural moral rights is, as Bentham said, "nonsense on stilts." Because of its emphasis on maximization, the utilitarian principle may be viewed as a matter of maximizing benefits minus costs. Hence, what may sound to some like a quaint 19th-century ethic may in fact be the basic normative principle behind much present-day government policy-making: cost-benefit analysis.[7] The utilitarian view may also be implicit in sayings like "We just have to do what's best, all things considered" or "We should choose the lesser evil."

So much for characterizing the utilitarian view. Objections to this view have been thoroughly elaborated in many places, and we will not review them here. Instead, we will consider how a utilitarian would approach some moral questions surrounding the AIDS issue.

Utilitarians place particular emphasis on the consequences of acts or policies.

Thus, if the only way to maximize utility would be to quarantine large numbers of AIDS carriers, the utilitarian principle would dictate doing so. Likewise, if mandatory screening would maximize utility, then that would be the right thing to do. It is plausible to think, then, that a utilitarian approach to certain questions about liberty-limiting policies might dictate the permissibility, even the obligatoriness, of such policies.[8] Thus, the legal tradition in the United States of allowing or requiring rather extreme measures, such as quarantine, when faced with a serious threat to public health, might well find a theoretical, moral friend in utilitarianism. Also, from a strict utilitarian perspective there are no moral rights (such as liberty or privacy) to be overridden, because no such rights exist. Hence, considerations of aggregate welfare reign supreme, and the *only* question to be settled is empirical: "What laws or policies will in fact maximize total net utility?"

Given the serious barriers to an effective mode of screening people in general (not just those in "high-risk" groups), mandatory screening of the adult population may well be ineffectual.[9] Considering also the negative consequences (resentment, costs, and so on), one might conclude that the adoption of such a policy would fail to maximize utility (although such a conclusion could be verified only after a detailed assessment in a strict utilitarian approach). Thus, the utilitarian principle may support a duty *not* to adopt a policy of mandatory screening. The question of what specific policies *would* be supported by utilitarian theory is not one that can be settled abstractly and speculatively. A defensible list of the specific consequences likely to occur from adopting a proposed policy (whatever it is) would be required, as well as a rational estimation of the aggregate net utilities of the different alternatives. Only then can we know which policies are supportable by appeal to the principle of utility. This point may be useful to recall when appraising the policies (actual or proposed) and laws discussed elsewhere in this volume.

Perhaps it needs to be said, in addition, that utilitarianism is not just a principle designed to specify when it is all right to limit the liberty of individuals. Rather, it is a general moral principle aimed at answering one of the fundamental questions of normative ethics, namely: "What ought we (I, the government, society) to do?" Because the answer is "whatever maximizes utility," the principle does not provide any theoretical moral limits on incursions into individual liberty or privacy. If massive incursions into individual liberty are the only way to maximize utility, then they are justified; and if anyone is morally troubled by this implication, the hard-nosed utilitarian may just say, "If you think it through, you'll get over it," or, "Too bad if you have contrary moral beliefs; they, alas, are just irrational." Conversely, if (for the reasons noted above) the consequences of such massive incursions would not maximize utility, they would be unjustified from the utilitarian point of view: Whether an act is right or wrong depends entirely on its actual consequences.

WE HAVE INTRODUCED five different, somewhat influential, allegedly legitimate grounds for restricting liberty—a starting point at least for anyone who wishes to consider seriously, in a principled manner, the justifiability of certain liberty-limiting laws and policies aimed at coping with the problems and questions surrounding AIDS.

The three essays that follow provide further exploration into the issue of grounds for restricting liberty. In Part III, various public policy proposals regarding AIDS are examined. Because AIDS can be transmitted through certain forms of sexual behavior, our beliefs about what constitutes permissible constraint of sexual behavior inevitably will influence our conclusions about permissible strategies and public policies for coping with AIDS. In such a situation, important questions of autonomy, intimacy, and privacy arise; the selections in Part IV directly focus, not on AIDS, but on views about sexual orientation, permissible sex, and the question of whether an emerging constitutional right of privacy or autonomy adequately expresses a defensible moral view about equality of basic rights.

Notes

1. To avoid detail, one might begin with Joel Feinberg's *Social Philosophy* (Englewood Cliffs, N.J.: Prentice-Hall, 1973). Feinberg's more recent four-volume work, *The Moral Limits of the Criminal Law* (New York: Oxford University Press, 1984–88), sets a new standard with its careful and thorough discussion of the moral constraints on the liberty-limiting intervention of the criminal law; in it, he describes more principles (and in greater detail) than we have noted here (for example, he discusses the benefit-promoting principle as well as a kind of moralistic paternalism).

2. James L. Fletcher, "Homosexuality: Kick and Kickback," *Southern Medical Journal,* Vol. 77 (1984): pp. 149–150.

3. In this regard note that, in the *Los Angeles Times* poll mentioned earlier in this chapter, 17 percent of the respondents said they believed that "the Bible is the actual word of God and is to be taken literally word for word." Also over 42 percent agreed with the statements "Politics and morality are inseparable. And, as morality's foundation is religion, religion and politics are necessarily related" (*Los Angeles Times,* July 27, 1986). Because adherents to the divine command theory often use biblical passages as evidence of what God commands, such an approach commits one to some very troublesome moral judgments. Some passages condone slavery (Exodus 21:2–11, 20–21, 26–27; Ephesians 6:5), subordination of women (Proverbs 21:13–24; Matthew 19:3–9; Luke 7:37–50; John 8:3–11; I Corinthians 14:34–35), divorce for any reason (Deuteronomy 24:1–4), hating one's father and mother (Luke 14:26; Matthew 10:35), and wholesale killing (Deuteronomy 20:10–14). Others condemn a good deal of heterosexual sex (I Corinthians 7:1–9), taking interest on loans (Deuteronomy 23:19–20), and planning for the future (Matthew 6:34). Thus, if one accepts each and every passage in the Old and New Testaments as being in some sense divinely inspired and "true," some quite radical conclusions follow regarding what is right and wrong. For a refreshing and skeptical treatment of this topic, read H. L. Mencken's too-often ignored *Treatise on Right and Wrong* (London: Kegan Paul, Trench, Trubner & Co., Ltd., 1934).

4. It is possible to defend versions of legal moralism without appealing to the divine command theory. For example, on some views about moral rights you may wrong others without harming them if you violate their rights. Thus, if your neighbors read your newspapers while you are gone, without your consent, they thereby violate your rights (even though you have not suffered any harm). Two key questions arise whenever an act is declared intrinsically wrong under any system of legal moralism: (1) Why is the act intrinsically wrong? and (2) Even if it is wrong, why is it all right to prohibit the act coercively? Certain insults that are gratuitous and unkind may be considered wrong, but it is doubtful that we should criminalize all of them. For an excellent discussion of versions of legal moralism, see Joel Feinberg, *Harmless Wrongdoing* (New York: Oxford University Press, 1988).

5. John Stuart Mill, *On Liberty* (London, 1859); from an excerpt reprinted in Richard Wasserstrom, ed., *Morality and the Law* (Belmont, Calif.: Wadsworth Publishing Company, 1971), pp. 1–2.

6. A discussion of paternalism toward incompetents may be found in Donald VanDeVeer, *Paternalistic Intervention* (Princeton: Princeton University Press, 1986), Chapter 7.

7. It is widely assumed that efficiency is desirable. If asked "What's so great about efficiency?", perhaps the only plausible answer is that steps in that direction lead to maximization of utility. Hence, a utilitarian ethical theory may underpin the assumption that efficiency is an important good. This seems to be another indication of the not fully recognized influence of the utilitarian theory.

8. Note that our initial statement of the principle of utility is a weakened version, couched in terms of what is *permissible*. As usually understood, the principle is expressed in terms of what is a *duty* (and, hence, is a bolder claim).

9. For a closer examination of this question, read the article by Kenneth Howe in Part III. (A grasp of some of the technical, statistical concepts is necessary to fully understand the problems with screening.)

Morals and the Criminal Law

LORD PATRICK DEVLIN

The Report of the Committee on Homosexual Offenses and Prostitution, generally known as the Wolfenden Report, is recognized to be an excellent study of two very difficult legal and social problems. But it has also a particular claim to the respect of those interested in jurisprudence; it does what law reformers so rarely do: It sets out clearly and carefully what in relation to its subjects it considers the function of the law to be.[1] Statutory additions to the criminal law are too often made on the simple principle that "there ought to be a law against it." The greater part of the law relating to sexual offenses is the creation of statute, and it is difficult to ascertain any logical relationship between it and the moral ideas which most of us uphold. Adultery, fornication, and prostitution are not, as the Report . . . points out, criminal offenses: Homosexuality between males is a criminal offense, but between females it is not. Incest was not an offense until it was declared so by statute only fifty years ago. Does the legislature select these offenses haphazardly, or are there some principles which can be used to determine what part of the moral law should be embodied in the criminal? There is, for example, being now considered a proposal to make A.I.D., that is, the practice of artificial insemination of a woman with the seed of a man who is not her husband, a criminal offense; if, as is usually the case, the woman is married, this is in substance, if not in form, adultery. Ought it to be made punishable when adultery is not? . . . What is the connection between crime and sin, and to what extent, if at all, should the criminal law of England concern itself with the enforcement of morals and punish sin or immorality as such?

The statements of principle in the Wolfenden Report provide an admirable and modern starting point for such an inquiry. . . .

Early in the Report . . . the Committee put forward:

> our own formulation of the function of the criminal law so far as it concerns the subjects of this inquiry. In this field, its function, as we see it, is to preserve public

order and decency, to protect the citizen from what is offensive or injurious, and to provide sufficient safeguards against exploitation and corruption of others, particularly those who are specially vulnerable because they are young, weak in body or mind, inexperienced, or in a state of special physical, official, or economic dependence.

It is not, in our view, the function of the law to intervene in the private lives of citizens, or to seek to enforce any particular pattern of behavior, further than it is necessary to carry out the purposes we have outlined.

The Committee prefaces its most important recommendation . . . ,

that homosexual behavior between consenting adults in private should no longer be a criminal offense, [by stating the argument . . .] which we believe to be decisive, namely, the importance which society and the law ought to give to individual freedom of choice and action in matters of private morality. Unless a deliberate attempt is to be made by society, acting through the agency of the law, to equate the sphere of crime with that of sin, there must remain a realm of private morality and immorality which is, in brief and crude terms, not the law's business. To say this is not to condone or encourage private immorality.

Similar statements of principle are set out in the chapters of the Report which deal with prostitution. No case can be sustained, the Report says, for attempting to make prostitution itself illegal. . . . The Committee refers to the general reasons already given and adds: "We are agreed that private immorality should not be the concern of the criminal law except in the special circumstances therein mentioned." They quote . . . with approval the report of the Street Offenses Committee, . . . which says: "As a general proposition it will be universally accepted that the law is not concerned with private morals or with ethical sanctions." It will be observed that the emphasis is on *private* immorality. By this is meant immorality which is not offensive or injurious to the public in the ways defined or described in the first passage which I quoted. In other words, no act of immorality should be made a criminal offense unless it is accompanied by some other feature, such as indecency, corruption, or exploitation. This is clearly brought out in relation to prostitution: "It is not the duty of the law to concern itself with immorality as such . . . it should confine itself to those activities which offend against public order and decency or expose the ordinary citizen to what is offensive or injurious." . . .

These statements of principle are naturally restricted to the subject matter of the Report. But they are made in general terms and there seems to be no reason why, if they are valid, they should not be applied to the criminal law in general. They separate very decisively crime from sin, the divine law from the secular, and the moral from the criminal. They do not signify any lack of support for the law, moral or criminal, and they do not represent an attitude that can be called either religious or irreligious. There are many schools of thought among those who may think that morals are not the law's business. There is first of all the agnostic or free-thinker. He does not of course disbelieve in morals, nor in sin if it be given the wider of the two meanings assigned to it in the *Oxford English Dictionary,* where it is defined as "transgression against divine law or the principles of morality." He cannot accept the divine law; that does not mean that he might not view with suspicion any departure from moral principles that have for generations been accepted by the society in which he lives—but in the end he judges for himself. Then there is the deeply religious person who feels that the criminal law is sometimes more of a hindrance than a help in the sphere of morality, and that the reform of the sinner—at any rate when he injures only himself—should be a spiritual rather than a temporal work. Then there is the man who, without any strong feeling, cannot see why, where there is freedom in religious belief, there should not logically be freedom in morality as well. All these are powerfully allied against the equating of crime with sin. . . .

I must admit that I begin with a feeling that a complete separation of crime from sin (I use the term throughout this lecture in the wider meaning) would not be good for the moral law and might be disastrous for the criminal. But can this sort of feeling be justified as a matter of jurisprudence? And if it be a right feeling, how should the relationship between the criminal and the moral law be stated? Is there a good theoretical basis for it, or is it just a practical working alliance, or is it a bit of both? That is the problem which I want to examine . . . .

Morals and religion are inextricably joined—the moral standards generally accepted in Western civilization being those belonging to Christianity. Outside Christendom other standards derive from other religions. None of these moral codes can claim any validity except by virtue of the religion on which it is based. . . . It may or may not be right for the State to adopt one of these religions as the truth, to found itself upon its doctrines, and to deny to any of its citizens the liberty to practice any other. If it does, it is logical that it should use the secular law wherever it thinks it necessary to enforce the divine. If it does not, it is illogical that it should concern itself with morals as such. But if it leaves matters of religion to private judgment, it should logically leave matters of morals also. A State which refuses to enforce Christian beliefs has lost the right to enforce Christian morals. . . .

It is true that for many centuries the criminal law was much concerned with keeping the peace and little, if at all, with sexual morals. But it would be wrong to infer from that that it had no moral content or that it would ever have tolerated the idea of a man being left to judge for himself in matters of morals. The criminal law of England has from the very first concerned itself with moral principles. A simple way of testing this point is to consider the attitude which the criminal law adopts toward consent.

Subject to certain exceptions inherent in the nature of particular crimes, the criminal law has never permitted consent of the victim to be used as a defense. In rape, for example, consent negatives an essential element. But consent of the victim is no defense to a charge of murder. It is not a defense to any form of assault that the victim thought his punishment well deserved and submitted to it . . . .

Now, if the law existed for the protection of the individual, there would be no reason why he should avail himself of it if he did not want it. The reason why a man may not consent to the commission of an offense against himself beforehand or forgive it afterwards is because it is an offense against society. It is not that society is physically injured; that would be impossible. Nor need any individual be shocked, corrupted, or exploited; everything may be done in private. Nor can it be explained on the practical ground that a violent man is a potential danger to others in the community who have therefore a direct interest in his apprehension and punishment as being necessary to their own protection. That would be true of a man whom the victim is prepared to forgive but not of one who gets his consent first; a murderer who acts only upon the consent, and maybe the request, of his victim is no menace to others, but he does threaten one of the great moral principles upon which society is based, that is, the sanctity of human life. There is only one explanation of what has hitherto been accepted as the basis of the criminal law and that is that there are certain standards of behavior or moral principles which society requires to be observed; and the breach of them is an offense not merely against the person who is injured but against society as a whole.

Thus, if the criminal law were to be reformed so as to eliminate from it everything that was not designed to preserve order and decency or to protect citizens (including the protection of youth from corruption), it would overturn a fundamental principle. It would also end a number of specific crimes. Euthanasia or the killing of another at his own request, suicide, attempted suicide and suicide pacts, dueling, abortion, incest between brother and sister, are all acts which can be done in private and without offense to others and need not involve the corruption or exploitation of others. Many people think that the law on some of these subjects is in need of reform, but no one hitherto has gone so far as to suggest that they should all be left outside the criminal law as matters of private morality. They can be brought within it only as a matter of moral principle. It must be remembered also that although there is much immorality that is not punished by the law, there is none that is condoned by the law. The law will not allow its processes to be used by those engaged in immorality of any sort. For example, a house may not be let for immoral purposes; the lease is invalid and would not be enforced. But if what goes on inside there is a matter of private morality and not the law's business, why does the law inquire into it at all?

I think it is clear that the criminal law as we know it is based upon moral principle. In a number of crimes its function is simply to enforce a moral principle and nothing else. The law, both criminal and civil, claims to be able to speak about morality and immorality generally. Where does it get its authority to do this, and how does it settle the moral principles which it enforces? Undoubtedly, as a matter of history, it derived both from Christian teaching. But I think that the strict logician is right when he says that the law can no longer rely on doctrines in which citizens are entitled to disbelieve. It is necessary therefore to look for some other source.

In jurisprudence, as I have said, everything is thrown open to discussion and, in the belief that they cover the whole field, I have framed three interrogatories addressed to myself to answer:

1. Has society the right to pass judgment at all on matters of morals? Ought there, in other words, to be a public morality, or are morals always a matter for private judgment?

2. If society has the right to pass judgment, has it also the right to use the weapon of the law to enforce it?

3. If so, ought it to use that weapon in all cases or only in some; and if only in some, on what principles should it distinguish?

I shall begin with the first interrogatory and consider what is meant by the right of society to pass a moral judgment, that is, a judgment about what is good and what is evil. The fact that a majority of people may disapprove of a practice does not of itself make it a matter for society as a whole. Nine men out of ten may disapprove of what the tenth man is doing and still say that it is not their business. There is a case for a collective judgment (as distinct from a large number of individual opinions which sensible people may even refrain from pronouncing at all if it is upon somebody else's private affairs) only if society is affected. Without a collective judgment there can be no case at all for intervention. . . .

The language used in the passages I have quoted from the Wolfenden Report suggests the view that there ought not to be a collective judgment about immorality *per se*. Is this what is meant by "private morality" and "individual freedom of choice and action"? Some people sincerely believe that homosexuality is neither immoral nor unnatural. Is the "freedom of choice and action" that is offered to the individual, freedom to decide for himself what is moral or immoral, society remaining neutral; or is it freedom to be immoral if he wants to be? The language of the Report may be open to question, but the conclusions at which the Committee arrives answer this question unambiguously. If society is not prepared to say that homosexuality is morally wrong, there would be no basis for a law protecting youth from "corruption" or punishing a man for living on the "immoral" earnings of a homosexual prostitute, as the Report recommends. . . . This attitude the Committee makes even clearer when it comes to deal with prostitution. In truth, the Report takes it for granted that there is in existence a public morality which condemns homosexuality and prostitution. What the Report seems to mean by private morality might perhaps be better described as private behavior in matters of morals.

This view—that there is such a thing as public morality—can also be justified by *a priori* argument. What makes a society of any sort is community of ideas—not only political ideas, but also ideas about the way its members should behave and govern their lives; these latter ideas are its morals. Every society has a moral structure as well as a political one; or rather, since that might suggest two independent systems, I should say that the structure of every society is made up both of politics and morals. Take, for example, the institution of marriage. Whether a man should be allowed to take more than one wife is something about which every society has to make up its mind one way or the other. In England we believe in the Christian idea of marriage and therefore adopt monogamy as a moral principle. Consequently the Christian institution of marriage has become the basis of family life and so part of the structure of our society. It is there not because it is Christian. It has got there because it is Christian, but it remains there because it is built into the house in which we live and could not be removed without bringing it down. The great majority of those who live in this country accept it because it is the Christian idea of marriage and for them the only true one. But a non-Christian is bound by it, not because it is part of Christianity, but because, rightly or wrongly, it has been adopted by the society in which he lives. It would be useless for him to stage a debate designed to prove that polygamy was theologically more correct and socially preferable; if he wants to live in the house, he must accept it as built in the way in which it is.

We see this more clearly if we think of ideas or institutions that are purely political. Society cannot tolerate rebellion; it will not allow argument about the rightness of the cause. Historians a century later may say that the rebels were right and the Government was wrong, and a percipient and conscientious subject of the State may think so at the time. But it is not a matter which can be left to individual judgment. . . .

I return to the statement that I have already made, that society means a community of ideas; without shared ideas on politics, morals, and ethics no society can exist. Each one of us has ideas about what is good and what is evil; they cannot be kept private from the society in which we live. If men and women try to create a society in which there is no fundamental agreement about good and evil they will fail; if, having based it on common agreement, the agreement goes, the society will disintegrate. For society is not something that is kept together physically; it is held by the invisible bonds of common thought. If the bonds were too far relaxed, the members would drift apart. A common morality is part of the bondage. The bondage is part of the price of society; and mankind, which needs society, must pay its price. . . .

You may think that I have taken far too long in contending that there is such a thing as public morality, a proposition which most people would readily accept, and may have left myself too little time to discuss the next question, which to many minds may cause greater difficulty: to what extent should society use the law to enforce its moral judgments? But I believe that the answer to the first question determines the way in which the second should be approached and may indeed very nearly dictate the answer to the second question. If society has no right to make judgments on morals, the law must find some special justification for entering the field of morality: If homosexuality and prostitution are not in themselves wrong, then the onus is very clearly on the lawgiver who wants to frame a law against certain aspects of them to justify the exceptional treatment. But if society has the right to make a judgment and has it on the basis that a recognized morality is as necessary to society as, say, a recognized government, then society may use the law to preserve morality in the same way as it uses it to safeguard anything else that is essential to its existence. If therefore the first proposition is securely established with all its implications, society has a prima facie right to legislate against immorality as such.

The Wolfenden Report, notwithstanding that it seems to admit the right of society to condemn homosexuality and prostitution as immoral, requires special circumstances to be shown to justify the intervention of the law. I think that this is wrong in principle and that any attempt to approach my second interrogatory on these lines is bound to break down. I think that the attempt by the Committee does break down and that this is shown by the fact that it has to define or describe its special circumstances so widely that they can be supported only if it is accepted that the law *is* concerned with immorality as such.

The widest of the special circumstances are described as the provision of "sufficient safeguards against exploitation and corruption of others, particularly those who are specially vulnerable because they are young, weak in body or mind, inexperienced, or in a state of special physical, official, or economic dependence." . . . The corruption of youth is a well-recognized ground for intervention by the State, and for the purpose of any legislation the young can easily be defined. But if similar protection were to be extended to every other citizen, there would be no limit to the reach of the law. The "corruption and exploitation of others" is so wide that it could be used to cover any sort of immorality which involves, as most do, the cooperation of another person. Even if the phrase is taken as limited to the categories that are particularized as "specially vulnerable," it is so elastic as to be practically no restriction. This is not merely a matter of words. For if the words used are stretched almost beyond breaking point, they still are not wide enough to cover the recommendations which the Committee makes about prostitution. . . .

All sexual immorality involves the exploitation of human weaknesses. The prostitute exploits the lust of her customers and the customer the moral weakness of the prostitute. If the exploitation of human weaknesses is considered to create a special circumstance, there is virtually no field of morality which can be defined in such a way as to exclude the law.

I think, therefore, that it is not possible to set theoretical limits to the power of the State to legislate against immorality. It is not possible to settle in advance exceptions to the general rule or to define inflexibly areas of morality into which the law is in no circumstances to be allowed to enter. Society is entitled by means of its laws to protect itself from dangers, whether from within or without. Here again I think that the political parallel is legitimate. The law of treason is directed against aiding the king's enemies and against sedition from within. The justification for this is that established government is necessary for the existence of society and therefore its safety against violent overthrow must be secured. But an established morality is as necessary as good government to the welfare of society. Societies disintegrate from within more frequently than they are broken up by external pressures. There is disintegration when no common morality is observed, and history shows that the loosening of moral bonds is often the first stage of disintegration, so that society is justified in taking the same steps to preserve its moral code as it does to preserve its government and other essential institutions. . . . The suppression of vice is as much the law's business as the suppression of subversive activities; it is no more possible to define a sphere of private morality than it is to define one of private subversive activity. It is wrong to talk of private morality or of the law not being concerned with immorality as such or to try to set rigid bounds to the part which the law may play in the suppression of vice. . . . There are no theoretical limits to the power of the State to legislate against treason and sedition, and likewise I think there can be no theoretical limits to legislation against immorality. You may argue that if a man's sins affect only himself it cannot be the concern of society. If he chooses to get drunk every night in the privacy of his own home, is anyone except himself the worse for it? But suppose a quarter or a half of the population got drunk every night, what sort of society would it be? You cannot set a theoretical limit to the number of people who can get drunk before society is entitled to legislate against drunkenness. . . .

In what circumstances the State should exercise its power is the third of the interrogatories I have framed. But before I get to it I must raise a point which might have been brought up in any one of the three. How are the moral judgments of society to be ascertained? By leaving it until now, I can ask it in the more limited form that is now sufficient for my purpose. How is the lawmaker to ascertain the moral judgments of society? It is surely not enough that they should be reached by the opinion of the majority; it would be too much to require the individual assent of every citizen. English law has evolved and regularly uses a standard which does not depend on the counting of heads. It is that of the reasonable man. He is not to be confused with the rational man. He is not expected to reason about anything and his judgment may be largely a matter of feeling. It is the viewpoint of the man in the street or—to use an archaism familiar to all lawyers—the man in the Clapham omnibus. He might also be called the right-minded man. For my purpose I should like to call him the man in the jury box, for the moral judgment of society must be something about which any twelve men or women drawn at random might after discussion be expected to be unanimous. This was the standard the judges applied in the days before Parliament was as active as it is now and when they laid down rules of public policy. They did not think of themselves as making law but simply as stating principles which every right-minded person would accept as valid. It is what Pollock called "practical morality," which is based not on theological or philosophical foundations but "in the mass of continuous experience half-consciously or unconsciously accumulated and embodied in the morality of common sense." He called it also "a certain way of thinking on questions of morality which we expect to find in a reasonable civilized man or a reasonable Englishman, taken at random."[2]

Immorality then, for the purpose of the law, is what every right-minded person is presumed to consider to be immoral. Any immorality is capable of affecting society injuriously and in effect to a greater or lesser extent it usually does; this is what gives the law its *locus standi.* It cannot be shut out. But—and this brings me to the third question—the individual has a *locus standi* too; he cannot be expected to surrender to the judgment of society the whole conduct of his life. . . .

[I]t is possible to make general statements of principle which it may be thought the legislature should bear in mind when it is considering the enactment of laws enforcing morals.

I believe that most people would agree upon the chief of these . . . principles. There must be toleration of the maximum individual freedom that is consistent with the integrity of society. It cannot be said that this is a principle that runs all through the criminal law. Much of the criminal law that is regulatory in character—the part of it that deals with *malum prohibitum* rather than *malum in se*—is based upon the opposite principle, that is, that the choice of the individual must give way to the convenience of the many. But in all matters of conscience the principle I have stated is generally held to prevail. It is not confined to thought and speech; it extends to action, as is shown by the recognition of the right to conscientious objection in wartime: This example shows also that conscience will be respected even in times of national danger. The principle appears to me to be peculiarly appropriate to all questions of morals. Nothing should be punished by the law that does not lie beyond the limits of tolerance. It is not nearly enough to say that a majority dislike a practice; there must be a real feeling of reprobation. Those who are dissatisfied with the present law on homosexuality often say that the opponents of reform are swayed simply by disgust. If that were so, it would be wrong, but I do not think one can ignore disgust if it is deeply felt and not manufactured. Its presence is a good indication that the bounds of toleration are being reached. Not everything is to be tolerated. No society can do without intolerance, indignation, and disgust; they are the forces behind the moral law, and indeed it can be argued that if they or something like them are not present, the feelings of society cannot be weighty enough to deprive the individual of freedom of choice. I suppose that there is hardly anyone nowadays who would not be disgusted by the thought of deliberate cruelty to animals. No one proposes to relegate that or any other form of sadism to the realm of private morality or to allow it to be practiced in public or in private. It would be possible no doubt to point out that until a comparatively short while ago nobody thought very much of cruelty to animals, and also that pity and kindliness and the unwillingness to inflict pain are virtues more generally esteemed now than they have ever been in the past. But matters of this sort are not determined by rational argument. Every moral judgment, unless it claims a divine source, is simply a feeling that no right-minded man could behave in any other way without admitting that he was doing wrong. It is the power of a common sense and not the power of reason that is behind the judgments of society. But before a society can put a practice beyond the limits of tolerance there must be a deliberate judgment that the practice is injurious to society. There is, for example, a general abhorrence of homosexuality. We should ask ourselves in the first instance whether, looking at it calmly and dispassionately, we regard it as a vice so abominable that its mere presence is an offense. If that is the genuine feeling of the society in which we live, I do not see how society can be denied the right to eradicate it. Our feeling may not be so intense as that. We may feel about it that, if confined, it is tolerable, but that if it spread it might be gravely injurious; it is in this way that most societies look upon fornication, seeing it as a natural weakness which must be kept within bounds but which cannot be rooted out. . . .

The limits of tolerance shift. This is supplementary to what I have been saying but of sufficient importance in itself to deserve statement as a separate principle which lawmakers have to bear in mind. I suppose that moral standards do not shift; so far as they come from divine revelation they do not, and I am willing to assume that the moral judgments made by a society always remain good for that society. But the extent to which society will tolerate—I mean tolerate, not approve—departures from moral standards varies from generation to generation. . . .

A third . . . principle must be advanced more tentatively. It is that as far as possible privacy should be respected. . . . The police have no more right to trespass than the ordinary citizen has; there is no general right of search—to this extent an Englishman's home is still his castle. . . .

This indicates a general sentiment that the right to privacy is something to be put in the balance against the enforcement of the law. Ought the same sort of consideration to play any part in the formation of the law? Clearly only in a very limited number of cases. When the help of the law is invoked by an injured citizen, privacy must be irrelevant; the individual cannot ask that his right to privacy should be measured against injury criminally done to another. But when all who are involved in the deed are consenting parties and the injury is done to morals, the public interest in the moral order can be balanced against the claims of privacy. The restriction on police powers of investigation goes further than the affording of a parallel; it means that the detection of crime committed in private and when there is no complaint is bound to be rather haphazard and this is an additional reason for moderation. These considerations do not justify the exclusion of all private immorality from the scope of the law. . . .

I return now to the main thread of my argument and summarize it. Society cannot live without morals. Its morals are those standards of conduct which the reasonable man approves. A rational man, who is also a good man, may have other standards. If he has no standards at all, he is not a good man and need not be further considered. If he has standards, they may be very different; he may, for example, not disapprove of homosexuality or abortion. In that case he will not share in the common morality; but that should not make him deny that it is a social necessity. A rebel may be rational in thinking that he is right, but he is irrational if he thinks that society can leave him free to rebel.

Notes

1. The Committee's "statement of juristic philosophy" (to quote Lord Pakenham) was considered by him in a debate in the House of Lords on December 4, 1957, reported in *Hansard Lords Debates,* Vol. ccvl at 738; and also in the same debate by the Archbishop of Canterbury at 753 and Lord Denning at 806. The subject has also been considered by Mr. J. E. Hall Williams in the *Law Quarterly Review* (January 1958), Vol. lxxiv, p. 76.
2. *Essays in Jurisprudence and Ethics* (Macmillan, 1882), pp. 278 and 353.

The Concept of a Moral Position

RONALD DWORKIN

We might start with the fact that terms like *moral position* and *moral conviction* function in our conventional morality as terms of justification and criticism, as well as of description. It is true that we sometimes speak of a group's "morals," or "morality," or "moral beliefs," or "moral positions," or "moral convictions," in what might be called an anthropological sense, meaning to refer to whatever attitudes the group displays about the propriety of human conduct, qualities, or goals. We say, in this sense, that the morality of Nazi Germany was based on prejudice, or was irrational. But we also use some of these terms, particularly *moral position* and *moral conviction,* in a discriminatory sense, to contrast the positions they describe with prejudices, rationalizations, matters of personal aversion or taste, arbitrary stands, and the like. One use—perhaps the most characteristic use—of this discriminatory sense is to offer a limited but important sort of justification for an act, when the moral issues surrounding that act are unclear or in dispute.

Suppose I tell you that I propose to vote against a man running for a public office of trust because I know him to be a homosexual and because I believe that homosexuality is profoundly immoral. If you disagree that homosexuality is immoral, you may accuse me of being about to cast my vote unfairly, acting on prejudice or out of a personal repugnance which is irrelevant to the moral issue. I might then try to convert you to my position on homosexuality, but if I fail in this I shall still want to convince you of what you and I will both take to be a separate point—that my vote was based upon a moral position, in the discriminatory sense, even though one which differs from yours. I shall want to persuade you of this, because if I do I am entitled to expect that you will alter your opinion of me and of what I am about to do. Your judgment of my character will be different—you might still think me eccentric (or puritanical or unsophisticated) but these are types of character and not faults of char-

From Ronald Dworkin, "Lord Devlin and the Enforcement of Morals," *The Yale Law Journal,* Vol. 75, pp. 994–99. Reprinted by permission of the Yale Law Journal Company and Fred B. Rothman & Company.

acter. Your judgment of my act will also be different, in this respect. You will admit that so long as I hold my moral position, I have a moral right to vote against the homosexual, because I have a right (indeed a duty) to vote my own convictions. You would not admit such a right (or duty) if you were still persuaded that I was acting out of a prejudice or a personal taste.

I am entitled to expect that your opinion will change in these ways, because these distinctions are a part of the conventional morality you and I share, and which forms the background of our discussion. They enforce the difference between positions we must respect, although we think them wrong, and positions we need not respect because they offend some ground rule of moral reasoning. A great deal of debate about moral issues (in real life, although not in philosophy texts) consists of arguments that some position falls on one or the other side of this crucial line.

It is this feature of conventional morality that animates Lord Devlin's argument that society has the right to follow its own lights. We must therefore examine that discriminatory concept of a moral position more closely, and we can do so by pursuing our imaginary conversation. What must I do to convince you that my position is a moral position?

(a) I must produce some reasons for it. This is not to say that I have to articulate a moral principle I am following or a general moral theory to which I subscribe. Very few people can do either, and the ability to hold a moral position is not limited to those who can. My reason need not be a principle or theory at all. It must only point out some aspect or feature of homosexuality which moves me to regard it as immoral: the fact that the Bible forbids it, for example, or that one who practices homosexuality becomes unfit for marriage and parenthood. Of course, any such reason would presuppose my acceptance of some general principle or theory, but I need not be able to state what it is, or realize that I am relying upon it.

Not every reason I might give will do, however. Some will be excluded by general criteria stipulating sorts of reasons which do not count. We might take note of four of the most important such criteria:

1. If I tell you that homosexuals are morally inferior because they do not have heterosexual desires, and so are not "real men," you would reject that reason as showing one type of prejudice. Prejudices, in general, are postures of judgment that take into account considerations our conventions exclude. In a structured context, like a trial or a contest, the ground rules exclude all but certain considerations, and a prejudice is a basis of judgment which violates these rules. Our conventions stipulate some ground rules of moral judgment which obtain even apart from such special contexts, the most important of which is that a man must not be held morally inferior on the basis of some physical, racial, or other characteristic he cannot help having. Thus, a man whose moral judgments about Jews, or Negroes, or Southerners, or women, or effeminate men are based on his belief that any member of these classes automatically deserves less respect, without regard to anything he himself has done, is said to be prejudiced against that group.

2. If I base my view about homosexuals on a personal emotional reaction ("They make me sick"), you would reject that reason as well. We distinguish moral posi-

tions from emotional reactions, not because moral positions are supposed to be unemotional or dispassionate—quite the reverse is true—but because the moral position is supposed to justify the emotional reaction, and not vice versa. If a man is unable to produce such reasons, we do not deny the fact of his emotional involvement, which may have important social or political consequences, but we do not take this involvement as demonstrating his moral conviction. Indeed, it is just this sort of position—a severe emotional reaction to a practice or a situation for which one cannot account—that we tend to describe, in lay terms, as a phobia or an obsession.

3. If I base my position on a proposition of fact ("Homosexual acts are physically debilitating") which is not only false, but is so implausible that it challenges the minimal standards of evidence and argument I generally accept and impose upon others, then you would regard my belief, even though sincere, as a form of rationalization, and disqualify my reason on that ground. (Rationalization is a complex concept, and also includes, as we shall see, the production of reasons which suggest general theories I do not accept.)

4. If I can argue for my own position only by citing the beliefs of others ("Everyone knows homosexuality is a sin"), you will conclude that I am parroting and not relying on a moral conviction of my own. With the possible (though complex) exception of a deity, there is no moral authority to which I can appeal and so automatically make my position a moral one. I must have my own reasons, though of course I may have been taught these reasons by others.

No doubt many readers will disagree with these thumbnail sketches of prejudice, mere emotional reaction, rationalization, and parroting. Some may have their own theories of what these are. I want to emphasize now only that these are distinct concepts, whatever the details of the differences might be, and that they have a role in deciding whether to treat another's position as a moral conviction. They are not merely epithets to be pasted on positions we strongly dislike.

(b) Suppose I do produce a reason which is not disqualified on one of these (or on similar) grounds. That reason will presuppose some general moral principle or theory, even though I may not be able to state that principle or theory, and do not have it in mind when I speak. If I offer, as my reason, the fact that the Bible forbids homosexual acts, or that homosexual acts make it less likely that the actor will marry and raise children, I suggest that I accept the theory my reason presupposes, and you will not be satisfied that my position is a moral one if you believe that I do not. It may be a question of my sincerity—do I in fact believe that the injunctions of the Bible are morally binding as such, or that all men have a duty to procreate? Sincerity is not, however, the only issue, for consistency is also in point. I may believe that I accept one of these general positions, and be wrong, because my other beliefs, and my own conduct on other occasions, may be inconsistent with it. I may reject certain biblical injunctions, or I may hold that men have a right to remain bachelors if they please or use contraceptives all their lives.

Of course, my general moral positions may have qualifications and exceptions. The difference between an exception and an inconsistency is that the former can be supported by reasons which presuppose other moral positions I can properly claim to hold. Suppose I condemn all homosexuals on biblical authority, but not all fornicators. What reason can I offer for the distinction? If I can produce none which supports it, I cannot claim to accept the general position about biblical authority. If I do produce a reason which seems to support the distinction, the same sorts of question may be asked about that reason as were asked about my original reply. What general position does the reason for my exception presuppose? Can I sincerely claim to accept that further general position? Suppose my reason, for example, is that fornication is now very common, and has been sanctioned by custom. Do I really believe that what is immoral becomes moral when it becomes popular? If not, and if I can produce no other reason for the distinction, I cannot claim to accept the general position that what the Bible condemns is immoral. Of course, I may be persuaded, when this is pointed out, to change my views on fornication. But you would be alert to the question of whether this is a genuine change of heart, or only a performance for the sake of the argument.

In principle there is no limit to these ramifications of my original claim, though, of course, no actual argument is likely to pursue very many of them.

(c) But do I really have to have a reason to make my position a matter of moral conviction? Most men think that acts which cause unnecessary suffering, or break a serious promise with no excuse, are immoral, and yet they could give no reason for these beliefs. They feel that no reason is necessary, because they take it as axiomatic or self-evident that these are immoral acts. It seems contrary to common sense to deny that a position held in this way can be a moral position.

Yet there is an important difference between believing that one's position is self-evident and just not having a reason for one's position. The former presupposes a positive belief that no further reason is necessary, that the immorality of the act in question does not depend upon its social effects, or its effects on the character of the actor, or its proscription by a deity, or anything else, but follows from the nature of the act itself. The claim that a particular position is axiomatic, in other words, does supply a reason of a special sort, namely that the act is immoral in and of itself, and this special reason, like the others we considered, may be inconsistent with more general theories I hold.

The moral arguments we make presuppose not only moral principles, but also more abstract positions about moral reasoning. In particular, they presuppose positions about what kinds of acts can be immoral in and of themselves. When I criticize your moral opinions, or attempt to justify my own disregard of traditional moral rules I think are silly, I will likely proceed by denying that the act in question has any of the several features that can make an act immoral—that it involves no breach of an undertaking or duty, for example, harms no one including the actor, is not proscribed in any organized religion, and is not illegal. I proceed in this way because I assume that the ultimate grounds of immorality are limited to some such small set of very general standards. I may assert this assumption directly or it may emerge from the pattern of my argument. In either event, I will enforce it by calling positions which can claim no support from any of these ultimate standards *arbitrary,* as I should certainly do if you said that photography was immoral, for instance, or swimming. Even if I cannot articulate this underlying assumption, I shall still apply it, and since the ultimate criteria I recognize are among the most abstract of my moral standards, they will not vary much from those my neighbors recognize and apply. Although many who despise homosexuals are unable to say why, few would claim affirmatively that one needs no reason, for this would make their position, on their own standards, an arbitrary one.

(d) This anatomy of our argument could be continued, but it is already long enough to justify some conclusions. If the issue between us is whether my views on homosexuality amount to a moral position, and hence whether I am entitled to vote against a homosexual on that ground, I cannot settle the issue simply by reporting my feelings. You will want to consider the reasons I can produce to support my belief, and whether my other views and behavior are consistent with the theories these reasons presuppose. You will have, of course, to apply your own understanding, which may differ in detail from mine, of what a prejudice or a rationalization is, for example, and of when one view is inconsistent with another. You and I may end in disagreement over whether my position is a moral one, partly because one is less likely to recognize these illegitimate grounds in himself than in others.

We must avoid the skeptical fallacy of passing from these facts to the conclusion that there is no such thing as a prejudice or a rationalization or an inconsistency, or that these terms mean merely that the one who uses them strongly dislikes the positions he describes this way. That would be like arguing that because different people have different understandings of what jealousy is, and can in good faith disagree about whether one of them is jealous, there is no such thing as jealousy, and one who says another is jealous merely means he dislikes him very much.

"Harmless Immoralities" and Offensive Nuisances

JOEL FEINBERG

I am not at all sure that there are any private immoral actions that do not cause harm, but I am quite sure that *if* there are such things, there is no justification for their suppression by the state and especially not for their proscription by the criminal law. On the other hand, there clearly are such things as actions that are very offensive to others, and I think the state is justified in preventing at least some of these when certain strict conditions have been satisfied. In coming to these conclusions (which I shall defend in what follows) I appear to have endorsed one and rejected another of the principles commonly proposed as justifications for political restriction of private liberty. Preventing offense, I maintain, is at least sometimes a ground for limiting liberty, whereas the "enforcement of morality as such" is never a valid ground.

I

There are perhaps as many as seven liberty-limiting principles that are frequently proposed by leading writers. It has been held that restriction of a person's liberty may be justified:[1]

1. to prevent injury to others (the *private harm principle*);
2. to prevent impairment of institutional practices and regulatory systems that are in

From *Issues in Law and Morality,* Proceedings of the 1971 Oberlin Colloquium in Philosophy, edited by Norman S. Care and Thomas K. Trelogan (Cleveland: Case Western Reserve University, 1973), pp. 83–97. © 1973 by Oberlin College. Reprinted by permission of Oberlin College.

the public interest, such as the collection of taxes and custom duties (the *public harm principle*);

3. to prevent offense to others (the *offense principle*);
4. to prevent harm to self (*legal paternalism*) . . . ;
5. to prevent or punish sin, [that is,] "to enforce morality as such" (*legal moralism*);
6. to benefit the self (*extreme paternalism*) . . . ;
7. to benefit others (the *welfare principle*).

The private harm principle, which of course is indissolubly associated with the name of John Stuart Mill, is virtually beyond controversy. Hardly anyone would deny the state the right to make criminal, on this ground, such harmful conduct as willful homicide, aggravated assault, and robbery. Mill often wrote as if the prevention of private harm were the *sole* valid ground for state coercion, but this must surely not have been his considered intention. He would not have wiped from the books such crimes as tax evasion, smuggling, and contempt of court, which need not injure to any measurable degree any assignable individuals, except insofar as they weaken public institutions in whose health we all have a stake, however indirect. I assume then that Mill held both the private and the public versions of the harm principle.

In some sections of *On Liberty*, Mill suggests that harm of one kind or another is the *only* valid ground for coercion, so that the prevention of mere offensiveness, as opposed to harmfulness, can never be sufficient ground to warrant interference with liberty. Yet in the final chapter of *On Liberty*, Mill seems to retreat on this issue too. There he refers to public acts that are "a violation of good manners and, coming thus within the category of offenses against others, may rightly be prohibited. Of this kind," he continues, "are offenses against decency, on which it is unnecessary to dwell. . . ."[2] Mill's view about offensiveness can be made consistent, however, in the following way. One subclass of actions, on his view, has a very special social importance. These actions are instances of expressing orally or in print opinions about matters of fact and about historical, scientific, theological, philosophical, political, and moral questions. . . . The free expression of opinion is of such great importance to the well-being and progress of the community that it can be validly restricted only to prevent certain very clear harms to individuals, such as libel, slander, incited violence, and, perhaps, invasions of privacy. The importance of free expression is so great and so special that only the necessity to prevent direct and substantial harm to assignable persons can be a sufficient reason for overriding the presumption in its favor. Mere shock to tender sensibilities can never be a weighty enough harm to counterbalance the case for free expression of opinion. But Mill did not consider public nudity, indecency, public displays of "dirty pictures," and the like, to be forms of "symbolic speech," or expressions of *opinion* of any kind. The presumption in favor of liberty is much weaker in the case of conduct that does not have the "redeeming social importance" peculiar to assertion, criticism, advocacy, and debate; and hence, even "mere offensiveness" in the absence of harm may be a valid ground for suppressing it. . . .

II

What is offensiveness and how is it related to harm? If we follow some legal writers and define *harm* as the violation of an interest, and then posit a universal interest in not being offended, it will follow that to suffer offense is to suffer a kind of harm. But there are some offenses that are (in a narrow sense) "harmless" in that they do not lead to any *further* harm, that is, they do not violate any interests other than the interest in not being offended. Thus, there is a sense of "offense" which is contrasted with harm, and in the interest of clarity, that is the sense we should employ.

Offensive behavior is such in virtue of its capacity to induce in others any of a large miscellany of mental states that have little in common except that they are unpleasant, uncomfortable, or disliked. These states do not necessarily "hurt," as sorrow and distress do. Rather, the relation between them and hurt is analogous to that between physical unpleasantness and pain. There are, after all, a great variety of unpleasant but not painful bodily states—itches, shocks, and discomforts—that have little in common except that they don't hurt but are nevertheless universally disliked.

No complete catalog of the unpleasant states caused by offensiveness is possible here, but surely among the main ones are: irritating sensations ([for example], bad smells and loud noises); unaffected disgust and acute repugnance caused, for example, by extreme vulgarity and filth; shocked moral, religious, or patriotic sensibilities; unsettling anger or irritation as caused, for example, by another's "obnoxious, insulting, rude, or insolent behavior;" and shameful embarrassment or invaded privacy, as caused, for example, by another's nudity or indecency.

Nuisance law protects people from loud noises, noisome stenches, and other direct and inescapable irritants to the senses, usually by providing civil remedies. An evil smell, of course, even when not harmful (in the narrow sense) can still be an annoyance, inconvenience, or irritation. Something like "unaffected disgust" is often evoked by behavior that is neither harmful nor in any ordinary sense "immoral," but is rather vulgar, uncouth, crass, boorish, or unseemly to an extreme. Normally, bad manners are considered beneath the attention of either morals or law, but when they are bad enough, some have plausibly argued, we can demand "protection" from them. Imagine a filthy and verminous man who scratches himself, spits, wipes his nose with the back of his hand, slobbers, and speaks in a raucous voice uttering mostly profanities and obscenities. If such a person spoke freely to passers-by on the public street, he just might be subject to arrest as a public nuisance, whether he harms anyone or not.

Still other offensive behavior tends to arouse outrage and indignation more than "unaffected disgust." Because the connection between open displays of disapproved conduct and indignation is so well known, engaging in such conduct is frequently a deliberate way of issuing a symbolic insult to a group of people. Sometimes open flaunting is in itself a kind of taunting or challenging and is well understood as "an invitation to violence." The flaunter deliberately arouses shocked anger and revulsion just as if he were saying with contempt, "That's what I think of you and your precious values!" The wearing and displaying of Nazi emblems in New York would enrage and challenge in this manner. So, alas, would a racially mixed couple strolling harmlessly, hand in hand, down the streets of Jackson, Mississippi. The latter kind of behavior, of course, can have a point and a motive independent of the desire to flaunt and taunt. Engaging in such behavior in public must be known to affront the sensibilities of those regarded as benighted; but its motive may not be to taunt so much as to display one's independence and contempt for custom while boldly affirming, and thus vindicating, one's rights.

When there is no point to the flaunted conduct independent of the desire to offend, still another model is sometimes appropriate, namely, that of desecration or sacrilege. The sacred, whatever else it may be, is no laughing matter. A person to whom "nothing is sacred" is a person able to mock or ridicule anything. But most of us are so constructed that some things are beyond mockery to us. It is difficult then to tolerate swastikas (with their symbolic suggestions of barbarity and genocide) or public flag burnings, or dragging venerated religious symbols in the mud. These things are so widely and intensely resented that some find it hard to think of reasons why they should be tolerated.

Still another kind of offensive behavior is that usually called "indecent." Indecency can have any of the motives and intended effects discussed above. Its distinctive feature is the public exhibition of that which, because of its extremely personal or intimately interpersonal character, had best remain hidden from view, according to prevailing mores. To be offended by indecency is not to be insulted or angered so much as to be acutely and profoundly embarrassed. Indecency, like other offensiveness, may be indirectly harmful when it exacerbates guilt, leads to incapacitating shock, sets a bad example, or provokes violence; but when the law forbids even "harmless indecency," its primary purpose is simply to protect the "unwilling witness of it in the streets."[3]

I have little doubt [then] that the offense principle should supplement the private and public harm principles in any full statement of the grounds for justifiable constraint. That principle, however, is as dangerous as it is necessary, and, as I shall argue in the section on obscenity below, it must be hedged in with careful qualifications.[4]

III

Are there any harmless immoralities? According to the utilitarian conception of ethics, harmfulness is the very ground and essential nature of immorality; but there is no doubt that our moral code is not (yet) wholly utilitarian. Certain actions are still widely held to be immoral even though they harm no one or, at most, only the actor himself. The question is whether the law should be used to force people to refrain from such conduct.

The central problem cases are those criminal actions generally called morals offenses. Offenses against morality and decency have long constituted a category of crimes (as distinct from offenses against the person, offenses against property, [and so on]). These have included mainly sex offenses—adultery, fornication, sodomy, incest, and prostitution, but also a miscellany of nonsexual offenses including cruelty to animals, desecration of the flag or other venerated symbols, and mistreatment of corpses. In a very useful article, Louis B. Schwartz maintains that what sets these crimes off as a class is not their special relation to morality (after all, murder is also an offense against morality, but it is not a "morals offense") but rather the lack of an essential connection between them and social harm. In particular, their suppression is not required by the public security.[5] Some morals offenses may harm the perpetrators themselves, but there is rarely harm of this sort the risk of which was not consented to in advance by the actors. Offense to other parties, when it occurs, is a consequence of the perpetration of the offending deeds *in public* and can be prevented by "public nuisance" laws or by statutes against "open lewdness" or "solicitation" in public places. That still leaves "morals offenses" when committed by consenting adults in private: Should they really be crimes?

Some arguments in favor of the statutes that create morals offenses are drawn from the private and public harm principles. There might be no direct unconsented-to harm caused by discreet and private, illicit sex relations, it is sometimes conceded; but indirectly harmful consequences to innocent parties or to society itself invariably result. The socially useful institutions of marriage and the family can be weakened, and the chaste life made more difficult. Such indirect and diffuse consequences, however, are highly speculative, and there is no hard evidence that penal laws would prevent them in any case. On the other hand, the harm principles might be used to argue *against* such laws on the grounds that some of the side effects of the laws themselves are invariably harmful. Laws against homosexuality, for example, lead to the iniquities of selective enforcement and to enhanced opportunities for blackmail and private vengeance. Moreover, "the criminal law prevents some deviates from seeking psychiatric aid. Further, the pursuit of homosexuals involves policemen in degrading entrapment practices, and diverts attention and effort that could be employed more usefully against the crimes of violent aggression, fraud, and government corruption, which are the overriding concerns of our metropolitan civilization."[6]

Indeed, the essentially utilitarian argument based on the need for prudent allocation of our social energies in fighting crime may, by itself, be a conclusive argument against the use of the criminal sanction to prevent private (and therefore inoffensive) conduct whose harmfulness is indirect and speculative at most. While seriously harmful crimes against person and property are everywhere on the rise, our police stations, criminal courts, and prisons are flooded with persons charged with drunkenness or marijuana possession, and other perpetrators of "crimes without victims," and if their numbers are not joined by swarms of fornicators, pornographers, and homosexuals, it is only because detection of such "criminals" is so difficult. Only an occasional morals offender is swept into the police nets out of the tens of millions who must violate some part of our sex laws, and these are usually members of economically deprived classes and minority races. Herbert Packer gives sound advice, then, when he cautions the rational legislator that "every dollar and every man-hour is the object of competition among uses," and that "he should not only put first things first, but also, what is perhaps harder, put last things last."[7] From the point of view of resource allocation in the fight against crime, "*merely* moral offenses," that is, those disapproved acts that neither harm nor offend (if there are such) are indeed "last things."

It is another matter to use the criminal law to prevent the offense caused to disgusted captive observers by unavoidable public behavior. In such cases, the offense principle can justify a statute forcing the offending parties to restrict their offensive conduct to private places. This would be to use the law to prevent indecency, however, not immorality as such. . . . Such a statute would be very little more restrictive of liberty than similarly grounded statutes against public nudity. Some conduct may be so offensive as to amount to a kind of "psychic aggression," in which case, the private harm principle would allow its suppression on the same grounds as that of physical assault. But even when all this is said and done, the harm and offense principles together will not support all "enforcement of morality as such," for they do not permit interference with the voluntary conduct of consenting adults in the privacy of their own rooms behind locked doors and drawn blinds.

For these reasons many writers have argued for the repeal of statutes that prohibit private immorality; but not surprisingly the same considerations have led others to abandon the view that the harm and offense principles provide an adequate guide to legislative policy. The alternative principle of "legal moralism" favored by the latter writers has several forms. In its more moderate version, it is commonly associated with the views of Patrick Devlin.[8] Lord Devlin's theory, as I understand it, is really a form of utilitarianism or, more exactly, an application of the public harm principle. The proper aim of the criminal law, he holds, is the prevention of harm, not merely harm to individuals but also, and primarily, harm to society itself. A shared moral code, Devlin argues, is a necessary condition for the very existence of a community. Shared moral convictions function as "invisible bonds" or a kind of "social cement" tying individuals together into an orderly society. Moreover the fundamental unifying morality (to switch the metaphor) is a kind of "seamless web":[9] To damage it at one point is to weaken it throughout. Hence, society has as much right to protect its moral code by legal coercion as it does to protect its equally indispensable political institutions. The law cannot tolerate politically revolutionary activity; nor can it accept activity that rips asunder its moral fabric. Thus, "The suppression of vice is as much the law's business as the suppression of subversive activities; it is no more possible to define a sphere of private morality than it is to define one of private subversive activity."[10]

H.L.A. Hart finds it plausible that some shared morality is necessary to the existence of a community, but criticizes Devlin's further contention "that a society is identical with its morality as that is at any given moment of its history, so that a change in its morality is tantamount to the destruction of a society."[11] Indeed, a moral critic might admit that we can't exist as a society without some morality or other, while insisting that we can perfectly well exist without *this* morality (if we put a better one in its place). Devlin seems to reply to this criticism that the shared morality *can* be changed even though protected by law, and when it does change, then the emergent reformed morality in turn deserves *its* legal protection.[12] The law then functions to make moral reform difficult, but there is no preventing change where the reforming zeal is fierce enough. How then does one bring about a change in prevailing moral beliefs when they are enshrined in law? Presumably one advocates conduct which is in fact illegal; one puts into public practice what one preaches; one demonstrates one's sincerity by marching proudly off to jail for one's convictions:

> There is . . . a natural respect for opinions that are sincerely held. When such opinions accumulate enough weight, the law must either yield or it is broken. In a democratic society . . . there will be a strong tendency for it to yield—not to abandon all defenses so as to let in the horde, but to give ground to those who are prepared to fight for something that they prize. To fight may be to suffer. A willingness to suffer is the most convincing proof of sincerity. Without the law there would be no proof. The law is the anvil on which the hammer strikes.[13]

In this remarkable passage, Devlin has discovered another argument for enforcing "morality as such," and incidentally for principled civil disobedience as the main technique for initiating and regulating moral change. A similar argument, deriving from Samuel Johnson, and applying mainly to changes in religious doctrine, was well known to Mill. Religious innovators deserve to be persecuted, on this theory, for persecution allows them to prove their mettle and demonstrate their disinterested good faith, while their teachings, insofar as they are true, cannot be hurt, since truth will always triumph in the end. Mill regarded this method of testing truth to be uneconomical, as well as ungenerous:

> To discover to the world something which deeply concerns it, and of which it was previously ignorant, to prove to it that it had been mistaken on some vital point of temporal or spiritual interest, is as important a service as a human being can render to his fellow creatures. . . . That the authors of such splendid benefits should be requited by martyrdom, that their reward should be to be dealt with as the vilest of criminals, is not, upon this theory, a deplorable error and misfortune for which humanity should mourn in sackcloth and ashes, but the normal and justifiable state of things. . . . People who defend this mode of treating benefactors cannot be supposed to set much value on the benefit.[14]

If self-sacrificing civil disobedience, on the other hand, is not the most efficient and humane remedy to grant to the moral reformer, what instruments of moral change are available for him? This question is not only difficult to answer in its own right, it is also the rock that sinks Devlin's favorite analogy between harmless immorality and political subversion.

Consider what subversion is. In most modern law-governed countries there is a constitution, a set of duly constituted authorities, and a body of statutes, or "positive laws," created and enforced by the duly constituted authorities. There will be ways of changing these things that are well known, orderly, and permitted by the constitution. For example, constitutions are amended; new legislation is introduced; legislators are elected. On the other hand, it is easy to conceive of various sorts of unpermitted and disorderly change, for example, through assassination and violent revolution, or through bribery and subornation, or through the use of legitimately won power to extort and intimidate. Only these illegitimate methods of change, of course, can be called "subversion." But here the analogy between positive law and positive morality begins to break down. There is no "moral constitution," no well-known and orderly way of introducing moral legislation to duly constituted moral legislators, no clear convention of majority rule. Moral subversion, if there is such a thing, must consist in the employment of disallowed techniques of change instead of the officially permitted "constitutional" ones. It consists not simply of change as such, but of illegitimate change. Insofar as the notion of legitimately induced moral change remains obscure, "illegitimate moral change" can do no better. Still, there is enough content to both notions to preserve some analogy to the political case. A citizen works *legitimately* to change prevailing moral beliefs when he publicly and forthrightly expresses his own dissent; when he attempts to argue, and persuade, and offer reasons; when he lives according to his own convictions with persuasive quiet and dignity, neither harming others nor offering counterpersuasive offense to tender sensibilities. On the other hand, a citizen attempts to change mores by *illegitimate* means when he abandons argument and example for force and fraud. If this is the basis of the distinction between legitimate and illegitimate techniques of moral change, then the use of state power to affect moral belief *one way or the other,* when harmfulness is not involved, would be a clear example of illegitimacy. Government enforcement of the conventional code is not to be called "moral subversion," of course, because it is used on behalf of the *status quo*; but whether conservative or innovative it is equally in defiance of our "moral constitution"—if anything is.

The second version of legal moralism is the pure version, not some other principle in disguise, but legal moralism properly so called. The enforcement of morality as such and the attendant punishment of sin are not justified as means to some further social aim (such as the preservation of social cohesiveness) but are ends in themselves. Perhaps J. F. Stephen was expressing this pure moralism when he wrote that "there are acts of wickedness so gross and outrageous that self-protection apart they must be prevented at any cost to the offender and punished if they occur with exemplary severity." [15] (From his examples it is clear that Stephen had in mind the very acts that are called "morals offenses" in the law.) That the act to be punished is truly wicked and outrageous must be the virtually unanimous opinion of society, Stephen goes on to add; and the public condemnation of acts of its kind must be "strenuous and unequivocal." [16]

Adequate discussion of Stephen's view requires that a distinction be made between the moral code actually in existence at a given time and place, and some ideal rational code. The former is often called "conventional" or "positive" morality, and the latter "rational" or "critical" morality. Whether or not a given type of act is wicked according to a given positive morality is a matter of sociological fact; whether or not it is "truly wicked" is a question for argument of a different kind and notoriously more difficult to settle. Stephen apparently identified critical morality in large measure with the Victorian positive morality of his time and place. A century later we can be pardoned, I think, for being somewhat skeptical about that. Once we grant that there is no necessary and self-evident correspondence between some given positive morality and the true critical morality, it becomes plain that the pure version of legal moralism is one or another of two distinct principles, depending on which sense of "morality" it employs.

Consider first, then, the view that the legal enforcement of positive morality is an end in itself. This means that it is good for its own sake that the state prohibit and punish all actions of a kind held wicked by the vast majority of citizens, even when such acts are harmless and done in private with all deference to the moral sensibilities of others. It is hard to argue against propositions that derive their support mainly from ethical intuition, but when one fully grasps the concept of a *positive morality,* even the intuitive basis of this moralistic proposition begins to dissolve. What is so precious, one wonders, about public opinion as such? Let us suppose that public opinion about moral questions is wrong, as it so often has been in the past. Is there still some intrinsic value in its legal enforcement derived from the mere fact that it *is* public opinion? This hardly seems plausible, much less intuitively certain, especially when one considers that enforcement would make it all the more difficult to correct the mistake. Perhaps it gives the public some satisfaction to know that conduct it regards (rightly or wrongly) as odious or sinful occurs very rarely even behind drawn blinds and that when it occurs, it is punished with "exemplary severity." But again it is hard to see how such "satisfaction" could have any intrinsic value; and even if we grant it intrinsic value for the sake of the argument, we should have to weigh it against such solid intrinsic evils as the infliction of suffering and the invasion of privacy.

The more plausible version of pure moralism restricts its scope to critical morality. This is the view that the state is justified in enforcing a truly rational morality as such and in punishing deviations from that morality even when they are of a kind that is not harmful to others. This principle too is said to rest on an intuitive basis. It is often said that the universe is an intrinsically worse place for having immoral (even harmlessly immoral) conduct in it. The threat of punishment (the argument continues) deters such conduct. The actual instances of punishment not only back up the threat, and thus help keep future moral weeds out of the universe's garden, they also erase the past evils from the universe's temporal record by "nullifying" them, or making it as if they never were. Thus, punishment contributes to the net intrinsic value of the universe in two ways: by canceling out past sins and preventing future ones. . . .

There may be some minimal plausibility in this view when it is applied to ordinary harmful crimes, especially those involving duplicity or cruelty, which really do seem to "set the universe out of joint." It is natural enough to think of repentance, apology, or forgiveness as "setting things straight," and of punishment as a kind of "payment" or a wiping clean of the moral slate. But in cases where it is natural to resort to such analogies, there is not only a rule infraction, there is also a *victim*— some person or society of persons who have been harmed. When there is no victim—and especially where there is no profit at the expense of another—"setting things straight" has no clear intuitive content.

Punishment may yet play its role in discouraging harmless private immoralities for the sake of "the universe's moral record." But if fear of punishment is to keep people from illicit intercourse (or from desecrating flags or mistreating corpses) in the privacy of their own rooms, then morality must be enforced with a fearsome efficiency that shows no respect for anyone's privacy. There may be some, like Stephen, who would derive great satisfaction from the thought that no harmless immoralities are being perpetrated behind anyone's locked doors (to the greater credit of the universe as a whole); but how many of these would be willing to sacrifice their *own* privacy for this "satisfaction"? Yet if private immoralities are to be deterred by threat of punishment, the detecting authorities *must* be able to look, somehow, into the hidden chambers and locked rooms of anyone's private domicile. And when we put this massive forfeiture of privacy into the balance along with the usual costs of coercion—loss of spontaneity, stunting of rational powers, anxiety, hypocrisy, and the rest—the price of securing mere outward conformity to the community's moral standards (for that is all that can be achieved by the penal law) is exorbitant.

In an extremely acute article,[17] Ronald Dworkin suggests (without fully endorsing) a version of pure legal moralism that shares some of the features of both versions discussed above. He distinguishes between genuine moral convictions and mere prejudices, personal aversions, arbitrary dogmas, and rationalizations. The actual moral convictions of a community, providing they constitute a genuine "discriminatory morality," Dworkin suggests, might well be enforced by the criminal law; but the "morality" that consists in mere emotional aversion, no matter how widespread, is a morality only in a weak "anthropological sense" and is undeserving of legal enforcement. Indeed, "the belief that prejudices, personal aversions, and rationalizations do not justify restricting another's freedom itself occupies a critical and fundamental position in our popular morality."[18] The consensus judgment in our community that homosexuality is wicked, in Dworkin's view, is not a genuine moral judgment at all, and "what is shocking and wrong is not [Devlin's] idea that the community's morality counts, but his idea of what counts as the community's morality."[19]

Dworkin's point is a good one against Devlin's position on sexual offenses, but I would go much further still. Even if there is a *genuine* moral consensus in a community that certain sorts of "harmless" activities are wrong, I see no reason why that consensus should be enforced by the criminal law and at least one very good reason why it ought not to be enforced: Even a genuine "discriminatory" popular morality might, for all of that, be *mistaken,* and legal enforcement inhibits critical dissent and prevents progressive improvement.

Notes

1. I use the word *justified* in the formulation of these principles in such a way that it does not follow from the fact that a given limitation on liberty is justified that the state has a duty to impose it, but only that the state *may* interfere on the ground in question if it should choose to do so. Cf. Ted Honderich, *Punishment: Its Supposed Justifications* (Hutchinson of London, 1969), p. 175. Moreover, as these principles are formulated here, they state sufficient but not necessary conditions for "justified" (that is, permissible) coercion. Each states that interference is permissible *if* (but not *only if*) a certain condition is satisfied. Hence the principles are not mutually exclusive; it is possible to hold two or more of them at once, even all of them together. And it is possible to

deny all of them. In fact, since all combinations and permutations of these principles are (logically) possible, there are 2^7 or 128 possible positions (and more) about the legitimacy of coercion represented by the list.

2. J. S. Mill, *On Liberty,* Chapter 5, paragraph 7.

3. H.L.A. Hart, *Law, Liberty, and Morality* (Stanford, Calif.: Stanford University Press, 1963), p. 45.

4. Traditionally, offensiveness has tended to arouse even more extreme penalties than harmfulness. The New York Penal Law, for example, until recently provided a maximum sentence of ten years for first degree assault and twenty years for sodomy; Pennsylvania's Penal Code provides a maximum of seven years for assault with intent to kill and ten years for pandering; California provides a maximum of two years for corporal injury to wife or child but fifteen years for "perversion." Mayhem and assault with intent to commit a serious felony get fourteen and twenty years, respectively, in California, but statutory rape and incest get fifty years each. Zechariah Chafee gives the best example I know of perverse judicial zeal to avenge mere offense: "The white slave traffic was first exposed by W. T. Stead in a magazine article, 'The Maiden Tribute.' The English law did absolutely nothing to the profiteers in vice, but put Stead in prison for a year for writing about an indecent subject" (Z. Chafee, *Free Speech in the United States* [Cambridge, Mass.: Harvard University Press, 1964], p. 151). It is worth noting, finally, that the most common generic synonym for *crimes* is neither *harms* nor *injuries,* but *offenses.*

5. For example, "One has only to stroll along certain streets in Amsterdam to see that prostitution may be permitted to flourish openly without impairing personal security, economic prosperity, or indeed the general moral tone of a most respected nation of the Western world" (Louis B. Schwartz, "Morals Offenses and the Model Penal Code," *Columbia Law Review* 63 [1963], p. 670).

6. *Ibid.,* p. 672.

7. Herbert Packer, *The Limits of the Criminal Sanction* (Stanford, Calif.: Stanford University Press, 1968), p. 260.

8. Patrick Devlin, *The Enforcement of Morals* (London: Oxford University Press, 1965).

9. The phrase is not Devlin's but rather that of his critic H.L.A. Hart, in *Law, Liberty, and Morality,* p. 51. In his rejoinder to Hart, Devlin writes: "Seamlessness presses the simile rather hard, but apart from that, I should say that for most people morality is a web of beliefs, rather than a number of unconnected ones" (Devlin, *Enforcement,* p. 115).

10. Devlin, *Enforcement,* pp. 13–14.

11. Hart, *Law, Liberty, and Morality,* p. 51.

12. Devlin, *Enforcement,* pp. 115ff.

13. *Ibid.,* p. 116.

14. Mill, *On Liberty,* Chapter 2, paragraph 14.

15. James Fitzjames Stephen, *Liberty, Equality, Fraternity* (London, 1873), p. 163.

16. *Ibid.,* p. 159.

17. Ronald Dworkin, "Lord Devlin and the Enforcement of Morals," *Yale Law Journal* 75 (1966).

18. *Ibid.,* p. 1001.

19. *Loc. cit.*

Part III

Law and Public Policy

Preview

What should a society do, asks Professor of Law Richard F. Duncan, when up to 2 million people are carriers of a disease that is (1) contagious; (2) incurable; (3) terminal; and (4) spreading rapidly?[1] Should we engage in mass screening to identify all the carriers? Should we quarantine or isolate them?[2] Should we quarantine only those with AIDS or ARC, or only noncompliant positives? Should people with AIDS or ARC or who are ACH be denied insurance or employment?

Some questions that involve rights issues—such as whether to close commercial sex establishments that facilitate dangerous sexual activity—become matters of public policy because of money. In an attempt to explain why the issue of closing (or regulating) gay bathhouses is a matter of public concern, Steven J. Stone says that "although sexual activity between consenting adults, heterosexual or homosexual, is essentially a private matter and an individual decision, the costs of health care are a societal responsibility."[3] It is interesting to note the extent to which questions of quarantine or screening are concerned with matters of dollars and cents.

The Lyndon LaRouche–sponsored AIDS initiative that appeared (and was defeated) on the November 1986 California ballot was interpreted as mandating quarantine, mass screening, and the firing of certain workers, notably teachers, health care employees, and food handlers. A recently concluded study by the Department of Public Policy at the University of California at Berkeley says that "the LaRouche Initiative, Proposition 64, if passed and fully implemented, could cost the state $7.9 billion, one quarter of the state's annual budget."[4] The study puts a "$2.5 billion price tag on quarantining 300,000 people. . . . There would be a further $1.5 billion lost in tax revenues and another $2.9 billion in unemployment benefits. The cost of testing everyone in the state would alone come to $1 billion."[5]

It is useful, warns June E. Osborn, M.D., "in order to appreciate the economic trouble to come, to think of *every single case* of AIDS as costing the same as a heart transplantation."[6] Private insurance companies (who, after all, are in business to make a profit) do not find it cost effective to test everyone who applies for insurance. In remarks reprinted in this volume, Donald Chambers, M.D., vice president and chief medical director of the Lincoln National Life Insurance Company, makes it clear that insurers do not wish to test everyone. A policy of selective testing not only raises questions of justice and fairness but also assumes that AIDS is confined to certain identifiable population groups. Note that Kenneth Howe, in his argument against mandatory screening, claims both that HIV is distributed among well-defined populations and that certain modes of transmission confine it to these populations. These assumptions, which underlie parts of the arguments both for and against screening, received scrutiny in the General Introduction.

Chambers also makes clear that insurers want to test only those who apply for private insurance, not those who have or will have group insurance. However, if employers use screening to refuse employment, many individuals will be denied group insurance as well. The United States military, a large employer, instituted a policy of testing all new recruits as of October 24, 1985, with the result that those who test positive will be barred from the armed services. The reason given by the Department of Defense for implementing the screening policy was the inability to test blood under battle conditions. Many people are unconvinced, however, suspecting instead (among other reasons) a desire to evade costs. Soldier-to-soldier blood transfusions during battle are rare. Moreover, the military blood supply is already protected by HIV screening of blood donors. Further, the policy is overbroad in that it applies to thousands of office workers and desk personnel.[7]

Jesse Helms, in his Senate testimony against the (now enacted) District of Columbia law prohibiting insurance companies from testing for HIV antibodies, said that AIDS is a health issue, not a civil rights issue. However, as we see from the following quotation, AIDS is certainly a financial issue for Helms:

> And who will be harpooned in the pocketbook? Not the insurance industry, Mr. President. The increased cost will be passed on to other policyholders in the form of higher premiums—the policyholders who may already have higher premiums because of being at risk of developing cancer, or at risk of a heart attack. Now, because of the D.C. AIDS law, they will have an even higher premium because someone else is at risk of contracting AIDS. This is unfair, Mr. President.[8]

Richard Mohr addresses exactly this type of argument when he says that, to demonstrate that rate increases are unfair, the insurance industry would have to show that raising rates violates some right or legitimate claim of its clients. Although it would be nice if no one's insurance premiums were increased, says Mohr, simply raising the price of insurance (like raising the price of milk) does not violate anyone's rights.

In a country like the United States, which has no national health care system, it is understandable that private financial interests would be central to public policy regarding the halting of an epidemic. In every other major Western country, according to Dennis Altman, "there exists some sort of national health insurance, so that people struck with catastrophic illness do not find themselves scrambling to pay for basic care. In most other affluent societies the sorts of basic welfare services required by the seriously ill are provided by the State."[9] As a former president of the American Public Health Association said of the Reagan administration, "They tend to see health in the same way that John Calvin saw wealth: It's your own responsibility and you should damn well take care of yourself."[10]

Kenneth Howe perceptively points out that debates about private financial interests are basically about cost shifting. Unless AIDS patients are abandoned, says Howe, the money for their cure will have to come from somewhere. Because the disease is now incurable, the test cannot be used by insurance companies to reduce health costs by detecting and treating AIDS early. Its only use, argues Howe, is to deny any access to private insurance, hence shifting the burden of cost from the private to the public sector. Thus, the public, as taxpayers, will have to pay health care costs; in addition, the public, as policyholders, will presumably absorb the cost of screening done by the insurance companies.

The lack of financial commitment and the tardiness of response on the part of the Reagan administration to the AIDS epidemic have been perceived by many as indifference, if not hostility, toward the victims of AIDS.[11] Of equal concern is a refusal to be candid about sex. As June E. Osborn puts it:

> The very messages that we must broadcast in order to abort the epidemic and buy time for further scientific advance require the use of words that are taboo in high places. We need urgently to pursue so-called psychosocial research—but we may not be "explicit," and we may not, in fact, send out messages that even seem to condone sexual and other practices that deviate from a governmentally sanctioned norm. No official document should use the phrase "safe sex," even if that currently appears to be the major promising route to safety for an important segment of the population.[12]

As Carol Tauer points out, countries such as Norway have engaged in imaginative educational efforts. For example, an Oslo billboard shows a cartoon face drawn on the top of a penis to illustrate a point about using condoms to prevent the transmission of AIDS. Other efforts, however, have been alleged to be in poor taste. For example, in New South Wales, Australia, a radio jingle about condoms to the tune of a '50s hit song, "Who's Sorry Now," was canceled by the minister for health.[13]

Education and counsel concerning risks, says Alvin Novick, are the appropriate goals of surveillance and research on AIDS. The worry is that the products of research may instead be political and social oppression. As Novick puts it, "The most threatening scenarios include the use of inappropriate or broadly imposed quarantine, the recriminalization of homosexual sexuality, or the inappropriate restriction of employment, access to housing, or other restrictions on the civil rights of persons in at-risk groups."[14] These fears are realistic. Knowing a little United States history regarding the imposition of overbroad and arbitrary quarantine is illuminating. At the turn of the century, the San Francisco Board of Health imposed a quarantine on twelve city blocks of (mostly) Chinese residents. Claiming it had found nine cases of bubonic plague, the board established a quarantine that affected more than 15,000 people. In *Jew Ho* v. *Williamson,*[15] a California Circuit Court found the quarantine to be "unreasonable, unnecessary, and applied in a discriminatory manner."[16]

As recently as June 1986, the U.S. Supreme Court smoothed the path for the continued criminalization (and even the recriminalization) of homosexual acts by upholding a Georgia statute outlawing consensual adult sodomy. This ruling and its relevance to AIDS is explored in detail in Part IV. Also in June 1986, the United States Department of Justice released a 49-page memorandum regarding the application of Section 504 of the Rehabilitation Act of 1973 to people who have AIDS or AIDS-related complex, or who have been infected with HIV. It concludes that

Section 504 prohibits discrimination based on the disabling effects that AIDS and related conditions may have on their victims. By contrast, we have concluded that an individual's (real or perceived) ability to transmit the disease is not a handicap within the meaning of the statute and, therefore, that discrimination on this basis does not fall within Section 504.[17]

Many, including the American Medical Association (AMA), have been outraged by the Justice Department's opinion, which the AMA (and others) interpreted as allowing companies to dismiss workers who have AIDS or ARC or who are ACH if a fear of contagion exists. The AMA has articulated its disagreement with the Justice Department's position in a friend-of-the-court brief filed with the Supreme Court in conjunction with *School Board of Nassau County* v. *Arline,* a case regarding the rights of a woman with tuberculosis. The AMA brief stated that

employment decisions about AIDS victims, like decisions about anyone handicapped by a communicable disease, should be based on reasonable medical judgments about their handicap and their risk to others, and not, as the Justice Department opinion would allow, on irrational fear of the handicapped individual's ability to communicate a disease.[18]

That irrationally based AIDS-related discrimination takes place is undoubtedly true. For example, the president of the Newark City Council proposed a law requiring AIDS tests for food workers—even though no proof exists that AIDS can be transmitted by food workers—because having such a law would give "some people a psychological lift."[19] In insisting on minimal rational standards for what can count as a moral position or a genuine moral conviction, Ronald Dworkin urges (see Part II): "Not every reason I might give will do . . . ." Among the reasons that "will not do" are those based merely on emotional reactions or false claims.

The Justice Department argued in its defense that it does not condone discrimination on the basis of perceived ability to communicate a disease; such a case is simply not covered in the Act. Section 504 states, "No otherwise qualified handicapped individual in the United States . . . shall, solely by reason of his handicap, . . . be subjected to discrimination . . . ."[20] Although there is no talk of "perception" here, in 1974, Congress enacted a definition of "handicapped individual" that made it clear that a person can be handicapped if he "is falsely perceived as being handicapped."[21] Thus, although the Justice Department, unlike the AMA, may have a point in trying to separate the issue of communicability from the notion of a handicap, one is left with a position that seems deliberately obtuse: If you are fired because someone falsely perceives you to be suffering from AIDS, you have been wrongly discriminated against, but if you are fired because someone falsely perceives that you will give him or her AIDS, you have not been wrongly discriminated against.

On March 3, 1987, the United States Supreme Court ruled 7–2 (in *School Board of Nassau County* v. *Arline*) that employers, schools, and other recipients of federal money may not discriminate against people who are physically or mentally impaired by contagious diseases, unless those people pose a serious risk of infection to others or could not do their work.[22] The majority, however, explicitly declined to decide whether Section 504 of the Rehabilitation Act of 1973 protects someone who tests positive as a carrier of HIV but has no symptoms or physical impairment. Still, the ruling, in its insistence that irrational fear of contagion is not a ground for dismissal, promises to provide a measure of protection against discrimination for unimpaired carriers of HIV.

While doing research for this book, we have come across those who are concerned about the possibility that a worker handling food might spit in a salad. Whatever one's worries, as Mark Senak, an attorney for the Gay Men's Health Crisis in New York, points out, "It's generally not professional people who have trouble. It's the file clerks who get trashed . . . ."[23] The media have devoted much attention to the question of whether male and female nurses with AIDS should be allowed to keep their jobs, but virtually no attention to the Florida surgeon who died of AIDS in 1983.[24] *The New England Journal of Medicine* reports that he operated on 400 patients from 1978 to 1983; as of August 1985, according to state health department records, no cases of AIDS have been found in these patients. Nonetheless, these assurances are problematic: Some have left Florida since their surgery and cannot be located, and, although the study is on-going at present, the follow-up time is inadequate. The report cites CDC guidelines on precautions to be taken by hospital personnel who have AIDS: "Personnel . . . should wear gloves for procedures that involve trauma to tissues or direct contact with mucous membranes or nonintact skin . . . ."[25]

Presumably CDC recommendations were followed in this case, although the account does not state so. The guidelines are invoked for the purpose of assuring us that there is not much to worry about. As Richard Goldstein has put it (although he was speaking of condoms and not rubber gloves), "But if a layer of latex is all that it takes to still the winds of doom, what kind of moral mystery does AIDS pose?"[26]

Many public policy issues would be simpler, and perhaps some would even disappear, if people in the United States shared with Europeans certain conceptions of rights. Carol Tauer puts policy issues in an alternative perspective when she asserts:

> It has been noted that persons at risk for AIDS in European countries display a relative lack of concern about possible loss of their civil rights. This phenomenon could perhaps be linked to the fact that homosexual activity is not illegal in these countries, and also perhaps to the national health care systems by which full medical coverage is provided to citizens of most European nations.[27]

The fact that certain types of sexual behavior capable of transmitting AIDS are felonies in many states in the United States makes those who commit the behavior reluctant to divulge names of sexual contacts or to volunteer to be tested for antibodies to the AIDS virus. Novick says, "Our knowledge depends on research, which, in turn, depends on voluntary cooperation."[28] In the United States, where the consequences of the exposure of one's sex life can be drastic, confidentiality takes on an enormous importance. This is not to say that confidentiality is unimportant in, say, Sweden. Rather, assurances of confidentiality in the United States are expected to carry too much of a burden in society's attempt to research and prevent the spread of an epidemic.

"The perils of anonymity," says Richard Mohr, "are another way in which the lack of gay civil rights has aggravated the AIDS crisis."[29] For any individual, the possession of civil rights within a community presupposes a certain degree of public awareness of his or her identity. (In Australia, for example, permanent residency status may be awarded to non-Australian lesbians and gay men who are "in genuine gay relationships" with Australians.[30]) Thus, maintaining a secrecy about one's homosexuality separates a person from the community in a very fundamental sense. As recent biographies point out, actor Rock Hudson, whose career depended upon the illusion of his heterosexuality, went to extreme lengths to conceal his gay life-style from the public; he revealed his homosexuality only when he was near death and unable to keep the media at bay. Dale C. Olson credited Hudson's openness about his struggle with AIDS with creating public understanding of the disease: "The actor humanized AIDS to those who viewed it as a disease of strangers who were homosexuals and intravenous drug abusers."[31]

Society's willingness to accept open communication with regard to AIDS is in fact a crucial point. In his concurring opinion in *Bowers* v. *Hardwick* (see Part IV), Chief Justice Warren Burger—arguing that millennia of moral and legal condemnation should not be cast aside—appeals to 18th-century English jurist Sir William Blackstone's *Commentaries,* where homosexual sodomy is described "as an offense of 'deeper malignity' than rape, a heinous act 'the very mention of which is a disgrace to human nature,' and 'a crime not to be named.'" It is no small irony to contrast these remarks with United States Surgeon General C. Everett Koop's urging that parents and teachers start education about AIDS "at the lowest grade possible."[32] According to Koop:

> Many people—especially our youth—are not receiving information that is vital to their future health and well-being because of our reticence in dealing with the subjects of sex, sexual practices, and homosexuality. This silence must end. We can no longer afford to sidestep frank, open discussions about sexual practices— homosexual and heterosexual. Education about AIDS should start at an early age so that children can grow up knowing the behaviors to avoid to protect themselves from exposure to the AIDS virus.[33]

On October 30, 1986, the National Academy of Sciences charged that the federal government's AIDS education programs have been "woefully inadequate"[34] and called for a $2-billion-a-year educational and research effort. It appears that some subjects, traditionally unmentionable in the United States, are rapidly becoming public. Stopping short of developing a series of Norwegian-style billboards, Baltimore's Health Education Resource Organization has published a series of slick new ads about AIDS prevention: "'Smart sportswear for the active man,' reads one, below a photo of red, yellow, and green condoms."[35] The growing number of deaths, the rising costs of medical care, and increasing awareness of sexually variant life-styles are initiating the kinds of questioning we see in Part III.

Notes

1. Richard F. Duncan, "Public Policy and the AIDS Epidemic," *The Journal of Contemporary Health Law and Policy,* Vol. 2 (Spring 1986), p. 169.

2. Generally, we will not attend to the distinction between two types of constraint: (1) temporary coercive isolation during a period of infectiousness, or "quarantine"; and (2) temporally open-ended coercive isolation, or "isolation."

3. Steven J. Stone, "Protecting the Public from AIDS: A New Challenge to Traditional Forms of Epidemic Control," *The Journal of Contemporary Health Law and Policy,* Vol. 2 (Spring 1986), p. 204, footnote 83.

4. Charles Linebarger, "If Passed, LaRouche Initiative Would Cost State Billions," *The Advocate* (September 30, 1986), p. 22.

5. *Ibid.*

6. June E. Osborn, "The AIDS Epidemic: Multidisciplinary Trouble," *The New England Journal of Medicine* (March 20, 1986), p. 780.

7. See Stone, *op. cit.,* pp. 198–99, footnote 48, and Leonard Cizewski, "HTLV-III Testing and the Military," *Changing Men: Issues in Gender, Sex and Politics,* Vol. 16 (Summer 1986), pp. 21–22.

8. Jesse Helms, *Congressional Record—Senate* (June 19, 1986), pp. S8008–09.

9. Dennis Altman, *AIDS in the Mind of America* (Garden City, N.Y.: Doubleday, 1986), p. 27.

10. *Ibid.,* p. 29.

11. See Altman, *op. cit,* pp. 26–29. See also Talbot and Bush, "While the Reagan Administration Dozes and Scientists Vie for Glory, the Deadly AIDS Epidemic Has Put the Entire Nation at Risk," *Mother Jones,* Vol. 29 (April 1985). For a dramatic account of early attempts to get attention and funding from the city of New York, see Larry Kramer's play, *The Normal Heart* (New York: New American Library, 1985).

12. Osborn, *op. cit.,* pp. 779–80.

13. Kendall Lovett, *Gay Community News* (March 22, 1986).

14. Alvin Novick, "At Risk for AIDS: Confidentiality in Research and Surveillance," *IRB: A Review of Human Subjects Research,* Vol. 6, No. 6 (Hastings-on-Hudson, N.Y.: The Hastings Center, November/December 1984), p. 11, and this volume.

15. 103 Fed. 10 (9th Cir. 1900).

16. Stone, *op. cit.,* p. 202.

17. U.S. Department of Justice, from a memorandum to Ronald E. Robertson, General Counsel, Department of Health and Human Services (Washington, D.C.: June 20, 1986), p. 1.

18. *The Louisville Courier-Journal* (July 13, 1986).

19. *The New York Times,* October 26, 1985; see also "The Constitutional Rights of AIDS Carriers," *Harvard Law Review,* Vol. 99, p. 1274, footnote 6.

20. U.S. Department of Justice, *op. cit.,* p. 15.

21. *Ibid.,* p. 47.

22. *The Washington Post* (March 4, 1987).

23. Mark Senak, quoted by Tamar Lewin in "Business and the Law: AIDS and Job Discrimination," *The New York Times* (April 15, 1986), p. 30.

24. Jeffrey J. Sacks, M.D., "AIDS in a Surgeon," a letter to the editor in *The New England Journal of Medicine,* Vol. 313, No. 6 (October 17, 1985), pp. 1017–18. See also letter by Stephen R. Mascioli, M.D., and Jeffrey Sacks's reply in the same journal (May 1, 1986), p. 1190.

25. *Ibid.,* p. 1017.

26. Richard Goldstein, "A Plague on All Our Houses," *The Village Voice Literary Supplement* (September 1986), p. 17.

27. Carol Tauer, this volume.

28. Novick, *op. cit.,* p. 11, and this volume.

29. Richard D. Mohr, "AIDS, Gay Life, State Coercion," *Raritan,* Vol. VI, No. 1 (Summer 1986), p. 56.

30. Proof of a "genuine gay relationship" is established by having lived with a partner for four years. Temporary resident visas are also available for the noncitizen partner in such a couple during the four-year waiting period. *Gay Community News* (September 21–27, 1986).

31. *Durham Morning Herald* (October 2, 1986).

32. C. Everett Koop, M.D., from a statement issued by the U.S. Public Health Service (Washington, D.C.: October 22, 1986), p. 4.

33. Koop, *op. cit.,* p. 3.

34. *The New York Times* (October 30, 1986).

35. *The Washington Post* (October 23, 1986).

AIDS, Quarantines, and Noncompliant Positives

DAVID J. MAYO

Introduction

[Ever s]ince lepers were told to keep themselves apart and live outside the city in the time of Leviticus, victims of contagious diseases have been subject to quarantine— that is, compulsory isolation from contact with others. Recently, quarantine has been discussed as a way of dealing with the threat AIDS poses to public health. For instance, Dr. Vernon Mark of the Harvard Medical School has suggested quarantining "carriers of AIDS who persist in spreading it by 'irresponsible' behavior" on an island in the middle of Massachusetts Bay that had formerly served as a leper colony.[1] Some AIDS quarantine proposals have considerable popular support: a July 1986 poll conducted by *The Los Angeles Times* found 46 percent of its respondents favoring a quarantine of AIDS victims.[2]

On the face of it, this might seem a reasonable strategy. AIDS is an infectious disease, which thus far is always fatal. Moreover, a highly reliable test is available for identifying persons who have been exposed and are probably carriers.

But while a serious public health threat is posed by AIDS, quarantine is a drastic measure. Compulsory isolation amounts to deprivation of liberty, which may be indistinguishable from imprisonment from the point of view of the person quarantined—particularly one who feels perfectly healthy. At one time quarantines were used quite freely in this country. As late as 1915 Mary Mallon (Typhoid Mary) was jailed in New York City after having infected 51 people with typhoid fever. She spent the remaining 23 years of her life there without ever having been convicted of a criminal offense.[3] More recently quarantines have become much less common, however, for both medical and moral reasons. Advances in medicine give us a better understanding of mechanisms of infectiousness and enable us to control infectious disease more effectively when it does occur. Increasing concern with civil rights since the Warren Court has raised questions of the constitutionality of quarantines. Quarantines represent a challenge to one's fundamental rights to free association, privacy (including the right to cohabit with one's spouse and family), and the right to interstate travel.[4] The implementation of an AIDS quarantine might also raise questions of due process and equal protection, if it would unfairly disadvantage gays, IV drug users, and hemophiliacs. The statutes that permitted the incarceration of Mary Mallon would certainly pose constitutional problems today.

In what follows I will address the desirability of three AIDS quarantine proposals, each of which would target a different group for quarantine. The first two I refer to as "mass" quarantine proposals, because they target large groups of people: (1) all persons with AIDS (or all persons with AIDS or ARC), and (2) all persons who test positive for antibodies to the human immunodeficiency virus (hereafter HIV) and hence are presumably infected and infectious. After arguing against both of these "mass" quarantine proposals on utilitarian and constitutional grounds and from considerations of justice, I will focus on a much more modest but still problematic proposal, a quarantine of all "noncompliant positives," that is, persons who are presumed infectious with AIDS on the basis of HIV sero-positivity (the presence in the blood of antibodies to the HIV) but who refuse to comply with the restrictions necessary to keep from infecting others. There I will argue that a quarantine of noncompliant positives avoids the most obvious difficulties of the other proposals, but that it is not without difficulties of its own.

Proposal #1: Mass Quarantine of All Persons with AIDS (and ARC)

As of this writing (October 1986), 12,000 AIDS patients are alive in the United States. Some are critically ill, but many feel well enough to work and—at least for the moment—lead relatively normal lives. The cost to these people of the disruption of being quarantined is obvious. Moreover, it would be equally obvious to anyone experiencing symptoms that might indicate AIDS, and hence would provide that person with strong motivation not to seek diagnosis and treatment.

Not only would such a quarantine have obvious costs; it would [also] have only marginal benefits in controlling the AIDS epidemic, since by and large AIDS patients are not the ones spreading the disease. The best medical evidence tells us that AIDS is not spread by casual contact, but only by intimate sexual contact or through blood exchange.[5] Thus, by and large, the people who infect others with the virus are those who engage in so-called "high-risk activities": particularly intercourse—especially anal intercourse—without a condom, and the sharing of needles. Since diagnosed AIDS patients know they are infectious and are informed of what activities can transmit AIDS, most of them will surely refrain from these activities. How many human beings would knowingly and willingly expose others to a lethal virus—especially one whose horrors they knew firsthand? Although there will be some exceptions, they will surely be rare.

Who then spreads AIDS? Like most infectious conditions, AIDS is usually spread by persons who don't realize they are infectious because they are still asymptomatic and feel healthy. It is a sad irony of infectious conditions generally that infected persons are apt to be most infectious before the onset of symptoms. AIDS differs from most infectious conditions . . . only in that it has an unusually long incubation period. (Apparently many who are infected with the HIV never do become ill.) Given CDC estimates, the number of people diagnosed with AIDS are outnumbered by those who are infectious but symptom-free on the order of 1:200, so at any given time the vast majority of those who are infectious feel completely healthy and are unaware they are infectious. By and large, these are the people who are responsible for most of the transmission of the HIV.

Undeniably there are some "noncompliant" AIDS and ARC patients who will persist in high-risk activities. Thus, even though quarantining all AIDS and ARC patients would have little statistical impact on the spread of the disease, it would have some impact. Some lives might be saved. This, however, is not sufficient to justify morally depriving all AIDS patients of their liberty. It would certainly be both unjust and an unconstitutional violation of due process, and/or of equal protection, to deprive a large group of people of their liberty on the grounds that a few of them may knowingly behave in ways that put others at risk—even the very serious risk of death.

If this seems counterintuitive, comparison with standards of evidence in the criminal law may be instructive. Imagine a case in which evidence—say, eyewitness accounts and extensive videotape—[has] established the physical appearance of a man [who] committ[ed] . . . a series of brutal murders that were distinctively similar. Imagine that a suspect matching the description "beyond a reasonable doubt" is apprehended and has no alibi, but is able to produce an identical twin bother—also with no alibi. So strong are our convictions about the injustice of punishing an innocent person that we embrace a legal system that dictates that both would go free, so long as neither could be shown "beyond a reasonable doubt" to be the guilty one. Even the high probability of the murderer now before us striking again would not justify incarcerating either, given our notions of criminal justice. How much less acceptable would it be, then, from the point of view of justice, for the state to incarcerate 12,000 people on the grounds that some unspecifiable few of them are liable to knowingly and willingly put others at serious risk?

Proposal #2: Quarantine All Persons Presumed Infectious on the Basis of . . . HIV Sero-Positiv[ity]

Since the HIV is usually spread by persons who are [infectious] but asymptomatic, perhaps a mass AIDS quarantine should apply to everyone who is infectious—or, more accurately, to those we can identify as probably infectious on the basis of test[s] for antibodies to the HIV. There is, of course, no certainty that all persons testing seropositive are in fact infected, nor that all those who are infected are infectious. Nevertheless, these tests remain powerful tools for predicting infectiousness. Purely from a public health standpoint HIV seropositives might seem the most logical group, quite in the tradition of quarantines, only with the modern advantage of being able to test for probable infectiousness in the absence of symptoms. If we think of quarantine as a way of slowing the spread of a disease through a population by isolating those who are already infected, this proposal probably represents the AIDS mass quarantine strategy in its most unadulterated form.

Before turning to objections to this proposal involving the moral and constitutional rights of innocent people whose lives would be unjustly affected, let us note first several insurmountable utilitarian difficulties. The most obvious involves the sheer numbers who would be quarantined. Current estimates tell us that between 1 and 2 percent of the U.S. population, or 2 to 5 million Americans, probably are HIV seropositive, [including not only] . . . many gays and IV drug users, but also most of the nation's hemophiliacs, as well as some spouses and children of all three of these groups. It is difficult to conceive even the sheer logistics of such a quarantine, much less the economic and other social implications.

This will not, after all, be a cooperative group. The vast majority will feel healthy, and their "quarantine" will not be for a mere 40 days, as the word originally implied, but very possibly for life. Thus "security" requirements for such draconian measures would be staggering.

A separate set of problems arises in connection with the task of identifying those to be quarantined in the first place. Since identification as seropositive would be tantamount to an indeterminate prison sentence, those who suspected they might be seropositive would want to avoid being tested. Thus, as some of its advocates have acknowledged,[6] such a quarantine program would in turn require a program of universal, mandatory testing. It is difficult to imagine how such a testing program could be implemented, especially given that a large segment of the population would be hostile to it. (William F. Buckley has suggested a program of universal testing with compulsory tattoo-identifications of all positives.[7]) Whatever form it took, it would meet with widespread hostility, resistance, and probably corruption. People will not flock to find out whether they are to be incarcerated indefinitely. And if universal testing could somehow be implemented, society would become divided into two antagonistic groups—the "clean" [versus] the "unclean" they would be trying to incarcerate.

Traditionally people have valued liberty so highly they have been willing to take great risks to preserve it. As one tries to envision programs of universal testing, and apprehension . . . for involuntary and potentially lifelong incarceration of large numbers of [people from] already stigmatized groups, one is led alternately to images of grade-B science fiction movies, with computers spewing forth the names of the "untouchables" who are to be rounded up, and thoughts of the French Resistance during World War II—a struggling underground dealing in false identification papers and working to hide those sought by the authorities or to smuggle them out of the country. The analogy with the Third Reich is perhaps apt, given Buckley's tattoo proposal.

In addition to these utilitarian difficulties, objections about the injustice—and the unconstitutionality—of mass quarantining of all HIV-positives should be obvious. Even the preliminary step of universal mandatory testing poses serious questions of unconstitutional invasion of privacy.[8] Quarantining everyone who *might* transmit the virus would involve morally and constitutionally intolerable impositions on the fundamental rights of at least a million seropositive Americans who pose no threat of infection either because they [are] willing to abstain from unsafe activities or because they [aren't] even infectious.

In fact, the number of noninfectious who would be quarantined on this proposal is much greater than might at first be thought, due to yet another difficulty with this proposal—that of test error. No test is perfect, and various costs result when mass quarantining is done on the basis of an imperfect test. Specifically, even a *low percentage* of "false positives" can result in a *high* number of cases if the total population being tested is large. The mathematics of the present case is surprising. Imagine that 1 percent of all Americans, or 2.4 million, are presently HIV seropositive. (Again, estimates from the CDC put the figure at 2 to 5 million.) Understand further that the test is presumed to be remarkably accurate—99 percent. This means that in addition to *correctly* identifying 1 percent of 240 million, or 2.4 million Americans as seropositive, it will also *misidentify* 1 percent of the remaining 99 percent of the 240 million, or 2,376,000 Americans as seropositive as well. Thus, the number of false positives will roughly equal the number of true positives the test will . . . identify, and roughly half of those quarantined will have been misidentified. Remember again our intuitions about punishing the innocent! (This, incidentally, is just a special case of the problem of the damage done by any program of compulsory mass testing where a cost is [exacted] for the individual with a false positive result, such as the drug testing program President Reagan recently mandated for civilian federal employees.[9]) Moreover, nearly 1 in 50 Americans would be quarantined!

There is a final practical difficulty connected with test error: It would keep the draconian quarantine from ending the epidemic. Those who test negative, believing that all positives had been quarantined, might well regard their own negative test results as license to participate once again in high-risk activities. Unfortunately this group would also include 1 percent (or 2.35 million) false negatives who were actually positive. This, of course, would prevent the quarantine from halting the spread of AIDS.

A Final Criticism: The Need for Cooperation and Trust

A final objection to both mass quarantine proposals is that they run exactly counter to the prevailing view of public health experts, that trust and cooperation between public health officials and persons at risk for AIDS must prevail if the spread of AIDS is to be slowed. Since no vaccine or cure for AIDS is available, the most promising strategy available for cutting down on the transmission of AIDS now is the reduction of high-risk activities, and this can be achieved only through cooperation and education of high-risk groups about what activities are unsafe. This task is already well under way in the gay community in some cities,[10] but is obviously frustrated by any antagonism between public officials and high-risk groups. Mutual trust is absolutely essential if individuals are to begin to listen to, believe, and finally act on the advice of health professionals about what activities are unsafe. That is virtually impossible when those at risk are—or believe they are—stigmatized as "outsiders." That is the nearly unanimous belief of those who actually work in public health with victims of stigmatizing diseases, particularly diseases associated with stigmatized behavior.[11] Moreover, AIDS research obviously requires the participation of HIV seropositives who do not have AIDS and other members of high-risk groups. However, many of these people fear that such cooperation may ultimately lead to breaches of confidentiality, which could cost them dearly as individuals in terms of future employment, insurance, and perhaps even their liberty. Serious public discussion of mass AIDS quarantine proposals obviously exacerbates and legitimatizes those concerns about confidentiality, and thus again frustrates cooperation just when it is needed most.

We have looked at . . . utilitarian arguments against mass AIDS quarantines, deontic arguments involving appeals to justice, and constitutional arguments. Any mass AIDS quarantine would involve enormous costs for those quarantined. It would prove socially divisive, expensive, and almost certainly counterproductive of the goal of slowing the spread of AIDS. Objections involving justice augment these utilitarian concerns: Any mass AIDS quarantine would inevitably involve unjust intrusions on the fundamental interests and rights of large numbers of innocent people, and would do so in ways that would be unconstitutional on a number of grounds.

Among those concerned about AIDS quarantines, there is obviously disagreement about how many of the people covered by mass quarantine proposals would be "innocent." This will obviously depend on one's views of homosexuality, promiscuity, and IV drug abuse, and of the extent to which people who have contracted AIDS "should have known better" in light of what was known at the time about the disease. Interesting as these questions are, however, they needn't concern us here, since each mass quarantine proposal would involve unjustly quarantining very large numbers of persons with AIDS who are "innocent" by even the most conservative moral standards, [such as] those born with AIDS, those who [were] unaware of their sexual partners' risky behavior, [and] those infected through purportedly virus-free blood transfusions.

Proposal #3: Quarantine of Noncompliant Positives

The final proposal, to quarantine only noncompliant positives, promises to escape many of the objections to the mass quarantine proposals. Since it would involve disrupting the lives of far fewer people, and would be correspondingly less divisive and expensive, it escapes the brunt of many of the utilitarian objections. Moreover, it hardly seems unjust to quarantine persons who knowingly and willingly put others at risk of death. They are not innocent morally and, at the very least, are morally and legally negligent. Finally, the merits of such a quarantine seem obvious: Preventing a noncompliant infectious person from engaging in unsafe activities may very possibly save lives. Let us begin, then, by looking more closely at just what such a quarantine would involve.

The first thing to notice is that the goal of this quarantine proposal is not to end the spread of AIDS, but merely to slow it. Again, [in] most [instances] AIDS is spread by persons who don't know they're infectious, and who therefore are not "noncompliant positives." Despite efforts to discourage *all* unsafe activities through AIDS education, some persons in high-risk groups—especially among the majority who do not know they are infectious—will not give them up.

Moreover, only a small fraction of noncompliant positives would ever actually be considered for quarantine, since in most cases they alone know they are noncompliant positives, and like most people doing terrible things they are not going to facilitate exposure of their own irresponsible behavior. Public health officials typically have no way of knowing of continued participation in high-risk activities by a person known to be positive, since such activities are by and large private, either intrinsically (in the case of sexual activities) and/or because they are illegal. While partners/victims of noncompliant positives will, of course, be aware of the activities, they will typically be unaware of the fact that their partners are positives. And in those rare cases where people learn they have been victimized, they may not step forward to complain or report it. At that point the irreparable harm may already have been done to them. Moreover, they may have their own reasons for wanting to avoid exposure—for instance, the nature, and perhaps the illegality, of the unsafe activities. (Some of the same reasons rape victims have for remaining silent may apply.) Thus, this quarantine proposal could really apply to only relatively few individuals.

Several commentators seem to suggest that since this kind of quarantine would have so little impact on the overall number of AIDS cases, it should not be taken seriously as a public health measure.[12] The idea here seems to be that unless such a quarantine could have an impact on the epidemic in statistical terms, it would be useless. But this surely would be a mistake. We do not regard laws prohibiting murder as useless even though they merely reduce and do not eliminate murders. Even if quarantine wouldn't have much impact in statistical terms, it still might save a few—or a few hundred—lives. And that is surely worth taking seriously.

Next let us consider some of the legal specifics of the proposed quarantine. What, exactly, would it involve legally, and how, if at all, would it differ from legislation already in place in most states? More needs to be said, after all, than that legislation is needed permitting us to lock up people who are noncompliant positives. Specifically two quite different legal models or approaches, civil [and] criminal, might come into play in connection with noncompliant positives, each with its own pros and cons.

The most obvious model is public health law, which, by and large, is civil law. Although there is some variation from state to state, public health regulations typically require physicians (and other health personnel) to report known cases of specified infectious conditions to the state health department or officer, and to see to it that the infected person does nothing that would infect others. (In the words of the Minnesota regulations, for instance, health personnel must "make certain that isolation precautions are taken to prevent the spread of disease to others.") Upon learning that such restrictions are being ignored, the physician may be required to report that fact to the public health officials, who may then turn to the courts to seek an injunction against the individual's continued participation in unsafe activities. The court may then order the least restrictive measures necessary to that end. This would typically involve a court order to refrain from high-risk activities and might also include an order to attend [a course of] instruction in what those activities are, or perhaps an AIDS support group for counseling.[13] If a noncompliant positive disregarded these orders as well, he might be found in contempt of court, at which point his behavior would become a matter for the criminal and not the civil law, and more restrictive measures might then be imposed—a fine or short jail sentence, for instance. (A noncompliant positive prostitute in Florida was given the choice at this point of a jail sentence or "house arrest" requiring her to wear an electronic monitor and to stay within 200 feet of her phone.[14]) Indefinite incarceration, which is, after all, what the proposed quarantine would amount to, would only be invoked as a last resort.

What would be needed *legislatively* to effect an AIDS quarantine of noncompliant positives might be very simple. State public health officials are generally given broad powers to do whatever is necessary—within constitutional limits—to control reportable infectious diseases, so it could be as trivial as adding AIDS to a list of reportable infectious diseases, which already includes other diseases ranging from malaria to leprosy. This was done in November, 1985 in Minnesota, where the state health commissioner may seek injunctive relief against infectious activity under the rubric "public nuisance." Alternatively, new legislation might specify quarantine as a specific option to be instituted only when all lesser remedies have failed. This was the form of legislation Connecticut enacted in 1984, for instance.[15]

Implementing such a quarantine in particular cases, however, would be considerably more difficult, given constitutional protections of certain fundamental interests. Each step of the legal process, from "doctor's orders," to court order[s], to convictions for contempt of court, to indefinite quarantine, is increasingly restrictive. As the restriction of liberty becomes more severe, higher *standards of need* must be met to avoid constitutional problems, such as fourth amendment problems of unreasonable search and seizure and fourteenth amendment problems of deprivation of liberty without due process. Moreover, as the steps move from the civil law to the criminal law, the *standards of evidence* become more strict. Typically in civil cases plaintiffs must prove their cases by "a preponderance of evidence." In criminal cases, however, the state must show that the defendant is guilty "beyond a reasonable doubt." Before a person could be indefinitely incarcerated, as Mary Mallon was in 1915, very high standards indeed would have to be met. Public officials would have to be able to establish "beyond a reasonable doubt" that the person was both seropositive and noncompliant. But each of these would be problematic.

Consider first the fact of an individual's HIV sero-positivity. Already there is a legal "tension" when a state legislates both "reporting laws," which require physicians to report certain medical conditions of their patients, and also "privacy laws," which cover a person's medical records. Again, some states . . . list HIV sero-positivity (along with other sexually transmitted diseases) as [a] reportable condition, and then ignore the spirit (and perhaps even the letter) of their own legislation by providing free anonymous HIV testing at public clinics to encourage members of high-risk groups to find out whether they are infectious. (Without the assurance of anonymity public health officials realize few would come in for such testing.) Personal physicians often feel a greater loyalty to their patient's interests in the confidentiality of their records than to the state's interest in knowing some of what is in them. With other sexually transmitted diseases, private physicians may routinely ignore reporting laws.[16] With AIDS, some physicians have even directed high-risk patients seeking HIV testing to the free public clinics where they can be tested anonymously. Thus, it is unclear how a person's sero-positivity would come to the attention of public health officials, much less be something they could demonstrate "beyond a reasonable doubt."[17]

Even if it could be demonstrated that a suspected noncompliant positive was in fact HIV seropositive, there would still remain the problem of establishing "beyond a reasonable doubt" that the person was persisting in unsafe activity. Only some sexual activities are "unsafe," for instance, and the difference between safe and unsafe activity may be as fine as a condom. The conflict with privacy is painfully obvious if we ask what, exactly, we expect a physician—or investigating public health officials—to do in order to establish that a married hemophiliac is noncompliant by continuing to engage in condom-free intercourse with his wife. In fact, nearly all of the cases of noncompliant positives which have been dealt with in the courts so far have involved prostitutes.

At this point someone might conclude that since public health law is too clumsy to provide an effective basis for the quarantining of any more than a few isolated noncompliant positives, perhaps we should abandon the civil law model as a basis for quarantining such individuals, and see what the criminal law has to offer. Why, one might ask, don't we just enforce existing criminal laws which proscribe high-risk behavior? IV drug abuse is illegal. So, in most cases, is prostitution, and, in some states, sodomy. Why the need for special AIDS quarantine legislation: Don't these criminal laws already on the books provide an alternative mechanism for dealing with noncompliant positives?

In some ways this might be easier—it would certainly be "cleaner," legally. However, in another way this suggestion just helps illustrate the severity of the problems we've been discussing. If anything has been proven by the millions of dollars the government has spent on "the war against drugs," it is that law enforcement agencies are powerless to make a dent in the problem of drug abuse by searching out significant numbers of individual drug abusers and making a case against them in court that is convincing "beyond a reasonable doubt." Similarly no state ever succeeded, although many have tried, in eliminating the "world's oldest profession," prostitution. Again, part of the reason for this is that there is a tension between aggressive enforcement of the criminal law and civil rights, and we as a society have opted to resolve this tension with a "rule of law," which requires very high standards of evidence in criminal cases, and with strict constitutional safeguards of certain fundamental interests. Attempts to eliminate sharing of needles, prostitution, and homosexuality through the criminal law will be no more successful when the motivation is the control of AIDS than they have been when the motivation was moral.

Conclusion

The difficulties with a quarantine of noncompliant positives differ from those of the mass quarantine proposals, but in the final analysis may be almost as grave. The legislation involved in a quarantine of noncompliant positives escapes most of the ethical and constitutional objections which would befall any attempts to legislate mass quarantines. Indeed, legislation which could, in principle, lead to the quarantine of noncompliant positives is already in place as part of the public health law of many states. However, as we have seen, in any particular case the escalating stages of restriction that can be imposed on a recalcitrant positive carry with them increasingly urgent constitutional safeguards and increasingly stiff standards of need and of proof. While it is conceivable that the courts may ultimately feel driven to deal with some few noncompliant positives by ordering their indefinite incarceration and be able to do so in a way that withstands constitutional challenges, this is unlikely to happen in more than a few isolated cases.

We conclude that proposals for the quarantining of large numbers of noncompliant positives are both constitutionally naive and counterproductive to slowing the spread of AIDS. They serve, as almost nothing else can, to increase distrust and breed antagonism between public health officials and members of high-risk groups, who must work together in mutual trust if AIDS research and AIDS education are to proceed.

Notes

1. Judy Foreman, "Mass. Neurosurgeon Suggests Quarantine for AIDS Carriers," *The Boston Globe* (November 21, 1986), p. 30. Quoted in Timothy Murphy, "Quarantines in an Epidemic," a paper presented at a conference at the University of California at San Francisco on *AIDS and Medical Humanities* in May 1986.
2. *The Wall Street Journal* (August 11, 1986), p. 34. An earlier survey reported 25 percent favored quarantining persons with AIDS. (*The Washington Post National Weekly Edition* [December 23, 1985], p. 37.)
3. Murphy, *op. cit.*, p. 3.
4. "The Constitutional Rights of AIDS Carriers," *The Harvard Law Review* 99, No. 6 (April 1986), p. 1282.
5. That is why the federal government, many states, corporations, schools, and other institutions are urging that AIDS patients should not be excluded from schools, public accommodations, or jobs—even food-handling jobs—unless these involve very special circumstances which could put others at risk, such as prostitution, performing surgery, or donating blood, sperm, or organs. Of course, the "best" evidence about how AIDS is spread, like *any* scientific evidence, is not *certain knowledge*. Worst-case scenarios can be fantasized which science cannot ever *disprove*; it is logically possible that the HIV may turn out to be transmitted through casual contact. However, public policy—indeed, even everyday individual rational activity—cannot be predicated on fantasy worst-case scenarios, but must instead be grounded in the best evidence available.
6. Dr. Vernon Mark has also suggested mandatory testing, as a prelude to a quarantine for noncompliant positives (see again Foreman, *op. cit.*, p. 30, footnote 1), and Lyndon LaRouche is on record as favoring a mass testing program (see "LaRouche-Supported Initiative on AIDS Policy in California Spurs Debate on Handling Disease," *The Wall Street Journal, op. cit.*, p. 34).
7. William F. Buckley, "Identify All the Carriers," *The New York Times* (March 18, 1986), p. A27.

8. "Nothing short of compelling necessity can [constitutionally] justify forcing individuals to submit to blood tests that might cause personal anguish [as would be associated with an AIDS test]. Only if a state could show that a mandatory blood test requirement were necessary to advance the public health could it justify such a measure. Yet it is difficult to conceive of a scenario in which the protection of public health would require compulsory AIDS blood tests, as AIDS is not spread by casual contact." "The Constitutional Rights of AIDS Carriers," *op. cit.,* p. 1287.

9. See Tom Wicker, "Push for Drug Testing Strains U.S. Values, for Dubious Success," *St. Paul Pioneer Press and Dispatch* (August 27, 1986), p. 9A.

10. The situation with regard to IV drug users provides an enlightening contrast to that of gays, who have a greater sense of community and political organization and some articulate spokespersons.

11. Allan M. Brandt, *No Magic Bullet: A Social History of Venereal Disease in the United States Since 1880* (New York: Oxford University Press, 1985).

12. Ronald Bayer, "AIDS, Power and Reason," a paper presented at a workshop on *Ethics and Bioethical Problems in Contemporary Society: An Intercontinental Exchange* in Siena, Italy, in June 1986.

13. In this regard see the correspondence between James Chin, chief of the infectious disease section of the Department of Health Services of the State of California, and Sharon Mosely, of the California Office of Legal Services. This correspondence appears as an appendix to Chris D. Nichols, "AIDS—A New Reason to Regulate Homosexuality?" *Journal of Contemporary Law* 11, No. 1 (1984), pp. 340–43.

14. Michael Mills, Constance Wofsy, and John Mills, "Special Report: The Acquired Immunodeficiency Syndrome: Infection Control and Public Health Law," *New England Journal of Medicine* 314, No. 14 (April 3, 1984), p. 934.

15. Alvin Novick, "Quarantine and AIDS," *Connecticut Medicine* 49, No. 2, pp. 81–83.

16. Sharon Rozan and Michael Liebowitz, *Politics of Gonorrhea* (Chicago, 1970).

17. In August 1986 the attorney general of Minnesota indicated he would seek legislation mandating testing for all convicted (male or female) prostitutes, with the understanding that those who test positive will have to undergo AIDS education and agree to refrain from unsafe activities as a condition of parole. *Minneapolis Star and Tribune* (August 26, 1986), p. 2B.

AIDS Testing:
An Insurer's
Viewpoint

DONALD CHAMBERS

While insurance companies are accustomed to making actuarial projections, we have never before been faced with the uncertainties posed by AIDS. At the top of our list of concerns is uncertainty over the magnitude of the seemingly ever-expanding reservoir of people in this country who are infected with the AIDS-causing virus. Even though experts had estimated that 400,000 persons had the virus, estimates now range up to 1 or 2 million persons. Whatever the number now, it is expected to double in the next twelve months, and perhaps continue to increase exponentially for several years to come.

One reason why attention should focus on these virus carriers is that they may be spreading the disease to others. In all probability, most of these people appear to be healthy and therefore unaware that they could, in fact, spread the virus.

There is growing reason to be concerned about the long-term prognosis of those who are infected with the virus. The often mentioned probability figures that "5 percent to 19 percent" of those who have the AIDS antibody will develop AIDS within 2–5 years may well underplay the level of seriousness of the carrier state. Dr. James Curran, of the CDC, was quoted in [the October 1985 issue of] *Atlantic [Monthly]* as stating that "everyone infected with the AIDS virus might at some point within his or her lifetime manifest diseases or disorders—perhaps cancers that have never before been encountered." Dr. Mathilde Krim, head of the AIDS Medical Foundation, said in [the October 1985] issue of *Harper's* magazine that "the percentage of those infected who may develop the full syndrome may be much higher than we think." Dr. Robert

Excerpted from two speeches given by Donald Chambers, M.D. (vice president and chief medical director of the Lincoln National Life Insurance Company): "The Financing of Health Care Costs Associated with Acquired Immune Deficiency Syndrome" (November 1, 1985), a statement presented by the Health Insurance Association of America to the Health Subcommittee on Energy and Commerce; and "AIDS" (Phoenix, Ariz., January 7–14, 1986), panel remarks delivered at the Executive Round Table Meetings. Reprinted by permission of the author.

C. Gallo of the National Cancer Institute was quoted by *USA Today,* in an October 17 article, as saying "many conditions could be associated with this virus; AIDS is just one of the diseases this virus may cause." In that same article, Dr. Curran said AIDS could be just the "tip of the iceberg" of conditions associated with the HTLV-III virus.

It is clear from these statements of experts that, in any analysis of the costs related to AIDS, a consideration must be made of not only AIDS victims themselves, but also present carriers and those at high risk for the disease.

The Cost of Treating AIDS Victims

As the Subcommittee is aware, there seems to be little data reported on the costs of treating AIDS patients. To date, there has been an estimated $1.25 billion of hospital costs incurred by the first 9,000 AIDS victims. According to the Centers for Disease Control, this has resulted in average hospital costs of $140,000 for each AIDS victim. This does not reflect the cost of outpatient visits to physicians and clinics. Not only is $140,000 low for health claims, it does not take into consideration disability and death claims, both of which have a significant impact on the insurance industry. The insurance company which I represent, Lincoln National Life Insurance Company, has identified some 40 group medical expense cases and of the 13 claimants who eventually died, total costs have averaged $60,000.

Insurance companies find it very difficult to compile such data; in many instances, an insurance claims examiner can only assume that a case is an AIDS case, since the word *AIDS* is generally not mentioned. Even on death certificates, it seems that doctors are reluctant to list AIDS as an underlying cause of death.

Despite these limitations, the Health Insurance Association of America is in the process of surveying its member companies to determine the cost of AIDS-related claims. Our AIDS survey will attempt to quantify the impact which AIDS-related health, disability, and death claims have on the insurance industry. In our continuing efforts to be of assistance, the HIAA would, of course, be happy to furnish the Subcommittee with our survey results when they are received.

Inpatient hospital costs are only a part of the overall costs of caring for the AIDS patient. Localities such as San Francisco are at the forefront of efforts to foster the use of home health care and other out-of-hospital, lesser-cost modalities. Insurance companies through large case management programs are exploring attractive alternative care and cost-saving opportunities such as home health care. These trends should be encouraged.

Insurance Implications

Whatever the health care costs are today, we know they will climb rapidly in the next few years, given the rapid rise in cases. At last count, some 160 million Americans under age 65 were covered by some form of group health insurance and millions more by individual health insurance. The health insurance industry is well aware of the liabilities it faces, and we are fully prepared to pay all AIDS-related claims under the terms of our *existing* contracts, just as we pay claims for all other medical conditions.

Mr. Chairman, I want to emphasize that as an industry we do have a fiduciary relationship with our policyholders, meaning among other things that we are pledged to set premium rates at a level that is consistent with the evaluation of risk for that client.

About 85 percent of insureds in this country are covered by group insurance, which is not individually underwritten, since the underwriting process applies to the group as a whole. On the other hand, individual insurance and group insurance for firms with fewer than 10 employees does involve individual underwriting, [that is,] the selection and classification of risk. All relevant health-related information is evaluated by the underwriter and an assessment of risk is made. Applicants are then asked to pay a premium that reflects their level of risk. For those whose risk is very high, no offer can be made.

The underwriting process involves making informed rational distinctions between persons in different risk groups, and in that way we strive to maintain equity. Each applicant is asked to pay his fair share. Low-risk applicants are not asked to subsidize high-risk applicants.

Current state legislative trends threaten to jeopardize the underwriting process by denying insurance companies the right to order and use AIDS antibody test results. California and Wisconsin have enacted laws strictly forbidding insurers from using antibody tests to determine insurability. This violation of sound underwriting *principles* is one to which the industry takes exception, as it marks an unprecedented departure from an insurer's traditional ability to underwrite with access to *all* pertinent medical information. Legislative sanctions of this type simply foster adverse selection—a process by which a disproportionate number of high-risk individuals are given incentive to purchase health insurance, resulting in a severely skewed and unfair subsidization of the high-risk group by the low-risk population. The industry feels it is incumbent upon us as insurers of the population at large to do all we can to detect the minority of applicants who have been infected with the AIDS virus. Testing applicants for the presence of the HTLV-III antibody does indeed provide the underwriter with a reliable tool on which to base his risk assessment.

In contrast, individuals are now being tested for the AIDS antibody when they donate blood or plasma. In addition, with the assistance of federal and state subsidies, individuals are being tested at alternative testing sites on an anonymous basis.

The manner in which blood donees are protected by requiring antibody tests of donors makes it clear that the general population must be protected from the AIDS virus. We are only asking that the same principle continue to be applied in the area of health insurance.

Confidentiality

With respect to the confidentiality of test result data obtained by blood banks, plasma centers, and alternative test sites, the insurance industry understands the necessity of maintaining public confidence in our nation's blood banking system. We want to take this opportunity to reiterate our pledge to not attempt to access this data.

We will also take every precaution to safeguard confidentiality of all AIDS-related information, including antibody test result data. Insurance companies have a long and accomplished track record in dealing with highly sensitive medical information—information dealing with such sensitive matters as chemical dependency, alcoholism, and syphilis. We will protect AIDS-related data in an equally secure fashion. The life and health insurance industry fully supports the model Privacy Protection Act adopted by the National Association of Insurance Commissioners . . . which addresses the consumers' need for confidentiality. . . .

Testing Poses a Dilemma for Insurance Companies

At first glance it seems perfectly obvious that insurance companies need and would elect to do antibody testing. There are a million or more people out there who have been infected and who run a substantial risk of developing serious illness, not to mention the 100,000-plus who have ARC and 8,000 or so with AIDS.

Although most high-risk persons have not been tested, they are keenly aware of their high-risk status and their need for adequate insurance coverage, especially health insurance. There can be no doubt that many of these people are presently applying for additional insurance coverage.

How can we detect HTLV-III carriers? How can we counteract the antiselection that we know is taking place? We can do antibody testing.

But until recently companies have not been rushing to initiate testing. There are several reasons why this is so.

For one thing, there has been a very effective and frankly intimidating offensive waged by gay rights and civil liberty groups who maintain that testing is unfairly discriminatory and that insurers will not be able to assure needed confidentiality of test results. California and then Wisconsin passed laws which prevented insurers from using antibody tests. Although certain measures of the Wisconsin bill have now been overturned, additional states are now threatening to pass similar and even more restrictive legislation.

Another reason for relative inaction by insurance companies revolves around very difficult and interrelated marketing, cost, and legal questions surrounding the matter of who should be tested. Most marketing people would prefer no testing. Underwriters might favor the use of tests in high-risk situations only—[for instance,] young to middle-aged unmarried males living in high-incidence areas of our country. But then lawyers are quick to point out that various state anti-discrimination laws forbid selective testing based on criteria such as sex and marital status. They say that if screening is to be done, then all applicants must be tested.

Companies cannot afford to test everyone, nor do they want to do so. But what kind of limited and affordable testing program can be established that is both legally acceptable and effective? This is a very difficult, if not impossible, question to answer.

These and other factors have prevented most companies from as yet adopting positive and meaningful strategies. . . .

Concluding Thoughts

The first is this. The issue of AIDS and insurance is very complex and highly explosive. It seems that our every move is subject to critical analysis. Each company owes it to itself and to the industry to act in an informed and responsible manner. Those companies that have not yet developed a solid level of expertise in this area are probably well advised to do so just as soon as possible. And I would hope that the ACLI and the HIAA will play an important role in helping companies to help themselves in this regard.

Secondly, I would suggest that the issue of antibody testing is of landmark proportions. If we are denied the right to use HTLV-III antibody and other AIDS-related information, will we then be barred from using still other tests for other diseases? Clearly this sort of movement could severely jeopardize our ability to underwrite all applicants in a fair and equitable manner.

AIDS in the Work Place: The Ethical Ramifications

RONALD BAYER
and GERALD OPPENHEIMER

. . . Living with the presence of AIDS will test the moral fiber of the nation. This is the social challenge of AIDS. Will it be met with compassion or anger? Will those who are ill and/or carry the virus be treated with dignity, or as pariahs, stripped of privacy and the right to function as members of the community? Finally, will reason rule, or will the country be swept along in an hysteria that encourages policies in both the private and public sectors that are cruel and ineffective? How these questions are answered will affect dimensions of social life extending far beyond those immediately touched by AIDS.

Among the most crucial issues to confront is the degree to which those who are sick or infected with the HTLV-III virus will find themselves excluded from employment, the benefits of health insurance protection, or access to life insurance. The problem often has been posed as a scientific, actuarial, or economic one, but it is at base social and moral. For society, the broad policy question at stake is how to guide and limit the decisions of employers and insurers so that equity and the fabric of social life will not fall victim to the alarm and panic that now seem to dominate the public discussion.

Reprinted from *Business and Health* by permission of the Washington Business Group on Health, 229½ Pennsylvania Ave., S.E., Washington, D.C. 20003.

Screening Possibilities, Problems

Although a lot remains to be learned, what is known about AIDS makes inappropriate much of the current discussion of restrictions on those who are ill and those who are carriers. It appears that the virus associated with it is spread through sexual contact, contaminated needles, and blood transfusions. It is not airborne. Close observation of those who are ill and their families has made it clear to virtually every scientist who has studied the disease that casual contact poses no risk to the public. Until a year ago, discussions of the appropriate response to AIDS centered on those who were sick or displayed symptoms of AIDS-related complex, a pattern of disorders that may include a generalized swelling of the lymph nodes and exhaustion but that does not meet the restrictive criteria for AIDS as defined by the CDC. [In March 1985], a test was developed to screen the blood supply by detecting the presence of antibodies to the new HTLV-III virus. Though designed explicitly for the elimination of contaminated donations from the blood system, the test had obvious implications for those who believed it necessary to protect the public from all who carry the AIDS-related virus.

The enzyme-linked immunoabsorbent assay—ELISA for short—detects the presence of antibodies stimulated by HTLV-III viral antigens. The results are scored along a continuum. A reactive result may indicate that the tested blood contains specific antibodies to HTLV-III proteins. The individual is said to be seropositive. This means that he or she has been infected with the HTLV-III virus and has produced an immunological response. At the low end of the reactivity scale, the results are considered borderline and arbitrarily not positive.

The ELISA test is very sensitive; that is, its results correspond very closely to the presence of HTLV-III antibody in AIDS patients. To confirm whether a positive test result is a true positive, a more technically difficult and expensive test called the Western blot can be performed. This costs $65 to $100 vs. $2 to $3 for ELISA. The Western blot test identifies antibodies to proteins of specific molecular weight. Another confirmatory test is the immunofluorescence assay.

When these tests were first developed, it was not known whether the presence of antibodies also indicated the presence of active virus. Many researchers now believe that at least two-thirds of seropositive individuals carry the live virus. All of those who carry the virus are now presumed to be infectious, and may be so for life.

Less than a year since the test was put into use by all blood banks, the worst fears of those who warned how the ELISA test might be used as a mass screening device by employers and insurance companies have been substantiated. Two states, Wisconsin and California, have barred the use of the test for such purposes, but powerful forces are seeking to institute widespread testing. Most significantly, the military decided to initiate antibody screening for all recruits as of . . . October [1985]. The justifications for this move will have implications for both the public and private sectors.

Despite the findings of the CDC that persons who have AIDS as well as those who carry the virus pose no risk to those with whom they work, the military has asserted that the health and well-being of those in the service require rejection of recruits who may develop AIDS. Furthermore, the military has argued that the ultimate medical cost associated with the care of those who develop AIDS justified its decision to exclude individuals who were at increased risk of becoming ill.

If concern about the health of military personnel, as well as fear of the cost of medical care, could serve the largest single employer in the U.S. as a justification for screening all recruits, how long will it be before employers throughout the country with more limited access to scientific data and more limited resources to cover the cost of medical care of their employees rely upon similar arguments? In its place, a more far-reaching decision by the Department of Defense has been announced: to test all active duty personnel and to discharge from the service anyone who admits during screening to drug use or homosexuality. The suspicion of some that AIDS testing represents a clinical device for barring homosexuals from military employment has by this set of decisions been given increasing credibility.

Employment Discrimination Issues

It is difficult to document the extent to which people have lost their jobs or been subject to employment discrimination or harassment as a result of developing AIDS. The Lambda Legal Defense Fund, serving the homosexual community, has documented cases and has undertaken the defense of complainants who have been victims of such acts. In Dade County, Fla., despite the arguments of the local health commissioner, county supervisors seek to promote the screening of all food handlers so that those who are antibody positive could be excluded from jobs. In New York City, some local leaders have called for the mandatory screening of all teachers, health care workers, and barbers in order to prevent the employment of those who carry the HTLV-III virus. There have been similar calls across the country and by some members of Congress.

The legality of discrimination against those who carry the HTLV-III virus or who are sick with AIDS is a complex matter. Until recently, the doctrine of "employment at will" permitted almost unlimited discretion to employers to refuse to hire or fire individuals for any reason or for no reason. Only union contracts and specific legislative provisions limited such plenary authority.

In most states, however, the refusal to hire an individual with a medical condition who is capable of performing a job, or the decision to terminate the employment of such an individual is deemed a violation of laws designed to protect the disabled and handicapped. Forty states forbid such discrimination against private employees; all but three protect disabled public employees. In addition, federal law requires all public agencies and private organizations that receive federal funds to avoid discrimination against the handicapped. Even so, the law regarding those with AIDS or those who carry the virus is extremely vague at this point.

Whatever the ambiguity of the law, it is possible to define the ethical standards that ought to be used in judging acts of discrimination [in] matters involving AIDS. Those standards can draw upon the evolution of legal prescriptions that protect women and racial minorities against discriminatory practices in the work place. Under the doctrine of bona fide occupational qualification, an employer may exclude individuals from jobs only if they fail to possess the skills to perform the required assignments. The assumption, for instance, that all women are incapable of performing certain heavy labor tasks cannot be accepted. Only when a class as a whole is by definition incapable of performing certain functions may it be systematically excluded. For example, discriminating against women in jobs for male locker room attendants would not be deemed a violation of civil rights law. This very high legal standard, which requires that firms practicing discrimination bear the burden of proof, could provide a moral yardstick against which to judge employment discrimination against those with AIDS as well as those who carry the antibody to HTLV-III.

What morally acceptable grounds would there be for an employer to refuse to hire someone with AIDS or AIDS-related complex? All scientific evidence indicates that fellow workers are not at risk from exposure to individuals who are sick, nor are members of the public who might be brought into contact with a worker with AIDS. So arguments based on the need to protect coworkers and the public have no rational justification. On the other hand, those who are sick may, in fact, be unable to perform certain duties or may pose undue hardships to a company because of prospects of repeated illness and related absences. An employer could reasonably determine on a case-by-case basis that a particular individual ought not be hired for reasons such as these.

The situation is different for those already employed who then become sick. Here the moral question posed for employers is whether they have an obligation to continue the employment of individuals whose capacities and work record are affected by AIDS. Generosity and decency could well dictate one response; narrow financial and efficiency-oriented calculations another. But two points need to be underscored. First, the status of having AIDS is in itself not grounds for dismissal; only the work-related consequences of AIDS provide such grounds. More important, there is no justification for adopting a more restrictive policy for those who have AIDS than exists for those with other illnesses, for example, cancer.

Whatever the complexities of the issues surrounding those diagnosed as having AIDS or AIDS-related complex, the situation is very different for those who carry the virus but are asymptomatic. They are infectious but pose no risk to others unless they engage in sexual activities, share needles with them, or donate blood. Since they are asymptomatic and may indeed never become ill, there can be no performance-related justification for refusing to hire or for firing such individuals.

Is there, then, no identifiable employer interest that could provide at least a preliminary argument for seeking to exclude, as a class, those who are antibody positive or who are sick with AIDS? Here the potential cost of health care for those who are ill or who may become ill emerges as a critical issue. Indeed, this matter has surfaced with increasing frequency. Leon Warshaw, the executive director of the New York Business Group on Health, has noted a sharp increase in inquiries about AIDS and medical costs. "Employers want to know if their health coverage costs will rise, and [if they] can . . . set up screening barriers to employment," Warshaw noted.

Concern about the potential cost of care was an essential element in the justification provided by the military for its planned screening program. And [in] June [1985], Hollywood, Fla., solicited bids for the screening of all municipal employees, in part because of a desire to protect the city's benefit plan from the "astronomical expenses" incurred by AIDS patients. A public outcry ultimately forced Hollywood to withdraw its proposal, but the effort is indicative of a level of concern throughout the country among public and private sector employers who often bear the full cost of health care of their workers.

What Is Justifiable?

That such fears have been articulated does not mean that the related concerns are empirically justifiable. Nor does it mean that there is a moral justification for implementing discriminatory employment practices. On empirical grounds, it would be necessary to determine the overall impact of the medical expenses for an employee with AIDS for a given health plan. Such a determination would require: better data than are now available on the actual cost of care associated with AIDS as well as AIDS-related complex; a much better diagnostic tool for determining who among those who are antibody positive will develop AIDS; and some assumptions about the number of individuals employed who might become ill. With so many factors still uncertain, the formulation of policy centered on the cost to employers for the health care of those who might develop AIDS must be highly conjectural.

But more is at stake. Americans have decided that protection against the cost of health care expenditures will be available primarily through employment-based health insurance. Can the U.S. as a matter of social policy and equity permit the exclusion from employment of those who might incur extraordinarily high health care expenditures? To do so would have the doubly troubling consequence of denying not only health care protection, but also the right to gainful employment. Can a disease like AIDS provide the moral justification for creating a dependent class, one that is barred from private and public sector employment and forced upon a welfare system?

Finally, will antibody testing serve as a clinical subterfuge for social screening? Epidemiologically, AIDS in the U.S. currently occurs predominantly among homosexual and bisexual men and intravenous drug users. Specifically, 61 percent are homosexual or bisexual with no concomitant intravenous drug use; 12 percent are both homosexual or bisexual and intravenous drug users; and 17 percent are heterosexual intravenous drug users. In a society that only recently has begun to extend a modicum of equal treatment to homosexuals, within which legal protections against employment discrimination for such individuals is rudimentary at best and where discrimination because of sexual orientation is still a matter of practice, it is not unreasonable to expect that antibody tests will be used to provide a clinical justification for an antihomosexual bias. That the existence of AIDS has with increasing frequency been used as an excuse for the reinstitution of sodomy statutes, as in Texas, should be alarming.

For these reasons, screening in the private sector poses a grave risk to those who are socially vulnerable, a risk that is not balanced by benefits to society in general nor to those who might be brought into contact with carriers of the HTLV-III virus. Indeed, the only consequences that could follow from the implementation of screening programs in the work place are those harmful to the goal of preserving compassion, equity, and reason during the AIDS epidemic.

Health Insurance Concerns

The AIDS issue is an open one for the insurance industry, too. Most telling in this regard is a paper prepared by a task force of insurance company medical directors for the American Council of Life Insurance and the Health Insurance Association of America. Though not yet adopted as an official statement, the report represents a critical commentary reflecting the industry's concerns. Proceeding from the assumption that AIDS may entail outlays of billions of dollars to cover medical expenses, loss of time, and death benefits, the task force warned of the potential effect upon an industry that has not allocated reserves for such a purpose. How severe the impact might be would depend, the report noted, on "how effectively applicants can be underwritten in the upcoming months and years."

According to the task force, only the appropriate use of the ELISA test could prevent an untoward outcome. Prohibiting the use of the ELISA test, the insurance group contended, would allow those who know themselves to be at risk to purchase insurance under conditions that would be harmful to the industry and that would be unacceptable from the point of view of equity.

Among the most troubling features surrounding AIDS for the health insurance industry is the confusion that characterizes the estimated cost of caring for each diagnosed case, with figures ranging from $25,000 to $140,000. The industry and those that regulate it will have to chart a course in the face of actuarial ambiguity.

To date, health insurers appear to have met their legal obligations to reimburse the contracted medical expenses of AIDS patients. However, payments have not been made when there has been a clear indication that AIDS was a preexisting condition, that is, one that was known to exist because of diagnosis or symptomology prior to obtaining insurance.

But what is a preexisting condition in the case of AIDS? Is a positive finding on the HTLV-III antibody test a preexisting condition? Is AIDS-related complex a preexisting condition for AIDS? Should these health states prevent affected individuals from gaining health insurance? Should their premiums be higher as a consequence? These matters have not yet been resolved.

Although the question of exclusion on the basis of preexisting conditions is of critical importance to the insurance industry, for most persons covered by group health insurance, particularly experience-rated groups, the preexisting condition clause is usually waived. Nevertheless, because the presence of those with AIDS in an insured group could affect its premium determination, employers might well consider the use of a preemployment screening mechanism to reduce such a prospect. The preexisting condition exclusion can affect individuals who directly purchase insurance on their own.

For those patients with AIDS who are covered by private health insurance, many problems remain. The treatment costs may exceed the maximum per hospitalization or lifetime benefits. Experimental drugs and procedures (and in the case of AIDS, much of the clinical approach may entail novel efforts) are not reimbursed by most insurance carriers. Out-of-hospital treatment including hospice care may not be paid in full.

Though private health insurers do not currently know the magnitude of the costs they will face in the future, they are trying to reduce their vulnerability by cautiously proposing the use of the HTLV-III antibody test as a required screening measure for all individual applicants seeking to purchase health insurance. In Wisconsin and California, where the state legislatures have mandated that the test results not be used as a condition of employment or insurability, carriers have threatened to exclude AIDS from coverage.

In eight states—Minnesota, Connecticut, Indiana, Florida, North Dakota, Montana, Wisconsin, and Nebraska—pools have been created to guarantee coverage to people whose initial applications for health insurance are refused because of risk factors or health conditions. Twenty other states are considering similar legislation. Premiums under such pooling arrangements vary, but they average about 150 percent of the median insurance rates. In six states with insurance pools, there is a six-month preexisting condition clause. Indiana and Nebraska have provided an option of coverage without such exclusion for an increase of 10 percent in the premium charged.

Before health insurance carriers can ask about AIDS on their application forms or require antibody testing, they will have to receive permission to do so from the relevant regulatory agencies in states where they sell policies. The uncertain predictive value of the HTLV-III antibody test, as well as political exigencies, may limit the number of states that allow such screening. In New York, for example, the state insurance department has held that "there is no test established that is a valid identifier of AIDS," though "if a test is developed that proves a person will get AIDS, that could be used to limit the person's insurance coverage."

The issue of antibody testing is both scientific and political. A decision about whether and how insurance companies could use such tests inevitably will be made under conditions where the narrower interests of carriers will be but one factor. Overriding social concerns about equity and the creation of a class of uninsured individuals dependent upon the welfare system could well prove determinative. From a societal perspective, the central issue is whether the costs of health care will be socialized and broadly distributed or borne by those who may become ill and by the welfare system. Were there a system of national health insurance, such a question would, of course, never arise.

Assumptions for
Life Insurance

The situation surrounding life insurance is a more complex matter. While assured access to health care is a broadly shared concern with strong popular as well as moral foundations, the right to life insurance has no such support. Indeed, those at especially high risk have always had difficulty in purchasing life insurance or have been confronted with premiums that for most would be considered prohibitive.

The life insurance industry fears that individuals, believing they are at increased hazard for AIDS because they know they are members of risk groups or are sero-positive, might seek to insure themselves at very high levels. Among the life insurance companies that have argued openly for the right to raise questions about indicators for AIDS have been Northwestern Mutual Life Insurance Company of Milwaukee (Wisc.) and the Lincoln (Neb.) National Corporation, both of which have sought permission from state insurance regulators to make such inquiries. Donald Chambers, medical director of Lincoln National, has made the claim most clearly: "It is immensely important to be able to use tools that are as accurate as possible when determining insurability. Unfortunately, if we are not allowed, for example, to use the antibody testing, we may be forced to make certain assumptions that we'd rather not make."

One such assumption is that all homosexuals or those suspected of being homosexual be treated as if they were antibody positive. As a result, some underwriters have suggested that applications from all unmarried men of a certain age, living in certain cities or in specific neighborhoods, be carefully scrutinized.

In some instances, insurers have asserted that those who are antibody positive will be declared uninsurable. Others have claimed that the antibody test or other risk factors will be used in determining actuarially appropriate premiums. Despite the position of Lincoln National, Mutual Life Insurance Company of Milwaukee, and the insurance industry's task force report, many large insurers have not announced plans for antibody screening.

As life insurance carriers seek to develop policies from their vantage point, private perspectives are forced to confront broader concerns about the social functions of life insurance in the U.S. as well as the demonstrable public interest in the norms that ought to govern the insurance industry. Underwriting rules should not be applied to exclude an entire class of applicants (unmarried men of a certain age), nor be used to reinforce stereotypes (only unmarried men have male sexual partners, or all homosexual men are promiscuous). Steven Rish, vice president for life and health operations of the Nationwide Insurance Company, articulated a corporate perspective when he asserted, "Insurance companies are businesses; they are not a social system." Precisely because this is the case, insurance companies, alone, cannot be permitted to set the terms under which coverage will be made available.

In the debates over unisex insurance rates and in the decision to eliminate gender-based calculations from retirement plans, overriding social considerations have been used to limit the implications of actuarial science. Such should be the case with life insurance protection for those at risk for AIDS. Should insurers be permitted to deny coverage to all those suspected of being homosexual or those whose antibody status suggests they are at increased risk for AIDS? Should insurers be permitted to set premiums at a level that would place life insurance protection out of reach because of cost? Should the pooling arrangements now available in some states for health insurance be used to socialize the burden of life insurance protection? These are matters that require broad public discussion—a discussion in which the principle of equity ought to be given a central role.

In the end, AIDS represents a fundamental challenge to American society. How it is met will not only tell a great deal about our society, but also about what kind of society it will become during the next trying years.

AIDS, Gay Men, and the Insurance Industry

RICHARD D. MOHR

Wisconsin, California, and the District of Columbia have barred insurance companies from using tests for the AIDS antibody to screen applicants for health and life insurance policies. At the urging of gay activists, Governor Cuomo has introduced such legislation in the New York assembly. Are such laws warranted and just? Though the relevant issues have been misunderstood on both sides, governments can legitimately and should bar insurance companies from using the AIDS antibody test.

The gay side tries to play down the ability of the test to predict the likelihood that someone will come down with AIDS. And as long as one sticks just to the individual this is true; after all, not everyone who smokes heavily will come down with lung cancer or die of heart disease. But the individual case is irrelevant to the determination of actuarial tables for insurance purposes. What is relevant is statistical probabilities *over groups*. And there is no denying that people who have the AIDS antibody revealed by the test are much more likely to come down with AIDS than those for whom the test is negative, just as smokers are much more likely to come down with lung cancer than nonsmokers. That one cannot say which individual smoker or which antibody carrier will become ill is irrelevant to the determination of insurance rates.

The insurance industry, however, is equally misguided. It claims that banning the use of the antibody test is unfair because the rates of the majority of people will go up even though they are not at risk for AIDS. It is true that rates will go up, but this does not establish that the government policy is unfair.

To establish that the law is unfair, the insurance industry would have to show that this rate increase will violate some right or legitimate claim of its clients. And this it

From *Gay Community News,* 62 Berkeley Street, Boston, Mass. 02116 (September 21–27, 1986), p. 5.

cannot do. While it is nice if costs, like taxes or the price of milk, are lower as the result of some government policy, no one's rights have been violated if some legitimate government purpose has the effect of raising taxes or the price of milk. Similarly, though it may irk the majority (and the insurance industry is counting on this), simply raising the price of insurance does not violate anyone's rights.

To make the point concretely, does an individual policyholder have a legitimate complaint against this insurance company if the insurance company has not pursued a policy of trying to screen out every imaginable risk group for every imaginable disease that might raise insurance rates? The answer is obviously not.

My rights against my insurance company have not been violated if it fails to ask women whether they have had multiple sex partners and thus have put themselves at increased risk for fatal cervical cancer. There is nothing wrong therefore—no rights are violated—if the government, for some legitimate reason, freezes insurance companies from asking that question. And it does have such a legitimate reason: to protect privacy. So too, then, if the government freezes the industry from asking after a person's antibody status, no individual policyholder's rights have been violated. And the government does have a legitimate reason to do so: to help raise gay people out of their refugee status, a status that has been aggravated by the AIDS crisis.

Insurance companies come to the AIDS crisis with dirty hands. Traditionally, they have as a matter of policy discriminated against gay people in issuing policies and in employment opportunities, and in practice they have done so especially effectively—because they snoop. They make their money from the statistical norm, and so they suppose that is also the moral norm. They mistakenly think they are promoting something normal, something American, when they have discriminated against gays. It is therefore especially appropriate—a matter of compensatory justice—that the insurance industry should shoulder some of the burden in the move toward social justice for gays.

Why Mandatory Screening for AIDS Is a Very Bad Idea

KENNETH R. HOWE

The initial hysteria about AIDS has diminished somewhat, as the means of transmission have become better understood and as the risk of contracting the disease has become associated with well-defined populations, such as male homosexuals, intravenous drug users, and hemophiliacs. At the same time, however, another threat from AIDS has grown—the prospect of the widespread use of mandatory screening, motivated by desires to protect the public health and the private interests of insurance companies and employers.

Five bills were introduced in Michigan legislative committees—one would permit screening by insurance companies and one would mandate screening as a condition of receiving a marriage license. In New York City, calls have been made for mandatory screening of teachers, health care workers, and barbers. The American Council of Life Insurance and the Health Insurance Corporation of America have assembled a task force on how to respond to the impact of AIDS on the insurance industry, working on the assumption that outlays might be in the billions. In October 1985 the military instituted a program to screen all recruits and active duty personnel. Recruits who test positive are rejected. Active duty personnel who test positive are restricted in duty; those who confess to homosexuality or drug use are discharged. Finally, in mid-1986 a LaRouche-backed initiative, "Proposition 64," calling for mass screening of the general population, garnered enough signatures to appear on the ballot in California.

If screening could identify all and only individuals who would develop AIDS or

Reprinted by permission of the author.

could transmit the AIDS virus, it would remain to be shown that (probably coercive) mandatory screening to detect all cases could be justified. This question can in general be avoided, however, by focusing on the fact that AIDS screening is riddled with error, which has important consequences. On the one hand, error results in falsely identifying individuals as having AIDS or being carriers (false positives), prompting anxiety about AIDS when the danger is not real and creating the potential for extending the undesirable consequences already suffered by AIDS patients to a larger segment of the population. On the other hand, error also results in falsely classifying individuals as not having AIDS or not being carriers (false negatives), creating a false sense of security and possibly contributing to the spread of the disease. In the context of screening donated blood, false positive donations are mistakenly discarded whereas false negatives contaminate the blood supply.

Although ethicists[1] and medical researchers[2] have . . . raised the problem of error in AIDS screening, ethical and technical considerations have not been combined to the extent that they should be. Not surprisingly, ethicists focus on the problem of balancing the rights of individuals against other private and public goods, whereas individuals schooled in the statistical properties of laboratory tests confine themselves to more-or-less ethically neutral technical reports. By showing how technical difficulties should stop mandatory screening from ever getting off the ground, some of the more troubling outcomes of diagnosed AIDS (encroachments on privacy, threats of quarantine, unwarranted exclusions from school or work, and so forth) can be avoided on a larger scale.

Statistical Properties of AIDS Screening Tests

Three tests, the enzyme-linked immunoabsorbent assay (ELISA), the Western blot, and the immunofluorescence assay (IFA), are currently used to detect antibodies associated with the AIDS virus. (The importance of the fact that the tests are not designed to screen for the virus itself, let alone the disease, will be discussed later.) The precise nature of these tests aside, what is important for present purposes is how they perform in terms of five statistical properties: precision, accuracy, sensitivity, specificity, and predictive value.

Precision.   The precision of a test is the degree to which it gives consistent or replicable results. Sources of imprecision include things such as procedures, materials, equipment, and individual laboratory technicians' interpretations. Precision may be measured by running a given test repeatedly and then calculating the variability of results—the lower the variability, the greater the precision.

Though always to be taken into consideration, imprecision seems not to present any especially severe problems for AIDS testing. Unclear results, which are fairly common, can usually be handled by simply rerunning the test in question. ELISA tests which are initially positive are routinely run a second time by the Red Cross.

Accuracy. Whereas test precision pertains to the consistency of results, accuracy pertains to what test results mean, [that is], what a test detects. Tests can be precise but consistently measure the wrong thing; and this is where AIDS screening becomes problematic. "AIDS screening" is actually a misnomer because none of the three tests detects either the AIDS virus or AIDS; they detect antibodies associated with the virus. The presence of the antibodies is taken to be a highly reliable indicator of the presence of the virus, which, in turn, is taken to be a highly reliable indicator of infectiousness. Extending this chain of inferences to AIDS itself is much more tenuous: Only an estimated 10 percent of individuals infected with the AIDS virus will ever develop the disease.[3] Thus, if the tests in question were otherwise error-free, a (true) positive test would entail only a 10 percent chance that AIDS would eventually be manifested.

Sensitivity and Specificity. The sensitivity of a test is the degree to which it yields positive results when the property of interest is present; the specificity of a test is the degree to which a test yields negative results when the property of interest is absent. More formally, the sensitivity of a test relative to a property, A, is the probability of a positive result *given* A; the specificity of a test relative to A is the probability of a negative result *given* not-A.

In general, the sensitivity and specificity of a given test are inversely related, depending on what test value serves as the cut point between positive and negative results. A certain set of values is unavoidably shared by the class of interest and its complement, due to both biologic variation and imprecision. With the ELISA test, for instance, as the cut point value is decreased, a greater percentage of positives are yielded. As a result, the test becomes more sensitive because it will label as positive samples that have the antibodies for the AIDS virus within the overlapping area of values. At the same time, however, the test becomes less specific because it will also label as positive samples within the area of overlap that fail to have the antibody, reducing the test's ability to correctly identify negatives.

Given this relationship between sensitivity and specificity, a choice has to be made regarding whether it is more important to emphasize sensitivity (and accept an increase in false positives) or specificity (and accept an increase in false negatives). The ELISA test (the most frequent first-used test) tilts toward specificity. On the other hand, and although the claims have been disputed,[4] a recent relatively large sample study[5] indicates that the ELISA test is also highly sensitive. According to the study, the three licensed tests [ELISA, Western blot, and IFA] have respective sensitivities and specificities of 93.4 percent and 99.8 percent, 99.6 percent and 99.2 percent, and 98.9 percent and 99.6 percent. The evidence suggests that, relative to laboratory tests in general, the ELISA has very good sensitivity and specificity.

Predictive Value. Sensitivities and specificities are established by knowing or assuming that the property tested for is present or not present. For instance, to say that the ELISA is 95 percent sensitive is to say that 95 percent of tests will be positive *given* that each individual tested has the antibody for the AIDS virus; to say it is 99 percent specific is to say that 99 percent of tests will be negative *given* that no individuals tested have the antibody for the AIDS virus. It is exceedingly important to recognize that the assumption (or knowledge) about the presence or absence of AIDS antibody in connection with sensitivity and specificity does not apply in either the screening or diagnostic context. Indeed, the status of the individual tested is precisely what needs to be determined.

This leads to the concept of predictive value, in which the relationship between what is assumed or known and what is to be determined is just the reverse of what it is for the concepts of sensitivity and specificity. The predictive value of a positive test is the probability that the property is present *given* a positive test; the predictive value of a negative test is the probability that the property is not present *given* a negative test. As a consequence of Bayes' Theorem, predictive values can be determined given the following information: The sensitivity and specificity of the test in question and the prevalence of the property of interest in the population tested ([or], in the case of the AIDS virus, the proportion of the population that has the antibody).

Predictive values are frequently confused with sensitivities and specificities, and this is a serious mistake. Prevalence is an extremely important component of predictive value and can overwhelm high sensitivity or specificity. The problem may be illustrated by imagining a fisherman who fishes a local bay for heavenly fish, which are numerous in the bay and very large. The fisherman has developed a highly "sensitive" and "specific" net by constructing it in such a way that it will capture almost all of the heavenly fish and allow almost all of the smaller and not very numerous junk fish to pass through the mesh. His net does not work perfectly because it sometimes gets tangled and because there is an overlap in size between unusually small heavenly fish and unusually large junk fish. Suppose one day this fisherman ventures out into the ocean where there are very few heavenly fish and very many junk fish. Although from among the fish that enter his net he will still capture the same high percentage of heavenly fish and the same low percentage of junk fish, he will capture a high percentage of very few heavenly fish and a low percentage of very many junk fish. Overall, and much to his dismay, he will net a much larger proportion of junk fish to heavenly fish than he had in the bay.

Precisely the same problem that the fisherman encountered by venturing out of his bay arises when the ELISA test, with its touted sensitivity and specificity, is applied to a group in which the prevalence of the AIDS antibody is low. For example, the Michigan Department of Public Health estimates that the prevalence of the AIDS virus in the population that excludes high-risk groups is .00001. Assume the ELISA is 98 percent sensitive and 99.5 percent specific and is used on this population. Under these assumptions, the ELISA has only 1 in 100,000 chances to be correctly positive, whereas it has 99,999 in 100,000 chances to go wrong—the result is that a whopping 99.8 percent of positives will be falsely positive.

The proportion of false positives can be substantially reduced by using the Western blot, the IFA, or both to confirm the results from the ELISA. (The ELISA–Western blot sequence is by far the most common procedure.) But just how much of a reduction can be obtained is uncertain because no "gold standard" exists that would permit the three tests to be independently validated.

With this brief overview of technical issues in hand, the advisability of AIDS screening with respect to its two general defenses, protecting the public health and protecting private interests, may now be evaluated.

Screening to Protect the Public Health

AIDS screening to protect the public health involves different considerations, depending on whether the population to be tested is high risk ([that is], has a high prevalence of the AIDS virus) or is low risk ([that is], has a low prevalence of the AIDS virus).

In the case of high-risk individuals, such as homosexual males and intravenous drug users, the predictive value of positive results will be much better than it is for the general population because of the relatively high prevalence of AIDS infections within these populations. (It should be observed that the predictive value of negative results will be adversely affected, [that is], high prevalence entails more false negatives.) Even so, a serious question arises regarding screening unwilling individuals. No one (I hope) would advocate hunting down such individuals and dragging them into testing facilities. If the aim is to protect these individuals' health, prevention through education about the practices that increase risk is likely to be the most effective strategy. Because no effective treatment for AIDS exists, testing individuals so that they might be cured and become noninfectious does not apply, and, for the same reason, the practice of contact tracing, associated with treatable infectious diseases, will not have its usual justification. Finally, it is unlikely that testing information would be of much value to the individuals themselves. Homosexual males, for instance, have a 10 percent chance of being infected prior to any testing, and the risk increases (statistically and in fact) in proportion to the number of sexual contacts. Knowledge about this risk should be sufficient (and apparently has been[6]) to motivate individuals who are so disposed to take necessary precautions. Moreover, the same advice would be given—avoid risky practices—no matter what the results of testing.

To examine the issue of AIDS screening for low-risk populations, consider the Michigan proposal to require screening as a condition of being granted a marriage license. Unlike the special problem posed by groups such as male homosexuals and drug users, applicants for marriage licenses constitute a captive population that is already required to undergo various medical tests.

As the risk (prevalence) of AIDS decreases for a group, so does the trustworthiness of positive test results. For example, if the ELISA is assumed to be 98 percent sensitive and 99.5 percent specific, it alone is used, and if the prevalence is assumed to be .0025 (the estimated prevalence for Michigan of combining low- and high-risk populations), then 70 percent of positive results will be false positives; if the ELISA alone is used and the low-risk prevalence of .00001 is assumed (a reasonable assumption for the marrying population), then 99.8 percent of positive results will be false positives. Since the percentage of false positives is unacceptable no matter which assumption is made about prevalence, confirmation by the Western blot is indicated.

Assume that the Western blot is conditionally independent of the ELISA ([that is], its errors are different from the ELISA's), its sensitivity is 90 percent, and its specificity is 99.9 percent (these are optimistic assumptions). Assume also that 140,000 individuals (the approximate number who marry each year in Michigan) are screened using the ELISA, that all positive ELISA results are confirmed with the Western blot, and that the prevalence is .0025 (the result of combining the high- and low-risk groups in Michigan). Given these assumptions, the expected result would be: 309 true positives, 1 false positive, 41 false negatives, and 139,649 true negatives. This looks like a dramatic improvement over the ELISA alone. However, it is reasonable to assume that the prevalence in the marrying population is likely to be much closer to that of the low-risk population (.00001). When this prevalence is assumed, the following results obtain: 1 true positive, 1 false positive, 139,998 true negatives, and 0 false negatives.

On the assumption they are at low risk, screening marriage license applicants is folly; at $10 per ELISA (what the American Red Cross of Michigan pays) and $65–100 per Western blot,[7] it would cost from $1.45 to $1.47 million to identify one individual at only a 10 percent risk of developing AIDS and at some unknown but lesser risk for passing it on to his or her spouse and offspring.

Assume, for the sake of argument, that Michigan's marrying population's risk is that of the combined high- and low-risk groups. This makes the question harder, but screening would still appear unjustified. First, it would cost from $1.47 to $1.5 million (using the above prices for the ELISA and the Western blot). Counseling individuals who initially test positive on the ELISA, at $50 each, would add an additional $50,000. It would seem that the overall public health could be more greatly improved by allocating resources in other ways. Furthermore, mandatory screening, by its nature, is ethically problematic, and the defenses that may sometimes justify it do not apply to AIDS screening. Because the individuals identified could not themselves be helped or rendered noninfectious, the public health argument would have to be that testing individuals about to be married and informing them of positive results could help halt the spread of AIDS by preventing the birth of infected babies. But, unless coercive measures were used to prevent procreation, the desired result would obtain only if infected individuals voluntarily decided not to marry or not to have children. Thus, AIDS screening for marriage licenses more closely resembles genetic screening than, say, screening for venereal diseases. Mandatory genetic screening is eschewed on the grounds that it involves too much uncertainty and poses too great a threat to privacy and autonomy relative to its expected benefit; mandatory screening for AIDS faces the same difficulty. The question is not whether it might have *some* beneficial effects, but whether, on balance, the beneficial effects outweigh the harmful ones.

It will be useful to compare the example of mandatory screening for marriage licenses with mandatory screening of donated blood. Both involve general populations, and the fact that screening donated blood is generally believed to be justifiable may be taken as an obvious counterexample to the arguments so far advanced against mandatory screening of general populations.

In purely utilitarian terms, screening donated blood seems little more justified than screening as a condition of being granted a marriage license. Transfusion-related AIDS, though documented, is rare, even prior to the implementation of blood screening. Thus, one could plausibly argue that the costs associated with ELISA screening, in dollars and in the fear and possible breaches of confidentiality for individuals who test positive, far outweigh the benefits to the public health. This argument, I believe, deserves to be taken seriously, especially in light of the facts that some false negatives will inevitably slip through the screen (the blood supply cannot be rendered *completely* safe) and that over 90 percent of positives will be false positives (nine out of ten pints of blood that are discarded will be mistakes). On the other hand, there are at least three considerations that render screening donated blood considerably more defensible than screening for marriage licenses.

These considerations involve the individuals to be tested, the individuals who handle donated blood, and the attitudes of the public at large. First, individuals have a much greater claim against government and other authorities regarding noninterference in marriage and childbearing than regarding the practice of donating blood. Opting out of donating blood to avoid screening has a much less profound effect on individuals' lives than opting out of getting married to avoid screening. Second, Red Cross workers and public health authorities, understandably, do not want to be vehicles for the transmission of the AIDS virus. Although rare, infection with AIDS via contaminated blood does occur. Unlike the case of mandatory screening for marriage, in which certain behaviors on the part of others are required to spread the infection, contaminated blood directly puts those who collect, distribute, and infuse it in the uncomfortable position of spreading the AIDS virus. Finally, given the persistence of tremendous public fears and misunderstandings, screening seems required to instill public confidence in the safety of the blood supply. No similar benefits would follow from intruding on individuals' marriage plans.

Screening to Protect Private Interests

Unlike screening to protect the public health, screening to protect private interests is motivated from private self-interest. Employers and insurers fear they will be required to absorb exorbitant costs in connection with AIDS victims, and there are signs they are beginning to assert their purported right to screen for AIDS in order to protect themselves against the projected costs.[8]

Because the motivation is self-interest, employers and insurers are likely to want to use the ELISA alone as a marker for high risk. At first sight, it may appear that this is similar to rating or excluding smokers, pilots, scuba divers, and so forth. However, because the false positives exceed the true positives by a significant margin, the *actual* source of risk, the AIDS virus, is unlikely to be present even given positive test results. This sort of high-risk rating for AIDS is like giving a nonsmoker whose parents smoke a high-risk rating because an individual's smoking habits are associated with his or her parents' smoking habits. Such rating schemes are clearly inequitable, and insurers and employers should not, in the name of their private interests, be allowed to affront justice in any way they see fit. To avoid this intolerable degree of injustice, then, employers and insurers would have to be required to perform confirmatory testing.

Again, the outcome of AIDS screening depends on the tests used and the prevalence of the AIDS virus in the population tested. As it turns out, in some situations AIDS screening may not even serve private financial interests. Consider the issue of health insurance. (Similar considerations apply to life insurance underwriters and to employers who must pay insurance premiums and accommodate lost work time.)

Screening 140,000 low-risk individuals with the ELISA alone (and making all the other assumptions associated with the parallel example in connection with screening for marriage licenses in Michigan) would cost at least $1.4 million and would detect at most one case of incipient AIDS. Using the Western blot as [a] confirmatory [measure] would increase the costs of screening by $46,000 to $70,000. Since the cost of treating one case of AIDS ranges from $25,000 to $140,000,[9] it would cost a health insurer considerably more to conduct a screening program than to pay for the expected medical costs associated with foregoing such a program.

If the prevalence is assumed to be that which results from combining the low-risk and high-risk Michigan populations, then the ELISA screening costs will remain the same at $1.4 million, and an additional $68,000 to $104,000 in costs would be incurred if ELISA positives were confirmed by the Western blot. From $100,000 to $560,000 would also be added, the expected treatment costs for the four AIDS cases that would result from 41 false negatives. The total cost of screening 140,000 individuals using the ELISA–Western blot sequence, where the prevalence equals .0025, would be $1.67 to $2.06 million. Without such a screening program, 309 infections would be expected, of which 10 percent, or 31, could be expected to develop into full-blown cases of AIDS. The cost of treating 31 AIDS patients ranges from $775,000 to $4.3 million.

As these scenarios suggest, whether it would be in the financial interests of health insurers to conduct AIDS screening turns importantly on the population tested and the costs of treating AIDS patients, and precise figures would be required to make this judgment in individual cases. But even when private interests can reap financial benefits from mandatory AIDS screening, the practice remains unjustified. The ultimate results would only be higher overall costs and cost shifting. Unless AIDS patients are abandoned, the money for their care will have to come from somewhere. Because AIDS screening could not be used to detect AIDS at some early, treatable stage, and thus reduce health care costs, its only use would be to exclude those at risk from private insurance or employment. This simply shifts the burden from the private to the public sector, and generates the additional, sizable cost of screening (which, no doubt, would be absorbed by policyholders). It is perfectly legitimate for government to override private interests when such interests clearly conflict with equity and the public welfare. Protection of the environment, the work place, and civil rights, as well as unisex life insurance benefits, . . . presumes that private interests are not to be left totally immune from government interference. Finally, regarding the fair treatment of insurance companies themselves, a ban on AIDS screening puts no insurance company at a competitive disadvantage, since all companies would be prevented from obtaining the information needed to exclude or rate individuals who tested positive for the AIDS antibody.[10]

Conclusion

Mandatory AIDS screening is a very bad idea. From a technical perspective, it is a wholly ineffective and inefficient means of protecting the public health.[11] From a more purely ethical perspective, it unnecessarily threatens the privacy and autonomy of high- and low-risk individuals alike and, because of the uses to which it would be put by private interests, offends any well-developed conception of justice.[12]

Notes

1. See Carol Levine and Ronald Bayer, "Screening Blood: Public Health and Medical Uncertainty," *The Hastings Center Report* (August 1985), pp. 8–11; and Ronald Bayer and Gerald Oppenheimer, "AIDS in the Work Place: The Ethical Ramifications," *Business and Health* (January 1986), pp. 30–34.
2. See the discussions by Michael J. Barry, Albert G. Mulley, and Daniel E. Singer; C. E. Miller; Steven Kleinman; and Stanley H. Weiss and James J. Goedert in "Letters," *Journal of the American Medical Association* 253(23) (June 1985), pp. 3395–97.
3. Estimates of the percentage of individuals infected with the AIDS virus who will develop AIDS or AIDS-related conditions (ARC) range from 1–2 percent to over 35 percent. The higher estimates are typically based on studies of the subset of male homosexuals consisting of highly promiscuous individuals. A number of confounding variables are associated with this subset—a large number of exposures due to a large number of sexual partners; a generally high rate of infection, especially with the Hepatitis B virus; and the use of "poppers"—that compromise their immune systems and probably render them more likely to develop AIDS and ARC if they are infected with the virus. Ten percent is estimated by Leibowitch (as reported by Lieberson) to be the upper limit of individuals infected with the virus that will ever show symptoms of any kind, when the entire population of infected individuals (versus a peculiar subset of male homosexuals) is the basis of the estimate. See Jonathan Lieberson, "The Reality of AIDS," *The New York Review of Books* (January 16, 1986), pp. 43–48; and Jean L. Mark, *Science* (January 31, 1986), pp. 450–51.
4. See "Letters," *op. cit.*
5. John C. Petricciani, "Licensed Tests for Antibody to Human T-Lymphotropic Virus Type III," *Annals of Internal Medicine* 103 (1985), pp. 726–29.
6. The effort to educate at-risk individuals in San Francisco appears to have been effective in reducing risky behavior. See Lieberson, *op. cit.*
7. See Ronald Bayer and Gerald Oppenheimer, "AIDS in the Work Place: The Ethical Ramifications."
8. See The American Council of Life Insurance, "The Acquired Immunodeficiency Syndrome and HTLV-III Antibody Testing," in *Taking Sides: Clashing Views on Controversial Bioethical Issues* (2nd ed.), edited by Carol Levine (Guilford, Conn.: Dushkin Publishing Group, 1987), pp. 316–21.
9. These figures are based on an estimate of the Centers for Disease Control, and costs are likely to be toward the low end of this range. The average cost of treating an AIDS patient at San Francisco General, which has the greatest experience, is $25,000 to $32,000. See Katie Leishman, "San Francisco: A Crisis in Public Health," *The Atlantic Monthly* (October 1985), pp. 18–40.

10. M. Scherzer, "The Public Interest in Maintaining Insurance Coverage for AIDS," in Carol Levine, *op. cit.,* pp. 322–26.

11. The advent of new and better tests, if they are forthcoming, will not render mass screening much more reasonable, for there isn't much room for technical advance. The ELISA and Western blot have good statistical properties themselves (especially when used in combination). The low prevalence of the AIDS virus in the general population is what renders screening so error-prone, and recent findings indicate that infection with the AIDS virus remains largely confined to identified high-risk populations and that the rate of increase of infections is declining within these populations. See James R. Carlson *et al.,* "AIDS Serology Testing in Low- and High-Risk Groups," *Journal of the American Medical Association* 253(23) (June 21, 1985), pp. 3405–08; and Merle A. Sande, "Transmission of AIDS," *New England Journal of Medicine* 314(6) (February 6, 1986), pp. 380–82.

12. I would like to thank Carol Hayes of the Michigan Department of Public Health for her assistance, and my colleagues in the Medical Humanities Program, Tom Tomlinson and Len Fleck, for their helpful comments.

At Risk for AIDS: Confidentiality in Research and Surveillance

ALVIN NOVICK

The Centers for Disease Control, through state and local health departments, are collecting data on the incidence of AIDS and its accompanying manifestations, and on the age, sex, race, residence, sexual orientation, and drug use of persons with AIDS. They seek additional data of a social, sexual, or medical nature in puzzling or atypical cases. AIDS is currently a reportable illness in almost all American communities. These data, taken together, serve to describe the AIDS epidemic chronologically, geographically, by at-risk groups, and by other demographic characteristics, and allow the identification of a range of clusters and nonrandom distributions.

They also allow the identification and subsequent analysis of cases in the category "other and no known risk group." These data may also reveal rare or novel opportunistic infections and malignancies. Currently patients are listed by name in local or state health departments, but their names are coded for submission to CDC.

Formal surveillance of persons suspected of having early or mild AIDS-related illnesses has not been widely undertaken, but such persons are being followed in research projects in several high-incidence areas. Currently, the medical tools for clear diagnosis of such persons are inadequate. With the identification of the LAV/HTLV-III virus as the probable infectious agent of AIDS,[1,2,3,4,5] however, great attention will be given to developing accurate and accessible tests for the live virus and for one or more antibodies to the virus in the blood (or other body fluids) of human subjects.[6] We may anticipate the development of active surveillance programs of persons who are seropositive, that is, show evidence of live virus. Some of these persons

From *IRB: A Review of Human Subjects Research,* Vol. 6, No. 6 (November/December 1984), pp. 10–11. Reprinted by permission of the author and publisher.

may already be enrolled in research projects. Others may be identified in the process of screening donated blood. Others may be actively sought by state or local agencies engaged in contact tracing.

New research projects for studying seropositivity in at-risk groups or in other subpopulations such as exposed health care workers or family members of persons who have AIDS or are seropositive will surely soon be undertaken. Thus, surveillance of persons with AIDS will probably soon be supplemented by programs surveying the incidence of the AIDS virus or of antibodies to the AIDS virus for public health reasons and for research. Personal, medical, sexual, and drug use data will surely be sought and compiled.

Furthermore, research projects are underway concerned with following the status of currently healthy gay men in order to describe the natural history of AIDS and of other AIDS-related clinical manifestations. Many other, mostly smaller, studies are investigating aspects of the behavioral epidemiology of AIDS in gay men, intravenous drug users, infants with pediatric AIDS, Haitian-Americans, exposed health care workers, blood recipients and donors, hemophiliacs, and others. These projects usually include healthy control subjects (often from at-risk groups) or persons who are currently healthy but may, in time, have AIDS or be seropositive for the AIDS virus or for antibodies to the AIDS virus.

Thus, the matter of the privacy and confidentiality of research subjects, of persons with AIDS, of persons who will come to be known as seropositive for antibodies to the AIDS agent, or of sex partners, of drug-injection equipment partners, or of other contacts of persons with AIDS or seropositive persons is already complex and will soon and rapidly become more so.

Seropositivity has not yet been widely studied. The epidemiology and natural history of the presence of live virus in persons are not yet established. We may, however, conjecture that those who are carrying the virus may transmit it even though it is virtually certain that many such persons are not themselves clinically ill and may never be. The epidemiology and natural history of the presence of antibodies to one or more components of the LAV/HTLV-III virus are also not established. In a small series of persons with AIDS-related complex, a majority were seropositive.[2,3] About half of those persons with AIDS, who have been studied, are seropositive, and at least a few persons who are clinically well are seropositive.[6] We do not yet know, however, whether the presence of antibodies to the AIDS agent correlates with prognosis, with the ability to transmit the agent to others, or with possible vulnerability to AIDS if accompanied by unknown environmental or host cofactors or by repeated exposure. Thus, neither individual medical management nor public health policies can be rationally based on seropositivity at present.

Properly designed research on AIDS is, of course, to the advantage of the general public and to persons in at-risk groups. However, in the realm of infectious disease, research includes surveillance; the results of surveillance of course determine some aspects of public health policy. Surveillance by its nature is invasive of privacy and its presumed products are potentially invasive of certain other civil rights or, at the very least, raise difficult issues where political and social controversy surely lurk, that is, quarantine, restrictions of personal behavior, and the like. Furthermore, while participation in research is usually voluntary and normally involves informed consent, at least some aspects of participation in surveillance are involuntary.

A peculiar feature of the AIDS epidemic in the U.S., of course, is that it has principally affected members of certain groups that were already subject to severe social sanctions—homosexual men, intravenous drug users, the female sex partners and infants of intravenous drug users, and recent Haitian-American immigrants. Taken together, persons in these groups make up about 95 percent of those with AIDS. They may well make up a similarly large portion of those who are seropositive.

Homosexual men have many substantial reasons to fear social exposure and oppression. In almost half of our states, homosexual sexuality is considered criminal, even in the privacy of one's home with a life partner who is a consenting adult. Homosexual men are widely subjected to discrimination on the basis of their sexual orientation. They are denounced by some religious and political figures, and even by health care professionals. Only a few American communities protect their basic rights. Even access to family support often requires agonizingly difficult camouflage.

Persons who use illicit drugs, and often their spouses and children, are socially and legally vulnerable. Haitian-Americans are often illegal immigrants with many realistic concerns about their rights, if exposed. Many Haitians, in addition, face the general difficulties and concerns of the poor, of foreigners, and of belonging to a community stigmatized by AIDS. Oppressed persons, such as all these groups, appropriately fear personal disclosure, which converts group oppression into severe personal hardship.

Surveillance requires data on private behavior. The identity of the persons concerned usually is not a necessary aspect of surveillance data and should be known only to their personal physician or their local health official. Persons in at-risk groups correctly perceive that lists of names generated by federal agencies would eventually—officially, carelessly, or maliciously—be shared and might be used to the detriment of those listed. Current laws, customs, precedents, and sensitivities are not sufficient to protect the privacy of research or surveillance data. If being listed federally threatens persons with AIDS (who are already known locally and are heavily stigmatized and whose official identification is mandated by local regulation), consider how much more threatening it will be to persons who come to be known as seropositive for antibodies to the AIDS agent, even though the clinical significance of such a finding is currently unknown. What of those who volunteer to be studied, while healthy and/or as control subjects, because they know themselves to be members of an at-risk group?

The risk to each of these men and women would be that their voluntary sharing of the details of their private lives could easily be used against them, with major social consequences. The risk to society is also massive, in allowing the modern precedent of the violation of private lives as the "reward" for cooperation in important research.

For research protocols, the ethical picture is now clear. Investigators should design their studies so as to guarantee the confidentiality of their highly vulnerable subjects. IRBs [International Review Boards] should require and monitor a very high level of sensitivity. Since such sensitivity does not occur spontaneously, it will require substantial advice, a general mood of concern, and the participation of risk-group advocates in the review and oversight of AIDS research.

Currently, surveillance protocols and the research associated with surveillance are usually not monitored by independent IRBs, if at all. At the very least, they should be brought under sensitive review and oversight (with the participation of risk-group advocates).

The appropriate product of surveillance and of research on AIDS is knowledge, leading to containing the epidemic by first understanding and then by reducing transmission. Education and counsel, concerning risks, are necessary and proper tools. The fears of persons in at-risk groups and their advocates, however, is that the products of surveillance and research on AIDS may be political and social oppression, as well as personal exposure and its consequences. The most threatening scenarios include the use of inappropriate or broadly imposed quarantine, the recriminalization of homosexual sexuality, or the inappropriate restriction of employment, access to housing, or other restrictions on the civil rights of persons in at-risk groups.

Clearly knowledge (and vigilance) are our best weapons against oppression. Our knowledge depends on research, which, in turn, depends on voluntary cooperation. If persons in at-risk groups were to withhold their cooperation, that would seriously impede progress. Thus, society's options are clear. The rights of the subjects of research or surveillance to confidentiality must be assured by law and regulation, by social expectation, and by greatly enhanced sensitivity. Identifying data must be closely and locally held, access restricted, and violations punished, if not successfully precluded. The development of federal lists or of other widely shared or vulnerable lists should be stopped or precluded.

Society has not yet made a clear statement or identified its own commitment to concern, respect, and compassion for the groups at risk for AIDS. Lacking such an ethical position, we must anticipate careless or malicious shortcomings. In addition, regulations can easily be changed or inverted, for evil as well as for good. For those reasons, we must be especially vigilant about planning our research and in honoring and protecting the confidentiality and privacy of our subjects.

Notes

1. Barré-Sinoussi, F., *et al.,* "Isolation of a T-Lymphotropic Retrovirus from a Patient at Risk for Acquired Immune Deficiency Syndrome (AIDS)," *Science* 220 (1983), pp. 868–71.
2. Popovic, M. *et al.,* "Detection, Isolation, and Continuous Production of Cytopathic Retroviruses (HTLV-III) from Patients with AIDS and Pre-AIDS," *Science* 224 (1984), pp. 497–500.
3. Gallo, R. C. *et al.,* "Frequent Detection and Isolation of Cytopathic Retroviruses (HTLV-III) from Patients with AIDS and at Risk for AIDS," *Science* 224 (1984), pp. 500–502.
4. Klatzmann, D. *et al.,* "Selective Tropism of Lymphadenopathy Associated Virus (LAV) for Helper-Inducer T-Lymphocytes," *Science* 225 (1984), pp. 59–63.
5. Feorino, P. M. *et al.,* "Lymphadenopathy Associated Virus Infection of a Blood Donor-Recipient Pair with Acquired Immunodeficiency Syndrome," *Science* 225 (1984), pp. 69–72.
6. Sarngadharan, M. G. *et al.,* "Antibodies Reactive with Human T-Cell Lymphotropic Retroviruses (HTLV-III) in the Serum of Patients with AIDS," *Science* 224 (1984), pp. 506–8.

AIDS and
Human Rights:
An Intercontinental
Perspective

CAROL A. TAUER

Background: Intercontinental Dimensions

Persons who suffer from AIDS or AIDS-related conditions fear not only the disease but also violations or deprivations of basic rights. They are concerned about invasions of their personal privacy and possible restrictions on their freedom of movement and activity. They worry that they may be denied employment, health or life insurance, housing, and even health care.

The United States and the various nations of western Europe differ in their responses to the social and ethical problems posed by AIDS. While all of these nations basically subscribe to the same international declarations of human rights (for example, the *Universal Declaration of Human Rights,* the *European Convention on Human Rights*), there are both conceptual and practical differences in their understanding of these statements.

In the international documents on human rights, we find support for three categories of rights which measures to control AIDS may threaten:[1] (1) the right of personal privacy and confidentiality regarding medical and sexual information; (2) the right to free movement within one's country and to associate where and how one chooses; (3) the right to pursue one's economic good, without limitation based on irrelevant grounds ([for example], sex, sexual preference). Providing some contrast

Reprinted by permission of the author.

to this perspective, the World Health Organization takes a more utilitarian stance in relation to its goal of promoting health as the right of all people. For WHO, health is fundamental to the attainment of international peace and security, and so cooperation in the control of disease, especially communicable disease, is essential.[2] In its 1976 document, *Health Aspects of Human Rights,* WHO explicitly adopts "the Benthamite principle of 'the greatest happiness of the greatest number'" and advocates curtailing personal liberty not only for the sake of the common good, but also to promote the health of the individual in question.[3]

Here we see exemplified in statements from one international forum, the United Nations, the underlying tension found in discussions of public policy on AIDS. What is the appropriate balance between the common good, in this case the public health, and the rights and liberties of individual persons? Each member nation is attempting to answer this question in the light of its own laws and traditions, and, as a result, a variety of different practices and policies are emerging.

But it is not only this question, complex as it is, which contributes to differing approaches to the AIDS crisis. A second crucial issue concerns the practice of medicine itself. Since AIDS is a disease, it is handled within a medical model, not only one of civil liberties. Thus, one's conception of the role and duties of the physician, the nature of the physician-patient relationship, and the physician's responsibility for the health of the individual and the public, will affect one's approach to AIDS. Again, each nation has different traditions and codes on these matters, which will influence its policy regarding AIDS.

In considering human rights and AIDS, this paper will focus on France and Great Britain, relating significant aspects of their responses to that of the United States. As of November 13, 1986, the largest numbers of AIDS cases reported in European countries were in France (997, not including the overseas departments), the Federal Republic of Germany (715), and the United Kingdom (512).[4] At this time, there had been over 26,500 cases in the U.S.; and the rate of infection in any European country (less than 20 per million population) was still low compared to the U.S. rate (greater than 110 per million).

In both France and Great Britain—in contrast to Italy, for example—very few of the AIDS patients are IV drug abusers. The overwhelming majority are homosexual or bisexual men, as in the United States; hence this paper will focus on the potential for violations of rights within that population.

While the approaches of these three countries illustrate cultural and political divergences rooted in history, two new trends also emerge: As an international bioethical community develops, engaging in discussion and sharing documents, there is movement toward a greater uniformity of response to bioethical problems. And secondly, in the United States there are signs of a movement away from the almost single-minded focus on individual rights and liberties of the recent past. Both of these factors will undoubtedly affect the AIDS debate in the coming years.

Confidentiality

Among the human rights which have a traditional link to medical ethics is the right of privacy. While privacy has many dimensions, the aspect of personal control of private information is perhaps the greatest concern of those at risk for AIDS and AIDS-related conditions. Violations of the confidentiality of private information not only trespass on an intimate domain, involving both medical data and information about sexual behavior, but, because of the nature of AIDS, they may also lead to denial of employment, insurance, and housing.

Medical professionals of all western societies have traditionally regarded confidentiality of information as a serious obligation. However, within the modern hospital in the United States, it is not unusual for as many as 100 people to have access to the medical records of the patient,[5] in addition to third-party payers of whatever sort. This situation is not unique to the U.S.; a dean of the Newcastle Faculty of Medicine observed that as many as 150 different people could have access to patient notes in hospital![6] Moreover, when a disease is reportable by law to either local or national health authorities, the cases (however they are identified) become part of a data bank, most likely computerized, over which no individual health professional has control.

The Centers for Disease Control, which mandate national reporting of AIDS cases in the United States, have developed a system for coding the identifications of the individuals involved. While authorities say there is no way to reconstruct a person's name from the coded identification, some members of the homosexual or gay community are dubious.[7] Furthermore, local departments of health at the state level have their own reporting regulations. Colorado and several other states even require the results of positive antibody tests to be identified by name, whereas California law explicitly prohibits such reporting unless there is written consent of the person tested.[8] The state of Minnesota, which predicts a major increase in cases, is experimenting with a curious policy: According to state law, positive antibody tests are to be reported by name; however, individuals may circumvent this requirement by being tested at an "alternative testing site" where they may remain anonymous.[9]

As of March 22, 1985, Great Britain included AIDS under some of the provisions of the law governing "notifiable diseases," but decided not to require the reporting of AIDS cases themselves.[10] Health officials said that a policy of voluntary reporting (without names) was operating effectively and was all that was needed.[11] British law gives particular legal protection to all records of sexually transmitted diseases which are held by National Health Service authorities. These records "shall not be disclosed" except to a medical practitioner for purposes of treatment or prevention.[12] In hospitals, records relating to venereal diseases are "locked away separate from the main hospital records,"[13] a unique provision which shows a high degree of sensitivity to the implications of disclosure.

French physicians invest medical confidences with a sacredness linked to a religious tradition, somewhat like the secrecy of the Catholic confessional. This view is expressed in French law, which protects "the professional secret" from disclosure in a court of law and does not even permit the patient to waive confidentiality in his own interest.[14] The duty of confidentiality with respect to all third parties is strongly asserted as part of "Code de déontologie médicale," the statement of medical ethics which is imposed by law on French physicians.[15]

While French law and practice seem to provide essentially absolute protection for medical confidentiality, British and American codes allow exceptions, either to protect a third party or for the sake of the common good. American case law contains precedents of a "duty to warn" a third party who is in danger of harm;[16] and currently there is much discussion as to how this duty would apply to the physician of a person who is infectious for the AIDS virus. The codes of both the British Medical Association and the General Medical Council permit disclosure for the sake of the public interest and, somewhat surprisingly, for purposes of approved medical research.[17] There appears to be quite a bit of leeway for the British physician to determine what may ethically be revealed, apart from special provisions such as the statutes on sexually transmitted diseases.

Physicians, like other professionals, customarily devise their own ethical codes and enforce them through self-regulation. Even when a professional code is included within statutory law, as in France, the duties are those already recognized by members of the profession in that country. Confidentiality, traditionally one of the most cherished values of the profession of medicine, is challenged today by public policy decisions which mandate its abrogation for a cause which is viewed as a greater good. Thus, required reporting of medical information implies that the good consequences which will follow as a result of gathering this information justify both overriding the patient's privacy right and endangering his related interests (for example, his interest in nondiscriminatory treatment when he seeks insurance).

There are two distinct purposes for which public health agencies may use the data they gather about cases of a communicable disease. Both purposes are preventive, but in different ways. The first purpose is epidemiological research, the tracing of patterns of a disease in order to identify causal agents, modes of transmission, ebbs and flows in the history of the disease. As a result of such research, recommendations on disease control are provided to the public, to physicians, and to local government agencies. The U.S. Centers for Disease Control and the British Communicable Disease Surveillance Centre gather their case data for this purpose. Much epidemiological study can be done without specific identification of the individuals involved, but some research requires that at least one investigator have this information. The protection of confidentiality in epidemiological research has been a topic of ethical concern for many years.[18]

But while continuing questions are raised, both Britain and the U.S. show a substantial history of epidemiological research. (See Gordis *et al.* for an impressive listing of results achieved by this work.) Because of its strong insistence on confidentiality, France has been slow to gather the data needed for studies of this type. French investigation of AIDS has therefore focused on virological and immunological research, while epidemiological work has been centered in the U.S. Recently, however, there have been signs of a convergence in bioethical standards. For example, a 1985 recommendation of the French national committee on bioethics, "Recommendations on Medical Registers for Epidemiologic Study and Prevention,"[19] stimulated a detailed response from the National Medical Council, . . . incorporating many of the confidentiality precautions suggested nine years ago by Gordis *et al.*[20] While France is clearly learning from the Anglo-American experience, its cautiousness and discretion can also be instructive to that tradition.

The second purpose for gathering case data is the exercise of direct intervention into the person-to-person transmission of a communicable disease. This intervention may involve the tracing and warning of contacts of an infectious person and/or surveillance of the activities of this person so as to prevent further possible transmission. While the epidemiological use of data presents a speculative danger of violation of confidentiality, its use for direct intervention (which requires a noncoded record of the person's identity) seems to present an immediate ethical dilemma. Whether this abrogation of confidentiality is justified by the lethal and catastrophic nature of AIDS is hotly contested in the U.S., while such measures seem generally to have been rejected in Great Britain and hardly even considered in France. In the U.S., state and local jurisdictions are in the process of developing a tangle of reporting regulations based on their perceptions of this second function for public health data.

Informed Consent and the Right to Know

The practice of medicine has traditionally been a paternalistic enterprise. In the past few decades it has become much less so in the United States, and there is now a clearer public recognition of patients' rights, both morally and legally. While the statutory assertions of these rights differ somewhat from state to state, as does case law, the American Hospital Association has promulgated a general statement which is universally accepted by hospitals. Among accepted rights are the right to informed consent to treatment, the right to know one's diagnosis and prognosis, and the right to refuse treatment, even life-sustaining treatment. In competent patients, these rights may not be overridden even for what a professional perceives to be the best interests of the patient.

In contrast, Great Britain and France have retained a more paternalistic view of the role of the physician, so that the physician's duty to promote the best interests of the patient generally takes precedence over the patient's rights related to autonomy. Correlatively, the standard for whether a physician has done his or her duty is established almost exclusively by the medical profession in France and Britain, and lawyers and judges defer to medical judgment and testimony in these matters. In the U.S., the courts often exercise an independent function on behalf of patients' rights, and standards such as that of "the reasonable patient" may be applied.

While the French code of medical ethics is part of statutory law, its formulation is entirely the work of the Conseil National de l'Ordre des Médecins.[21] This "Code de déontologie médicale" is expressed in terms of physician duties, and the only right the patient is specifically granted is that of choosing his or her own physician. While the physician is instructed to respect the wishes of the sick person as far as possible, an extraordinary control over information is retained: "For legitimate reasons, which the physician recognizes in conscience, a sick person may be left in ignorance of a grave diagnosis or prognosis."[22]

Although there is now a multidisciplinary national committee on bioethics in France, the charge of this committee restricts it to matters related to biomedical research; clinical issues remain under the jurisdiction of the medical council.[23] Since the committee interprets its charge rather broadly, its documents show substantive interchange with the medical council ([for example], see above on confidentiality and epidemiological research). Another currently debated issue involves Phase I drug trials, in which drugs are given their initial testing for toxicity, dosage, and mode of administration. In the United States, these trials are customarily conducted with healthy volunteers (usually paid). Such a practice has been repugnant to the French medical profession: "There is no justifiable scientific or medical reason for exposing to risk a subject who has no medical reason to participate in a trial and who can expect no benefit from it. Hence we condemn . . . all phase I trials conducted on normal subjects."[24] Most French jurists have also supported the view that a healthy subject does not have the right to consent to such involvement, even with full information, understanding, and voluntariness.[25] But the national ethics committee is providing a forum for consideration of a change in this stance; and there is evidence that such trials, with careful safeguards, may become ethically acceptable, as they are in the U.S.[26]

In his perceptive study *The Unmasking of Medicine,* Ian Kennedy has detailed the paternalistic bias of the British medical profession, ranging from control of the "sick note," by which the physician certifies that an absent worker truly was ill, to permission for an abortion, where physicians are unavoidably involved in psychosocial judgments.[27] A recent legal case in Britain has thoroughly examined American case law on informed consent and rejected some of its conclusions. The case, that of Mrs. Amy Sidaway, involved her complaint that her physician had not told her the risks of her surgery. The Court of Appeal decided against her, stating that "the doctrine of informed consent [forms] no part of English law," and that "most [people] prefer to put themselves unreservedly in the hands of their doctors. . . . [This] is simply an acceptance of the doctor-patient relationship as it has developed in this country." Final appeal to the House of Lords supported this view; the Lords determined that what to volunteer to disclose was a matter for the physician's clinical judgment. However, they did allow for a court finding contrary to medical testimony in extreme or blatant cases of nondisclosure, and they also stressed the physician's obligation to answer fully and truthfully any questions which the patient actually asked.[28]

Paternalistic practice in France and Britain represents not only the way the doctor-patient relationship has developed in each country, but, in general, the way the class structure has developed. In Britain, social classes 1 to 5 are defined on the basis of occupational and educational level, with class 1 the professional class. A camaraderie among doctors, lawyers, and professors results from their having enjoyed basically the same background and education; hence they are supposedly able to understand each other's language. On the other hand, those who belong to classes 4 or 5 could not be expected to understand technical information, so are assumed to put their trust in the professional's judgment.[29] In France the class structure is also much more clearly defined than in the U.S., and the rural and working classes have a standard of living and level of culture well below those of the bourgeoisie, which includes the professional class.

European notions of the status and role of the professional have had the practical consequence of determining who controls certain types of information. In *Un Virus Étrange Venu d'Ailleurs,* Jacques Leibowitch describes the current openness of information and discussion about AIDS as the Americanization of the disease. It is not merely that the U.S. Centers for Disease Control have decided what is to count worldwide as AIDS, a matter complained of by a variety of European scientists and clinicians.[30] But also socioculturally, "the disease carries the cultural insignia of its origin," presumably the United States.[31] Continuing in Leibowitch's words:

> To tell, to make known, to announce the disease and death—to inform the patient of the medical procedures that will follow, to obtain his informed consent, to expose and to discuss while exposing—North America has its cultural features. In France, we had another tradition. To say nothing, to know nothing; a father protects us with his mysteries. . . . [Now] everyone will know: Good-bye, mystery; hello, terror.[32]

Testing or Screening for AIDS Antibodies

The American patient's "right to know" is an enunciated extension of a general right claimed by the U.S. citizen. With regard to health matters, this claim is supported by U.S. public health officials, who take the position that full knowledge contributes to prudent personal health decisions. The Centers for Disease Control have based their recommendations regarding general testing for AIDS antibodies on that assumption.

Emphasizing that such tests should be voluntary and accompanied by thorough counseling, the CDC recommends that serologic testing "be routinely offered to all persons at increased risk when they present [themselves] to health-care settings." These recommendations enumerate first the behaviors counseled for those who test negative, and, second, the behaviors counseled for those who test positive.[33] While these behaviors are similar in many respects, the CDC seems to imply that knowledge of one's antibody status will be determinative if one needs to make changes in life-style and behavior.

Local health authorities have made similar recommendations. For example, the Minnesota State Department of Health has published notices with the heading, "Don't Guess about It," encouraging persons who may be infected to take advantage of free testing and counseling. In many localities of the U.S., general testing sites were first made available in order to dissuade persons seeking serologic testing from using blood donation centers for this purpose. But presently, the use of these testing sites is being encouraged on the typically American presupposition that more information is better than less in making individual medical or life-style decisions.

In contrast to the United States, British public health authorities are not urging general serum antibody tests, even for members of high-risk groups. The value of routine testing is questioned by the Chief Medical Officer, Department of Health and Social Security, as well as by staff of the National AIDS Counseling Training Unit.[34] After considering the purposes for which such test results might legitimately be used, these authorities conclude that the possible benefits are highly speculative. There is no concrete evidence that knowledge of test results actually leads to greater behavior change than mass education and focused counseling programs, nor that it would in any other way contribute to halting the spread of the disease. Thus these officials believe that there is no justification for risking the harms ([for example], stigmatization, loss of employment or insurance) to which the test might lead.

Here British health authorities take a position similar to that of many gay organizations in the United States. For example, the Gay Men's Health Crisis (New York City) nationally distributed an advertisement with the headline, "The Test Can Be Almost as Devastating as the Disease."[35] But there is disagreement within the gay community, and some gay groups, especially in urban centers of continental Europe, are urging use of the test.[36]

Lack of British enthusiasm for routine testing does not mean that there is indifference in the situations in which a confirmed positive test result would call for a clear response. Miller *et al.* . . . list settings within which screening ought to be done: with donors of blood and blood products, organs for transplant, semen, and growth hormone[s]; before and during the pregnancy of a woman at risk; and probably with hemodialysis patients. The slowness with which Britain instituted screening of blood donations (not widely introduced until October 1985) should not be attributed to lack of concern. Rather, the delay was due to great care and extensive investigation in order to locate, among available testing methods, the best one ([that is, the method] with the fewest false positives and with nearly zero false negatives).[37]

Discussion of serological testing in official sources in France is largely limited to its use with blood donors. The national committee on bioethics has proposed a policy on screening blood donors, noting the absolute necessity of such screening to ferret out infection of blood with SIDA (AIDS).[38] The proposal carefully delineates the counseling which must accompany a positive finding: The physician of the blood center must impress upon the seropositive person that he has a heavy responsibility to his family and/or other sexual contacts in order to stop the spread of the disease. The document shows the expected French discretion regarding intimate information; the physician must adjust his discourse to each individual situation, and no reporting requirement is mentioned or recommended.

Government-Sponsored Education Programs

Given their decision not to promote identification of cases of AIDS infections, British health authorities have been consistent in putting resources into mass education and focused counseling programs instead. Chief Medical Officer Acheson specifically includes adolescents, undeclared homosexual and bisexual men, and, in fact, all sexually active men and women among those whom government-sponsored educational programs must reach. He also notes that the national press, radio, and television will provide sexually explicit information if necessary, and that public response (to effectiveness and offensiveness) will be periodically evaluated.[39]

The first stage in the government's educational campaign included full-page advertisements in the national newspapers on March 16 and 17, 1986, advertisements in the gay press, and posters and leaflets provided to groups like the Terrence Higgins Trust (a gay organization formed to deal with AIDS), at a total cost of £2.5 million.[40] The national press advertisements were highly explicit, stating that "rectal sex . . . should be avoided," that "using a sheath [condom] reduces the risk of AIDS and other diseases," and that "any act that damages the penis, vagina, anus, or mouth is dangerous."[41]

While U.S. public health authorities have consistently advocated mass educational programs, their efforts have generally had to be more restrained. They have been able to provide some funding to those who work with the gay community and with IV drug users for the development of clear and direct educational programs. But material provided for mass consumption is directed either at those who will read fairly technical explanations of the disease and its transmission, or at those who are sophisticated enough to read between the lines of a vague, generalized warning. Adolescent, disadvantaged, and semiliterate persons are not apt to be informed by scientific or euphemistic discussions.

Several reasons for this restraint may be cited: (1) The Reagan administration has objections to government funding for sexually explicit materials, particularly regarding homosexual activity, and, as a result, a number of CDC programs have not been implemented.[42] (2) There is a strong antipornography movement, and some citizens are highly vocal about educational materials which they view as too explicit sexually.[43] (3) There is a widespread but unconfirmed belief that informing young people about sexual practices will only lead them to experiment with them. (4) Activities which are described in educational materials are often illegal; for example, sodomy is criminal by the laws of about half the states.

One may expect that the tide will turn as a result of Surgeon General C. Everett Koop's report on AIDS, issued October 22, 1986. In this report, Koop calls for AIDS sex education, beginning in the elementary grades, as the central focus of public health efforts against AIDS.[44] This focus is strongly supported by the study of the Institute of Medicine, National Academy of Sciences, which was made public one week later.[45] It is too early, however, to assess the effects of these recommendations.

In France, the reluctance to expose the disease is almost universal. While the gay community in the United States has been a leader in the educational effort there, in France there has been a tendency among gay people to deny the seriousness of the disease. An American reporter describes Parisian gays as "charmed by what they perceived to be the *vraiment New Yorkaise* overreaction to the situation. . . . Eyebrows arched wryly at the discussion of safe sex."[46] Association AIDES has found great resistance in its efforts to institute programs to educate patrons of gay bars and bathhouses in Paris.[47]

Gay people of other countries, however, have been particularly critical of French authorities for their meager financial commitment to AIDS education (while France is the European country hardest hit). It was not until late 1985 that the government allocated its first $30,000 for AIDS education, an amount less than one San Francisco foundation spends locally in a month.[48] When Dr. Luc Montagnier of the Pasteur Institute recently wrote an informational pamphlet, the decision was made to produce it as a glossy 94-page pamphlet which would be sold for $4, thus excluding many people who needed the information but would not or could not pay that sum.[49]

A country which has been most highly praised for its government's commitment to education on AIDS, as well as for its national office to coordinate all AIDS policy decisions, is the Netherlands. The director of this office, Jan Van Wijngaarden, attributes its success to the integration of homosexuality into Dutch society and the lack of bigotry among the Dutch public.[50]

Reports have also been received about imaginative educational efforts in Norway. For example, an Oslo billboard shows a cartoon face drawn on the top of the male organ to illustrate a text about using condoms to prevent the transmission of AIDS. Publicity of this type shows a realization that masses of people will only be attracted, hence informed and affected, by media presentations which are clever, contemporary, and graphic.[51]

Quarantine and Other Restrictive Policies

The ethical conflict between the common good and the rights or freedoms of individuals is perhaps illustrated most clearly in the situation where a restriction on movement or association is imposed or contemplated by public authorities. The quarantine, with its long and controversial history, provides an example of a public health measure which can be highly restrictive, and which in some forms is being proposed for the control of AIDS.

In Britain, the Public Health Act of 1984 has been interpreted specifically for its application to AIDS. The section on detention was amended thus:

> A justice of the peace may on the application of any local authority make an order for the detention in hospital of an inmate of that hospital suffering from acquired immune deficiency syndrome if the justice is satisfied that on his leaving . . . proper precautions to prevent the spread of that disease would not be taken by him.[52]

Two applications of the statute have been reported in British journals, both involving rather unusual circumstances. In one case, a hospitalized AIDS patient was put under detention orders for three weeks by Manchester magistrates. The Manchester medical officer described this man as "bleeding copiously and trying to discharge himself [from hospital]." The legal correspondent reporting to the *British Medical Journal* raised the obvious question: What if it were risky sexual behavior, rather than bleeding, which endangered others? Detention for such cause would seem to be within the intent of the law. Yet, as the correspondent notes, "To apply the law in this way would clearly raise grave political difficulties for the central government as well as for any local authority concerned."[53]

Interestingly, the other reported case of detention in England also involved bleeding. In this case, the patient was on a psychiatric ward, and at one point he cut his hands and deliberately smeared blood around his room and into a corridor. The police were called, and the person is now being detained in a prison setting.[54]

Thus far in the United States, actual quarantine or isolation has been seriously considered only in relation to prostitutes who are AIDS carriers. A restrictive measure which has had more impact on the gay community in general involves the closing or regulation of gay bathhouses or other meeting places where casual or anonymous sex is a common activity. San Francisco experienced a series of orders and injunctions; in the end, the California Superior Court prohibited legal closing of such establishments, but ordered safeguards like removal of cubicle doors, inspection by monitors every ten minutes, and expulsion of patrons observed in acts of high-risk sex.[55] New York has adopted an emergency regulation which provides for closing establishments which allow anal or oral sex acts on their premises.[56] While gay rights groups are most incensed at this ruling, it has also been applied to heterosexual gathering places.

French public policy has not yet confronted the issue of quarantine or even of regulation of bathhouse activity. In Paris, the police are reportedly engaging in increased harassment of the gay community, using the threat of AIDS as their justification, but apparently on legitimate grounds (for example, to identify minors practicing prostitution or frequenting bathhouses.)[57]

Perhaps the most comprehensive policy among European nations has been established by Sweden. By including AIDS under the provisions of its venereal disease laws, as it did in late 1985, Sweden could be interpreted to require compulsory testing of persons in high-risk groups, and for those with seropositive tests, reporting to health authorities, naming of all sexual partners, prohibition of risky conduct (sexual or drug-related), and, in certain cases, confinement to hospitals. At least one person with a seropositive test has been so confined because he continued to share needles with other drug users and to have sex without taking necessary protective precautions.[58]

Clearly a common thread in laws about AIDS, among states in the U.S., Great Britain, and Sweden, is *some* explicit provision for the mandatory restriction of persons who are judged to be an imminent threat to the health of others. However, major problems exist concerning not only the implementation but also the efficacy of such laws. As with [that of] some American states, British law focuses on persons who actually have AIDS, while scientists believe that those who have been infected with the virus, but have not (yet) developed the disease, may actually be more infectious than those who are ill. One must ask whether a policy calling for legal restriction has any meaning without required testing of large population groups; and since that sort of program is not seriously contemplated by public officials (except perhaps in Sweden), the legal enactments may be more token than efficacious. At most, they seem to provide legal protection for government officials who may wish to restrain an individual whose behavior is particularly blatant, harmful, and perhaps malicious.

Protections for Civil Rights

Each nation has its own tradition with respect to the protection of civil rights. Both the role of the law, whether constitutional, statutory, or case law, and the attitudes of the citizens, differ from country to country; and these differences engender subtle variations in the national concern for the civil rights of AIDS victims.

As members of the European Community, both France and Great Britain have subscribed to its *Convention on Human Rights* and have accepted the provision whereby an individual citizen may appeal to the Commission of Human Rights in Strasbourg if the citizen believes his or her rights under the Convention have been violated by his or her State. It has been suggested that grievances against the National Health Service with regard to confidentiality could be brought before this body, and cases on detention for psychiatric illness have already been decided.[59]

In Article 8, the *European Convention* gives explicit protection to the individual's private and family life, home and correspondence, and states that public authorities may not interfere with the exercise of this right unless it is necessary for some greater societal good.[60] This privacy right has been applied by the European Court against national laws prohibiting homosexual acts between consenting adults in private. Although the rest of the United Kingdom had decriminalized such activity in 1967 (Sexual Offenses Act), Northern Ireland had not. An individual's appeal to the European Commission in the early 1980s resulted in the Court's judgment that the law in Northern Ireland did, in fact, violate Article 8 of the Convention and had to be changed.[61]

It has been noted that persons at risk for AIDS in European countries display a relative lack of concern about possible loss of their civil rights. This phenomenon could perhaps be linked to the fact that homosexual activity is not illegal in these countries, and also perhaps to the national health care systems by which full medical coverage is provided to citizens of most European nations.[62]

While a privacy right is not specifically enunciated in the United States Constitution, it has been found to be implicit in other protections asserted there. Thus, it has been applied to issues in child-rearing and education, marriage, contraception, abortion (*Roe* v. *Wade*), and termination of medical treatment (*In re Karen Ann Quinlan*). However, recently the U.S. Supreme Court rendered a decision specifying a point beyond which the privacy right did not apply. On June 30, 1986, the Court asserted that individual states were entitled to make laws which prohibit sodomy. While most such state laws apply to both homosexual and heterosexual acts (anal and possibly oral sex acts), the Court's opinion clearly focuses on a possible state interest in prohibiting homosexual sodomy.[63] Although the ruling makes no mention of AIDS, it is possible that the majority justices had this disease in mind, for they seem concerned about decisions states may wish to make to safeguard public welfare. And it is known that at least one amicus brief urged the Court to consider AIDS as a good reason for states to have laws against sodomy.[64]

Though the rights of gay persons are protected in some jurisdictions of the U.S., particularly in liberal urban centers, there is no general protection for the homosexual person as such, as there is for the person of a minority race as such. Until recently, however, there was a belief that the rights of those with AIDS or AIDS-related conditions would be safeguarded under the federal Rehabilitation Act of 1973. Under this law, it is illegal for agencies and programs which receive any federal funds to discriminate against those who are handicapped or perceived to be handicapped, provided these persons are otherwise qualified (for example, to do a particular job). As of June 7, 1986, civil rights lawyers in the Justice Department supported a broad application of the Act to AIDS victims.[65] But shortly thereafter, a different position was taken by the Justice Department itself.

In a ruling of June 22, 1986, the Justice Department asserted that a person may not be excluded from a job or a program on grounds that he or she suffers from the disabling effects of the disease AIDS, but may be excluded if there is concern that he or she might spread the disease.[66] While adverting to the U.S. Public Health Service's assurances that AIDS is not spread by casual contact, the ruling calls the weight of this opinion into question by putting the burden of proof on the person who claims to have been dismissed unfairly. This decision is currently binding on the executive branch, which is the executor of regulations for federally funded agencies and programs.

However, the ruling will have little effect in cities and states which have already ruled that persons with AIDS or positive antibody tests are protected by local anti-discrimination laws. For example, Minnesota and its two major cities have indicated that the Justice Department ruling is irrelevant there.[67] Nonetheless, the Justice Department's conservative interpretation of the application of the Rehabilitation Act presages a national scenario of inconsistent policies, with discrimination excusable in some jurisdictions if an employer is irrationally fearful regarding the transmission of AIDS.

Notes

1. See I. Brownlie, Ed., *Basic Documents on Human Rights,* 2nd ed. (Oxford: Clarendon Press, 1981).
2. World Health Organization, "Preamble to the Constitution of the World Health Organization" (1946), in *The First Ten Years of the World Health Organization* (Geneva: WHO, 1958).
3. World Health Organization, *Health Aspects of Human Rights* (Geneva: WHO, 1976), p. 42.
4. Information provided by the WHO Control Program on AIDS, Geneva.
5. Mark Siegler, "Confidentiality in Medicine: A Decrepit Concept," *New England Journal of Medicine* 307 (1982), pp. 1518–21.
6. Alexander W. Macara, "Confidentiality—A Decrepit Concept? Discussion Paper," *Journal of the Royal Society of Medicine* 77 (1984), p. 579.
7. Charles Marwick, "'Confidentiality' Issues May Cloud Epidemiologic Studies of AIDS," *Journal of the American Medical Association* 250 (1983), pp. 1945–46.
8. Michael Mills, Constance Wofsy, and John Mills, "The Acquired Immunodeficiency Syndrome: Infection Control and Public Health Law," *New England Journal of Medicine* 314 (April 3, 1986), pp. 931–36.

9. Department of Health (Minnesota), "Rules Governing Communicable Diseases," *Disease Control Newsletter,* Insert 12, No. 5 (June, 1985); Walter Parker, "AIDS Screening Tests Offered Anonymously," *St. Paul Pioneer Press and Dispatch* (November 13, 1985), pp. 1A and 4A.

10. The Public Health (Infectious Diseases) Regulations 1985 (Statutory Instrument 1985, No. 434), England and Wales.

11. Rodney Deitch, "Government's Response to Fears about Acquired Immunodeficiency Syndrome," *Lancet* (March 2, 1985), pp. 530–31.

12. The National Health Service (Venereal Diseases) Regulations 1974 (Statutory Instrument 1974, No. 29), England and Wales.

13. E. D. Acheson, "AIDS: A Challenge for the Public Health," *Lancet* (March 22, 1986), p. 665.

14. John Havard, "Medical Confidence," *Journal of Medical Ethics* 11 (1985), pp. 8–11; Daniel W. Shuman, "The Privilege Study: The Psychotherapist-Patient Privilege in Civil and Common Law Countries," *Proceedings, Sixth World Congress on Medical Law* (Ghent, Belgium, 1984), pp. 73–77.

15. "Code de déontologie médicale," Décret No. 79–506 du Juin 1979, *Journal Officiel de la Republique Française* (June 30, 1979).

16. California Supreme Court, *Tarasoff* v. *Regents of the University of California,* 131 Cal. Rptr. 14 (decided July 1, 1976).

17. Raanan Gillon, "Confidentiality," *British Medical Journal* 291 (1985), pp. 1634–36; Huw W.S. Francis, "Of Gossips, Eavesdroppers, and Peeping Toms," *Journal of Medical Ethics* 8 (1982), pp. 134–43.

18. Leon Gordis, Ellen Gold, and Raymond Seltser, "Privacy Protection in Epidemiologic and Medical Research: A Challenge and a Responsibility," *American Journal of Epidemiology* 105 (1977), pp. 163–68; Charles Marwick, "Epidemiologists Strive to Maintain Confidentiality of Some Health Data," *Journal of the American Medical Association* 252 (1984), pp. 2377–83; W. E. Waters, "Ethics and Epidemiological Research," *International Journal of Epidemiology* 14 (1985), pp. 48–51.

19. Comité Consultatif National d'Éthique pour les Sciences de la Vie et de la Santé, "Avis sur les registres médicaux pour études épidémiologiques et de prévention," *Journées Annuelles d'Éthique 1985* (Paris: INSERM, 1985), pp. 13–14.

20. Louis René, "Secret médical et collecte de renseignements médicaux à usage épidémiologique," *Lettre d'Information du Comité Consultatif* No. 4 (April 1986), p. 3.

21. Conversation with Catherine Labrusse-Riou, member of the Comité Consultatif National d'Éthique (June 25, 1986).

22. "Code de déontologie médicale," Titre I, Articles 6 and 7; Titre II, Article 42: "Pour des raisons légitimes que le médecin apprécie en conscience, un malade peut être laissé dans l'ignorance d'un diagnostic ou un pronostic grave."

23. Conversation with Catherine Labrusse-Riou.

24. Pierre Arpaillange, Sophie Dion, and Georges Mathe, "Proposal for Ethical Standards in Therapeutic Trials," *British Medical Journal* 291 (1985), pp. 887–89.

25. *Ibid.,* p. 887.

26. Assistance Publique Hôpitaux de Paris, "Recommendations concernant les essais therapeutiques sur des voluntaires sains," *Lettre d'Information du Comité Consultatif* No. 3 (January 1986), p. 2.

27. Ian Kennedy, *The Unmasking of Medicine* (London: Granada, 1983).

28. Robert Schwartz and Andrew Grubb, "Why Britain Can't Afford Informed Consent," *Hastings Center Report* 15, No. 4 (August 1985), pp. 19–25; Diana Brahams, "Doctor's Duty to Inform Patient of Substantial or Special Risks When Offering Treatment," *Lancet* (March 2, 1985), pp. 528–30.

29. Schwartz and Grubb, *op. cit.,* p. 22.

30. J. Seale, "AIDS Virus Infection: Prognosis and Transmission," *Journal of the Royal Society of Medicine* 79 (February 1986), p. 122; Jean-Baptiste Brunet *et al.,* "Epidemiological Aspects of Acquired Immune Deficiency Syndrome in France," *Annals of the New York Academy of Sciences* (*A.I.D.S.*), Vol. 437, p. 334.

31. Jacques Leibowitch, *A Strange Virus of Unknown Origin,* trans. by Richard Howard, introduction by Robert C. Gallo (New York: Ballantine Books, 1985), p. 93.

32. *Ibid.*, pp. 92–94.
33. Centers for Disease Control, "Additional Recommendations to Reduce Sexual and Drug Abuse-Related Transmission of Human T-Lymphotropic Virus Type III/Lymphadenopathy-Associated Virus," *Morbidity and Mortality Weekly Report* 35 (March 14, 1986), pp. 152–55.
34. Acheson, *op. cit.*, pp. 662–66; David Miller *et al.,* "HTLV-III: Should Testing Ever Be Routine?" *British Medical Journal* 292 (April 5, 1986), pp. 941–43.
35. Advertisement in *GLC Voice* (Minneapolis, November 4, 1985), p. 10.
36. Michael Helquist, "The State of the Science: Taking the Test in Europe," *Coming Up!* 7, No. 4 (January 1986).
37. See, for example, "Notes and News: HTLV-III Antibody Screening," *Lancet* (August 31, 1985), p. 513.
38. Comité Consultatif National d'Éthique pour les Sciences de la Vie et de la Santé, "Avis concernant les problèmes éthiques posés par l'appréciation des risques du SIDA par la recherche d'anti-corps spécifiques chez les donneurs de sang," *Lettre d'Information du Comité Consultatif* No. 1 (July 1985), p. 1.
39. Acheson, *op. cit.*, p. 664.
40. "Notes and News: Public Information Campaign on AIDS," *Lancet* (March 22, 1986), p. 694.
41. "Are You at Risk from AIDS?" full page notice in the *Observer* (March 16–17, 1986).
42. Marlene Cimons, "AIDS Education Plans Halted to Avoid Uproar over Explicit Advice," *Minneapolis Star and Tribune* (December 4, 1985), p. 11A.
43. See, for example, Joe Kimball, "Officials Balk at Paying for AIDS Ad with Unclothed Man," *Minneapolis Star and Tribune* (June 17, 1986), pp. 1B and 5B; Lewis Cope, "Ad Blitz about AIDS Begins," *Minneapolis Star and Tribune* (August 9, 1986), pp. 1C and 6C.
44. "Surgeon General Calls for Early AIDS Education, Opposes Compulsory Tests," *Minneapolis Star and Tribune* (October 22, 1986).
45. "Huge AIDS Effort Urged," *St. Paul Pioneer Press and Dispatch* (October 30, 1986), pp. 1A and 4A.
46. Otis Stuart, "Ghosts," *New York Native* No. 139 (December 16–22, 1985), pp. 33 and 37.
47. Gerard Koskovich, "Letter from Paris," *The Advocate* No. 441 (March 4, 1986), pp. 31–32.
48. Randy Shilts, "Dutch Speedy, Others Lag on AIDS Warnings," *San Francisco Chronicle* (January 3, 1986).
49. "Lack of Funds Hampers European Efforts to Halt Spread of AIDS," *New York Times* (November 11, 1985).
50. Shilts, *op. cit.*
51. Jim Klobuchar, "Sermonette Would Play Well in Oslo," *Minneapolis Star and Tribune* (July 31, 1986), p. 1B. For an illustration of the use of advertising techniques to educate physicians about control of staph infection when standard educational efforts failed, see "When Wonder Drugs Don't Work," NOVA Broadcast (London: BBC-TV, 1986).
52. The Public Health (Infectious Diseases) Regulations 1985 (Statutory Instrument 1985) No. 434, Section 3.
53. "Detaining Patients with AIDS," *British Medical Journal* 291 (October 19, 1985), p. 1,102.
54. C. Thompson *et al.,* "AIDS: Dilemmas for the Psychiatrist," *Lancet* (February 1, 1986), pp. 269–70; responses in *Lancet* (March 1, 1986), pp. 496–97.
55. Mills, Wofsy, and Mills, *op. cit.*, p. 935.
56. "N.Y. Rule Curbing Gay Sex Practices Becomes Law," *Minneapolis Star and Tribune* (December 21, 1985).
57. "In Search of 'Moral Danger,'" *The Body Politic* (July 1985), p. 25.
58. "Swedish Government Considering Drastic Action to Stop AIDS," *Equal Time* (November 13, 1985) (reprinted from *New York Native*); Shilts, *op. cit.;* "HTLV-III Carrier Detained in Swedish Hospital," *American Medical News* (February 7, 1986), p. 8.
59. A. H. Robertson, *Human Rights in Europe* (Manchester: Manchester University Press, 1977); Paul Sieghart, *The International Law of Human Rights* (Oxford: Clarendon Press, 1983).
60. Brownlie, *op. cit.*, p. 343.
61. "Just Satisfaction under the Convention: Dudgeon Case," *European Law Review* 8 (1983), p. 205.

62. Helquist, *op. cit.*
63. "Excerpts from the Court Opinions on Homosexual Relations," *New York Times* (July 1, 1986), p. A18.
64. William F. Woo, "AIDS Epidemic and the Georgia Ruling," *St. Louis Post-Dispatch* (July 6, 1986). For a full discussion of this issue, see Chris D. Nichols, "AIDS—A New Reason to Regulate Homosexuality?" *Journal of Contemporary Law* 11 (1984), pp. 315–43.
65. Robert Pear, "AIDS Victims Gain in Fight on Rights," *New York Times* (June 8, 1986), pp. 1 and 19.
66. Robert Pear, "Rights Laws Offer Only Limited Help on AIDS, U.S. Rules," *New York Times* (June 23, 1986), pp. A1 and A13.
67. "AIDS Decision Scorned," *Minneapolis Star and Tribune* (July 22, 1986), p. 10B.

Part IV

Sexual Autonomy and the Constitution

Preview

If the legal distinctions between the intimacies of marriage and homosexual sodomy are lost, it is certainly possible to make the assumption, perhaps unprovable at this time, that the order of society, our way of life, could be changed in a harmful way.—Michael J. Bowers (the attorney general of Georgia)[1]

"People *should* make [basic life] choices in as imaginative, creative, exploratory, and inventive a way as human wit can devise, consulting one's personal desires, wants, needs, competences, and how one most harmoniously wishes them concurrently and complementarily to develop and be satisfied over a lifetime. Perhaps people fear freedom in this sense, preferring conventional solutions. That is their right. But such choices deserve no special moral approbation; they do not help us more rationally and courageously to choose our lives. In this sense, the constitutional right to privacy protects not only the autonomy rights of individuals, but facilitates the social and moral good that experiments in living afford to society at large—refreshing and deepening the social imagination about the role of children in human life, about the improper force of 'masculine' and 'feminine' stereotypes in human love and work, and about the varieties of human sexual arrangements."—David A.J. Richards (professor of law at New York University)[2]

As Professor Richards has noted, one can see in the Devlin-Hart debate of the late 1950s a repetition of many of the arguments that were used a century ago in the debate between Stephen and Mill. Today, we can see the Stephen-Devlin legacy in Bowers's manifestation of concern that important changes in moral ideas will threaten or harm society, while the Mill-Hart tradition is reflected in Richards's celebration of choice and his optimistic assertion that the social changes resulting from unconventional choices will benefit society.

On June 30, 1986, the U.S. Supreme Court decided *Bowers* v. *Hardwick*.[3] In a 5–4 decision, the Court held that the Constitution does not confer a fundamental right upon homosexuals to engage in sodomy, and, hence, the individual states may legally prohibit such acts.

Michael Hardwick, the respondent in this case, was arrested for sodomy in his own bedroom.[4] The police arrived at Hardwick's door to see him about an unrelated charge—a ticket for public drunkenness that Hardwick claims he had long since paid. Hardwick (a gay bartender) received the ticket as he was leaving his place of work. According to Hardwick, he left at 6:00 A.M. because he had been working on a sound system. Although he did not pay the fine on the appointed date, he did settle the matter in person at a later time. Thus, Hardwick was not expecting to be visited by the police. A houseguest answered the door and let the officer in. Not knowing that Hardwick had company, the guest said that Hardwick was in his room. The officer went to Hardwick's bedroom, caught him in the act of consensual fellatio, and arrested him. Although the charges were later dropped, Hardwick sued Michael J. Bowers, the attorney general of Georgia, in hopes of achieving Supreme Court review of a law that had, he thought, "inadequate rationale." According to the Georgia statute:

> A person commits the offense of sodomy when he performs or submits to any sexual act involving the sex organs of one person and the mouth or anus of another.

It is important to note at the outset that the issue before the Court in *Bowers* v. *Hardwick* was whether to affirm a lower court ruling that Georgia, in order to keep its sodomy statute, would have to demonstrate that it promoted a compelling state interest. However, Michael Hardwick's winning the case would not have made Georgia's sodomy law unconstitutional; it simply would have required Georgia to show that its sodomy statute serves some legitimate state objective and is the most narrowly drawn means of achieving that end.

Bowers is an example of legal moralism *par excellence*. As we have seen, Patrick Devlin takes the view that morality is ultimately a matter of feeling—in particular, feelings of disgust, indignation, and intolerance on the part of ordinary people. Moreover, he claims that moral views should be legally enforced if these feelings are sufficiently intense (reach "concert pitch," as H.L.A. Hart puts it). These feelings need not be based on any rational considerations. In essence, the majority of the Court said that there is no fundamental right to homosexual sodomy because people have strongly disapproved of it and have done so for a very long time.

For example, the majority says, "Sodomy was a criminal offense at common law and was forbidden by the laws of the original thirteen States. . . . In fact, until 1961, all 50 States outlawed sodomy, and today, 24 States and the District of Columbia continue to provide criminal penalities for sodomy performed in private and between consenting adults."[5] Chief Justice Burger says, "Decisions of individuals relating to homosexual conduct have been subject to state intervention throughout the history of Western Civilization."[6]

Bowers, in his petitioner's brief, states, "No universal principle of morality teaches that homosexual sodomy is acceptable conduct. To the contrary, traditional Judeo-Christian values proscribe such conduct. Indeed, there is no validation for sodomy found in the teaching of the ancient Greek philosophers Plato or Aristotle. More recent thinkers, such as Immanuel Kant, have found homosexual sodomy no less unnatural."[7]

In the *Laws* (the work of Plato cited by Bowers), Plato—himself a homosexual—

characterizes homosexual sex as unnatural, whereas in earlier dialogues he portrayed the intensity and delights of homosexuality,[8] even suggesting that homoerotic
experience is an important prerequisite for knowing the essence of Beauty.[9] In the
Laws, his last work, Plato maintained that heterosexuality—with its procreative
end—was inherently orderly; he approved of the use of the law to enforce what he
saw as natural, namely, orderly sexuality. Some commentators on Plato have charged
him with inconsistency. Others have said that Plato got increasingly conservative in
his old age. However, another possible interpretation exists.

Plato, in the *Laws,* was legislating for a public that, by and large, did not consist of
philosophers. Not above considerable elitism and (some say) a bit of totalitarianism,
Plato thought—as does Petitioner Bowers—that marriage, family, and procreation
were institutions designed to promote social control. Bowers says that

> homosexual sodomy is the anathema of the basic units of our society—marriage
> and the family. To decriminalize or artificially withdraw the public's expression of
> its disdain for this conduct does not uplift sodomy, but rather demotes these sa-
> cred institutions to merely other alternative life-styles. One author has described
> that result as the promotion of indifference toward these foundations of social
> order, where historically there has been endorsement.[10]

Unlike the attorney general of Georgia, Plato made an honorable pederastic exception for philosophers—an exception not needed (in the *Laws*) for members of
the general public, who lived their lives in the realm of opinion, not the realm of
knowledge.

Both Bowers and Richards—the authors of the opening quotations—cite the philosopher Kant, but to opposite ends. Bowers rightly states that Kant disapproved of
sodomy.[11] Richards cites Kant as a founder of the idea of human rights, as one "who
best articulated its radical implications for the significance of respect for moral personality."[12] Richards extends the Kantian idea of the importance of autonomy (self-
determination) to sexuality: "Sexuality . . . is not a spiritually empty experience that
the state may compulsorily legitimize only in the form of rigid, marital procreational
sex, but one of the fundamental experiences through which, as an end in itself,
people define the meaning of their lives."[13] Rights, typically, protect certain basic interests or desires of people even if so doing makes the majority unhappy. (It is not
insignificant that in the United States we do not periodically vote on whether to keep
the Bill of Rights.) Being able to love, according to Richards, is central to human
lives. Moreover, "freedom to love means that a mature individaul must have autonomy to decide how and whether to love another."[14]

Despite Kant's talk about rights as guarantees of proper respect for moral personality or rational autonomy, Kant did not see the implications of his theory for sexual
autonomy. Of course, whenever one is developing a new theory, one may fail to see
the whole range of its possible applications. Kant, for example, never asked whether
nonhuman animals were capable of rational autonomy. In the *Lectures,* he referred
to them as "man's instruments."[15] Kant also thought women quite lacking in rational

ability and therefore did not see that they had any need for the rights of "man." Thus, both Bowers and Richards are right in citing Kant. Kant was a very conventional man. He was also one of the originators of a theory of rights with radical implications for moral and social thought.

The Supreme Court, in *Bowers,* does not take a critical view of history. It does not consider the possibility that popular prejudices can undermine individual rights in societies that are deeply rooted in sexism, heterosexism, and racism. However, the Court has not always thought of history as buttressing moral claims. Twenty years ago, Section 20–59 of the Virginia law stated:

> If any white person intermarry with a colored person, or any colored person in-termarry with a white person, he shall be guilty of a felony and shall be punished by confinement in the penitentiary for not less than one nor more than five years.[16]

In *Loving* v. *Virginia*[17] a unanimous Court found Virginia's ban on interracial mar-riages a product of "invidious racism." In that case, the Court was unpersuaded ei-ther by tradition or by the trial court's statement that "Almighty God created the races white, black, yellow, malay, and red, and he placed them on separate continents. And but for their interference with his arrangement there would be no cause for such marriages. The fact that he separated the races shows that he did not intend for the races to mix."[18] The Court was also unpersuaded by the fact that antimiscegenation statutes had been common in Virginia since colonial times and that Virginia was one of sixteen states that prohibited interracial marriage. Nonetheless, when Michael Hardwick claimed that "the presumed belief of a majority of the electorate in Georgia that homosexual sodomy is immoral and unacceptable" is an "inadequate rationale to support the law," the Court said simply, "we do not agree."[19]

Justice Blackmun, in his dissenting opinion in *Bowers,* had the following com-ments on using the history of ideas as support for contemporary moral argument: "Like Justice Holmes, I believe that 'it is revolting to have no better reason for a rule of law than that it was laid down in the time of Henry IV. It is still more revolting if the grounds upon which it was laid down have vanished long since . . . .'"[20] In this regard, it is important to give serious attention to the later essays of Susan Nicholson and David Richards, who, in interestingly different ways, show how and why the pro-creative model of sexuality has been rejected.

There is an important feature of Devlin's legal moralism that is relevant to the outcome of *Bowers.* Devlin noted that "the limits of tolerance shift." Although, in his view, we are justified in passing laws on no other basis than deeply held feelings of disapproval, when the limits of tolerance shift, we should change the laws. Polls in 1986 conducted by *Time* and *Newsweek* magazines showed an absence of majority approval for the outlawing of any of a variety of specific sexual practices, including oral and anal sex, between consenting adults.[21] Thus, one might argue that the Su-preme Court does not even realistically apply legal moralism of the sort articulated by Devlin.

It is also important to note, for example, that the trend of states to repeal laws against sodomy or interracial marriage has been interpreted as cutting both ways. Virginia, as we have seen, was one of sixteen states that prohibited interracial marriage in 1967. Fifteen years earlier, thirty states prohibited interracial marriage. This data was taken by the Court as showing that the limits of tolerance shift. A similar trend vis-à-vis sodomy laws was used by the Court to show that many people still oppose sodomy.[22]

From a point of view like Devlin's, there is no theoretical limit to the legal enforcement of morality. Principles—such as Mill's principle of liberty or the right to privacy—are designed to function as just such limits. Blackmun, in his dissent, laments the "overall refusal" of the Court to "consider the broad principles that have informed our treatment of privacy in specific cases."[23]

The word *privacy* does not appear in the Constitution. Nonetheless, a series of Supreme Court decisions has established a right of privacy. It is said to exist in the penumbra of certain Amendments (the relevant Amendments are listed at the beginning of Part IV) and, more philosophically, in the concept of liberty itself. (The word *liberty* is in the Constitution.)

A number of cases have established the constitutional status of a right of privacy. *Griswold* v. *Connecticut*[24] held that a right of privacy protects the use of contraceptives by married people. In this case, much was made of the fact that if contraceptives were illegal, police could enter the bedroom and search for them. *Eisenstadt* v. *Baird*[25] held that unmarried people, under the equal protection clause, also have the right to use contraceptives. *Roe* v. *Wade*[26] held that the right of privacy encompasses a woman's decision to have an abortion. *Stanley* v. *Georgia*[27] upheld the right to private possession of obscene material. Although a First Amendment case, the Court stressed the importance of one's privacy in one's own home. In the words of Justice Marshall, "[Stanley] is asserting the right to read or observe what he pleases—the right to satisfy his intellectual and emotional needs in the privacy of his own home."[28]

One way to explain the connection between the concepts of *privacy* and *liberty* is to borrow some thoughts from J. S. Mill. As we have seen in the introduction to Part II, Mill advanced roughly the following principle of liberty: People (competent adults, not children) should be allowed to voice their opinions and direct their lives as they see fit as long as no one else is wrongfully harmed. It follows from this principle that what one does to oneself, as long as no harm comes to another, is one's own business. A private action then is one that concerns only the actor and does not wrongly harm others. Mill adds that if more than one party is involved, all parties must give their consent. Thus, what consenting adults do, as long as others are not wrongly harmed, is private: It is their own business and not the business of the law. Given this view, it would be natural to suppose that the right of privacy would include sexual intimacies between consenting adults in their bedroom. The recognition of a right to sexual autonomy—something very much like Mill's view—was believed by many, including David Richards and Justice Blackmun, to be the Court's view in its development of privacy law. Thus, many were surprised that the Court did not extend the right of privacy to the facts in *Bowers*.

Nan Hunter, an ACLU attorney, says, "*Hardwick* . . . is a statement of unmasked contempt. . . . The ordinary processes of law—identification of governing principles, extrapolation to newly presented sets of facts, and logical application and extension to build a rational continuity of principle—just didn't seem to matter, to even merit a full explanation."[29]

With respect to prior cases on privacy, the Court said, "None of the rights announced in these cases bears any resemblance to the claimed constitutional right of homosexuals to engage in acts of sodomy. . . . No connection between family, marriage, or procreation on the one hand and homosexual activity on the other has been demonstrated. . . ."[30] Of this, Hunter says, "That's it. No reasoning, no attempt to build an intellectually defensible principle or grounding for this distinction—as if gay people don't create families, belong in families, raise children, or have the staying power for those 9.4-year-long average marriages that are the bedrock of civilized society."[31]

The complaint here is not simply that the Court did not extend the right of privacy to consensual sexual conduct between adults in their bedroom, but that the Court did not even recognize the right of privacy as the fundamental right at issue. Blackmun, in the opening sentence of his dissent, says: "This case is no more about 'a fundamental right to engage in homosexual sodomy,' as the Court purports to declare, than *Stanley* v. *Georgia* . . . was about a fundamental right to watch obscene movies. . . ."[32] To push the point, the legislature in Kansas passed a law in 1986 banning sex toys in general and vibrators in particular.[33] If a challenge to this law should ever reach the Supreme Court, no one would expect the Court to find in the Constitution a fundamental right to own a vibrator.[34] Because the legislation was part of a pornography package, we might anticipate that the right of freedom of expression and/or the right of privacy would count as a fundamental right at issue.

A law is subjected to strict scrutiny by the courts when it burdens a fundamental right. In *Roe* v. *Wade,* the abortion decision, the Court held that a right to privacy was being asserted, that privacy was a fundamental right, and that the states could not show a compelling interest in interfering with this right. As a result, many states had to rewrite their laws; in particular, laws restricting abortions in the first three months of pregnancy were invalid. The important point here is that recognition of a fundamental right triggers heightened judicial scrutiny. Very good reasons (a "compelling interest," in the language of law) must be given by a state if a law is to survive this heightened scrutiny. If widespread strict antiabortion laws are any evidence of widespread disapproval of abortion, such evidence carried no weight with the Supreme Court in *Roe.*

In a case where no fundamental right is recognized, almost any reason, however weak, will do. As we have seen in *Bowers,* moral beliefs were used as reasons without meeting any rational requirements such as those suggested by Ronald Dworkin. For example, Dworkin would not count as genuine moral convictions those claims based only on arguments from authority such as appeals to the beliefs of Plato, Kant, and the Judeo-Christian tradition. Moreover, all four dissenters in *Bowers* accused the Court of misunderstanding the moral beliefs of the Georgia electorate. Justice

Stevens, in his dissent,[35] argued that the Court cannot use the moral beliefs of the Georgia electorate to support its holding (which is addressed only to homosexuals) because Georgia voters believe that *all* sodomy, not just homosexual sodomy, is immoral and unacceptable.

There is clear evidence that Georgia broadened its sodomy law in order to be more inclusive in its condemnation of lesbian and heterosexual acts. Until 1968, Georgia defined sodomy as "the carnal knowledge and connection against the order of nature, by man with man, or in the same unnatural manner with woman."[36] In *Thompson* v. *Aldredge,*[37] the Georgia Supreme Court found that sodomy under the laws of Georgia did not prohibit lesbian cunnilingus. In *Riley* v. *Garrett,*[38] the Georgia Supreme Court held that Georgia's criminal definition of sodomy did not prohibit heterosexual cunnilingus. In *Riley,* the Georgia Court said, "there is no apparent reason why the legislature would have intended to punish a man and a woman for doing something which would not be punishable if done by two women."[39] It concluded with a quotation from *Thompson:* "The fact that the unnatural sexual act here involved is finally as loathsome and disgusting as the acts proscribed by the Code does not justify us in reading into the statutory prohibition something which the General Assembly either intentionally or inadvertently omitted."[40]

Stevens argued that the holding in *Bowers* makes sense only if (1) homosexuals have a lesser interest in liberty than do heterosexuals, or (2) selective application of the Georgia law is justified. Stevens dispensed with argument (2) above: Selective application of the law is not what Georgia wanted, as is plainly shown by the history and text of its sodomy law. The first possibility, says Stevens, is untenable: "From the standpoint of the individual, the homosexual and the heterosexual have the same interest in deciding how he will live his own life, and, more narrowly, how he will conduct himself in his personal and voluntary associations with his companions."[41]

Criminalizing sodomy, according to Richards, constitutes a failure to appreciate the importance of sexual experience in human lives apart from its procreative end:

> Sexuality has for humans the independent status of a profound ecstasy that makes available to a modern person experiences increasingly inaccessible in public life: self-transcendence, expression of private fantasy, release of inner tensions, and meaningful and acceptable expression of regressive desires to be again the free child—unafraid to lose control, playful, vulnerable, spontaneous, sensually loved. While people may choose to forego this experience, any coercive prohibition of it amounts to the deprivation of an experience central in human significance.[42]

It is interesting to note that the United States government has thought it reasonable to provide heterosexual male soldiers with recreational sex. Like "soda pop and ice cream," says Susan Brownmiller, the U.S. military in Vietnam thought of "women's bodies as a necessary provision . . . to keep our boys healthy and happy."[43] Brothels controlled and regulated by the U.S. military existed within the base camps. Such brothels, reports Brownmiller, "were built by decision of a division commander, a two-star general, and were under the direct operational control of a brigade commander with the rank of colonel. Clearly, Army brothels in Vietnam existed by the grace of Army Chief of Staff William C. Westmoreland, the United States Embassy in Saigon, and the Pentagon."[44] High rates of venereal disease motivated the government funding of brothels on base. One company commander reported that he "kept six girls sequestered on his part of the base and had them shot full of penicillin every day."[45]

We do not know to what extent, if any, the Supreme Court's antisodomy ruling was influenced by the AIDS crisis. We do know that two friend-of-the-court briefs addressing AIDS were filed. One is by David Robinson, Jr., a law professor at George Washington University, who argued that the Georgia sodomy law is justified as a health measure. A second brief, filed jointly by the American Psychological Association and the American Public Health Association, called Robinson's claim "simply not true." These organizations asserted that the Georgia statute disserves the legitimate objectives of improving the public health and individual mental health.

Even if sodomy statutes were not typically overbroad (including sex acts unrelated to the transmission of AIDS) and underbroad (failing to include sex acts related to the transmission of AIDS), it is unclear that criminalizing sodomy would effectively deter sex acts that may transmit AIDS. Such statutes do nothing to foster social cooperation, deepening, as they do, a sense of injustice on the part of gays. As Kleinberg puts it, "The recent Supreme Court decision regarding sodomy laws is an enormous insult to a community in crisis. . . ."[46] Such considerations aside, had the Court ruled in Hardwick's favor, Georgia could have made its case—on the basis of public health or whatever—for its sodomy statute. In his friend-of-the-court brief, Robinson argues that Georgia should not be subjected to standards of precision in a health crisis. Referring to AIDS, Robinson says, "We are faced with a public health catastrophe of historic proportions. The States must be able to act with incomplete information, for the alternative is inaction, and inaction itself poses grave peril. To ask that legislatures act with the surgical precision which would be required by the Court of Appeals is to seek the impossible and to state that the law is to be helpless while thousands continue to be infected and to die."[47] It could be argued, however, that hard intellectual work is exactly what is now needed. At a time when we have little available except education to combat both the disease and public fear of the disease, it would seem reasonable to ask legislators, as well as anyone else, to engage in careful and rigorous thought.

Notes

1. Brief for Petitioner, *Bowers* v. *Hardwick* 106 S.Ct. 2841 (1986), p. 38.
2. David A.J. Richards, *Sex, Drugs, Death, and the Law: An Essay on Human Rights and Overcriminalization* (Totowa, N.J.: Rowman & Littlefield, 1982), p. 61.
3. 106 S.Ct. 2841 (1986).
4. The facts surrounding Hardwick's arrest are found in an interview with him in *The Advocate* (September 2, 1986), pp. 38–41, 110. See also Donahue Transcript #07116 (Cincinnati: Multimedia Entertainment, Inc., 1986).

5. 106 S.Ct. 2841, 2844, 2845 (1986).

6. 106 S.Ct. 2841, 2847 (1986).

7. Petitioner's Brief, *op. cit.,* p. 20.

8. See, for example, the *Symposium* and the *Phaedrus.*

9. Gregory Vlastos, foremost authority on Plato, gives this interpretation. See "The Individual as an Object of Love in Plato," *Platonic Studies* (Princeton: Princeton University Press, 1973). See, in particular, Appendix II (*Sex in Platonic Love*), pp. 38–42.

10. Petitioner's Brief, *op. cit.,* pp. 37–38.

11. Immanuel Kant, *Lectures on Ethics,* trans. Louis Infield (Cambridge: Hackett Publishing Company, 1979), p. 170.

12. Richards, *op. cit.,* p. 31.

13. *Ibid.,* p. 52.

14. *Ibid.,* p. 55.

15. Kant, *op. cit.,* p. 240.

16. *Loving* v. *Virginia,* 388 U.S. 1 (1967).

17. 388 U.S. 1, 3 (1967).

18. *Ibid.*

19. 106 S.Ct. 2841, 2846 (1986).

20. 106 S.Ct. 2841, 2848 (1986).

21. "Sex Busters," *Time* (July 21, 1986), p. 22. See also "Poll Shows Americans Disapprove of Ruling," *The Advocate* (August 5, 1986), p. 11.

22. In a footnote, Justice Stevens comments, "Interestingly miscegenation was once treated as a crime similar to sodomy." 106 S.Ct. 2841, 2857 (1986).

23. 106 S.Ct. 2841, 2852 (1986).

24. 381 U.S. 479 (1965).

25. 405 U.S. 438 (1972).

26. 410 U.S. 113 (1973).

27. 394 U.S. 557 (1969).

28. 394 U.S. 557, 565 (1969).

29. Nan D. Hunter, "Banned in the U.S.A.: What the Sodomy Ruling Will Mean," *The Village Voice* (July 22, 1986), pp. 15–16.

30. 106 S.Ct. 2841, 2844 (1986).

31. Hunter, *op. cit.,* p. 15.

32. 106 S.Ct. 2841, 2848 (1986).

33. "Sex Busters," *op. cit.,* p. 21.

34. Thanks to Beth Timson for this point.

35. Justice Stevens was joined in his dissent by Justices Brennan and Marshall. This dissenting opinion is not reprinted in this volume due to considerations of space.

36. Georgia Criminal Code 26–5901 (1933).

37. 187 Ga. 467, 200 S.E. 799 (1939).

38. 219 Ga. 345, 133 S.E.2d 367 (1963).

39. 219 Ga. 345, 347, 133 S.E.2d 367 (1963).

40. 219 Ga. 345, 347, 348, 133 S.E.2d 367 (1963).

41. 106 S.Ct. 2841, 2858 (1986).

42. Richards, *op. cit.,* p. 53.

43. Susan Brownmiller, *Against Our Will* (New York: Bantam Books, 1976), p. 94.

44. *Ibid.,* p. 98.

45. *Ibid.*

46. Seymour Kleinberg, "Life After Death," *The New Republic* (August 11 and 18, 1986), p. 28.

47. Brief of David Robinson, Jr., as *Amicus Curiae* in Support of Petitioners, pp. 41–42.

Selected Amendments from the Bill of Rights

Amendment I

Congress shall make no law respecting an establishment of religion, or prohibiting the free exercise thereof; or abridging the freedom of speech, or of the press; or the right of the people peaceably to assemble, and to petition the Government for a redress of grievances.

Amendment IV

The right of the people to be secure in their persons, houses, papers, and effects, against unreasonable searches and seizures, shall not be violated, and no warrants shall issue, but upon probable cause, supported by oath or affirmation, and particularly describing the place to be searched, and the persons or things to be seized.

Amendment V

No person shall be held to answer for a capital, or otherwise infamous crime, unless on a presentment or indictment of a grand jury, except in cases arising in the land or naval forces, or in the militia, when in actual service in time of war or public danger; nor shall any person be subject for the same offense to be twice put in jeopardy of life or limb; nor shall be compelled in any criminal case to be a witness against himself, nor be deprived of life, liberty, or property, without due process of law; nor shall private property be taken for public use, without just compensation.

Amendment VIII

Excessive bail shall not be required, nor excessive fines imposed, nor cruel and unusual punishments inflicted.

Amendment IX

The enumeration in the Constitution, of certain rights, shall not be construed to deny or disparage others retained by the people.

Amendment X

The powers not delegated to the United States by the Constitution, nor prohibited by it to the States, are reserved to the States respectively, or to the people.

Amendment XIV, Section 1

All persons born or naturalized in the United States, and subject to the jurisdiction thereof, are citizens of the United States and of the State wherein they reside. No State shall make or enforce any law which shall abridge the privileges or immunities of citizens of the United States; nor shall any State deprive any person of life, liberty, or property, without due process of law; nor deny to any person within its jurisdiction the equal protection of the laws.

Sinful Sex

SUSAN T. NICHOLSON

Abortion as a Sin of Sex

The Roman Catholic condemnation of abortion is complex in that typically it has two sources: (1) an ethic of sex, and (2) an ethic of killing. For reasons to be explained subsequently, this study focuses on abortion as it relates to the Catholic ethic of killing. Nevertheless, it is instructive to identify those aspects of Catholic sexual doctrine which are relevant to abortion.

Many non-Catholics and Catholics alike associate abortion with nonmarital sexual relations. Women who abort are frequently perceived as destroying evidence of and evading responsibility for their nonmarital sexual activity. Correlatively, restrictive abortion laws are urged as a deterrent to, or punishment for, such supposed sexual immorality. A standard rebuttal of this position consists in pointing out that a large percentage of women who abort have conceived as a result of marital sex.

It perhaps is not generally recognized that this rebuttal does not touch the singularly Roman Catholic association of abortion with sexual sin. Throughout its history, Roman Catholic leadership has sought to maintain, in one form or another, a link between sexual activity and procreation.[1] In its present form, church doctrine forbids the separation of the unitive (love-fostering) aspect of sexuality from the procreative aspect. This principle underlies the papal reaffirmation of the immorality of artificial birth control (Paul VI, 1968), and by it, all abortion stands equally condemned. Abortion deliberately deprives a preceding sexual act of its procreative aspect while leaving its unitive aspect intact. Abortion, thus, is held to be wrong, and the marital status of the sexual couple is irrelevant to this species of sexual sin.

It follows that even if the fetus were not a human being, Catholics would still view abortion as evil. This explains why the condemnation of abortion did not falter during those periods when Church fathers rejected the notion that a human being was present from conception onwards.

Reprinted by permission of *The Journal of Religious Ethics.*

Catholic insistence on the procreative function of sexuality is sometimes believed to arise from a desire for a high Catholic birth rate. This interpretation is inconsistent, however, with the superior position accorded virginity in Catholic doctrine. In the medieval period, some theologians accorded special honor to the virginity or complete sexual abstinence even of married couples. . . .

I suggest that the emphasis upon the procreative aspect of sexuality reflects instead a hostility toward sexual pleasure. For all but the last hundred years of the Church's history, theologians generally considered it at least venial, and perhaps mortal sin, to engage in sexual relations for the purpose of experiencing sexual pleasure. By insisting that sex be procreative, Catholic moralists were able to limit sharply the extent and variety of sexual pleasure, and to "excuse" what pleasure remained by reference to the child-rearing services the sexual couple rendered the species.

One effect of this theological *animus* toward sexual pleasure was the elimination of any basis for a connection between sexual pleasure and the expression of love. If one cannot legitimately seek sensuous pleasure in sexual experience, then the arousal and gratification of sensuous desires cannot be an embodiment of a virtuous love. Thus, while love was a vaunted Christian virtue, and although marital love was required of those engaging in sexual acts, the obedient Catholic couple was one who in an important sense experienced *sex without love*.

This stunning impoverishment of life was imposed upon Catholics by exclusively male and predominantly celibate theologians for almost 19 centuries. It was not, in fact, until 1852 that a Catholic theologian, Gury, thought to suggest that a legitimate function of marital sex might be the promotion of love . . . . As noted, present Church doctrine gives equal weight to the unitive and procreative aspects of marital sex. In refusing to grant complete independence to the unitive aspect, however, the Catholic Church is still captive to its traditional antipathy to erotic love. A brief historical sketch will illustrate the role of this antipathy in the Roman Catholic condemnation of abortion.

Early Church theologians taught that intercourse was immoral unless engaged in for the purpose of procreation. According to [John T.] Noonan . . . , this rule, lacking any explicit biblical basis, was borrowed from the teaching of the Roman Stoics, Musonius Rufus and Seneca. This places the intellectual heritage of the Catholic sexual ethic in a philosophical movement whose adherents sought to make themselves invulnerable to misfortune by freeing themselves of attachment to whatever was not under their control. A "tranquil flow of life" was thus achieved at the cost of a deadening of affect in certain areas. This theme is apparent in the works of the two best known Roman Stoics, Epictetus (c. A.D. 50–c. A.D. 130) and Marcus Aurelius (A.D. 121–A.D. 180).

Epictetus taught that one who would be free must learn to desire only what was totally within one's power. Marcus Aurelius strove for equanimity by observing that no matter what men might do to him, they could not alter the justice, purity, wisdom, and sobriety of his mind. Attaching value only to what was thus completely subject to his control, Marcus Aurelius was led to an affirmation of the Socratic view that it is not within the power of an evil man to harm a good one.

Like the *Apology* (28d–30a, 41d) in which Socrates makes this surprising claim,[2] Marcus Aurelius's *Meditations* is pervaded by a strong sense of impending death. Death is, of course, the final misfortune, and the dissolution of the body in death is undeniable. From a psychological point of view, both the trilogy relating the trial and death of Socrates and *Meditations* give the impression that the authors have reacted to the agonizing brevity of bodily existence by denying themselves the experience of human goods in which the body plays a conspicuous role. Socrates is never more lyrical in describing the philosophical flight from the body, nor more vivid in portraying the manner in which bodily pleasures imprison the soul, than in the dialogue which takes place on the day he knows he is to die.[3]

I am suggesting that the restrictive Roman Catholic sexual ethic might plausibly be viewed as originating in a self-protective withdrawal from whatever is subject to loss. Sexual pleasures are especially to be abjured, as they are capable of evoking the most intense attachment to the body and to another human being, neither of which is totally within one's control. Pleasure in sexual experience must consequently be extirpated, or at least strictly curtailed. Faced with inevitable human loss, a most stringent prophylactic is proposed: Anticipate that loss by a self-imposed deprivation.

It is Noonan's view that the rule of procreative intent arose and was reaffirmed in early Christianity partially in reaction to two rival religious movements—Gnosticism and Manicheanism—which rigorously condemned procreation. Both the Gnostics and the Manichees were suspected by the orthodox Christian of assigning non-procreative sexual activity a central place in their religious rites. It was believed, for example, that the Gnostics engaged in ritual meals of human semen and menses, the semen having been procured by *coitus interruptus,* masturbation, or homosexual acts . . . . A reaction to Manichean doctrine would appear to be especially likely in the case of St. Augustine, who had himself been an earlier devotee of the Manichean movement.

Whatever its origins, insistence on a subjective procreative intent in sexual activity was incorporated into the teaching of St. Augustine (354–430), where it was to exercise a dominant influence on the Church for the next ten centuries . . . . Adoption of the procreative requirement as formulated by Augustine implies the immorality of the following:

1. Sexual acts other than intercourse
2. Intercourse which was believed to be, or was deliberately made to be, incapable of procreation
3. Intercourse which was believed to be capable of procreation but which was not performed solely for that purpose[4]

The first category includes all sexual activity between persons of the same sex, heterosexual activity such as anal or oral sex, and *coitus interruptus*. The second category includes intercourse with a person believed to be sterile, as well as intercourse during what was erroneously believed to be a monthly sterile period in women. It also includes the use of whatever was believed to have contraceptive properties, such as herbal potions and salves.

It is evident that Augustine's teaching originated in an aversion to sexual pleasure rather than in a concern that there be more births. In fact, he was indifferent even to the survival of the species. In a work in which he encouraged continence both without and within marriage, he raised the rhetorical question: "What if all men should be willing to restrain themselves from all intercourse, how would the human race survive?" Augustine . . . answered easily, "Would that all men had this wish. . . . Much more quickly would the City of God be filled and the end of time be hastened."

Augustine gave a Christian perspective to the earlier pagan denigration of sexual desires by explaining "concupiscence" as an effect of the original sin inherited by the descendants of Adam . . . . Augustine's contempt for sex nourished, or was nourished by, his low regard for women. "I feel," he wrote, "that nothing more turns the masculine mind from the heights than female blandishments and that contact of bodies without which a wife may not be had." . . . And while admitting that women were useful in generating, Augustine could not see what help a woman would be to a man apart from that . . . .

The following passage from Augustine's *Marriage and Concupiscence* is particularly relevant to our discussion.

It is one thing not to lie except with the sole will of generating: This has no fault. It is another to seek the pleasure of the flesh in lying, although within the limits of marriage: This has venial fault. I am supposing that then, although you are not lying for the sake of procreating offspring, you are not for the sake of lust obstructing their procreation by an evil prayer or an evil deed. Those who do this, although they are called husband and wife, are not; nor do they retain any reality of marriage, but with a respectable name cover a shame. They give themselves away, indeed, when they go so far as to expose the children who are born to them against their will; for they hate to nourish or to have those whom they feared to bear. Therefore, a dark iniquity rages against those whom they unwillingly have borne, and with open iniquity this comes to light; a hidden shame is demonstrated by manifest cruelty. Sometimes this lustful cruelty, or cruel lust, comes to this, that they even procure poisons of sterility and, if these do not work, extinguish and destroy the fetus in some way in the womb, preferring that their offspring die before it lives, or if it was already alive in the womb to kill it before it was born. Assuredly if both husband and wife are like this, they are not married, and if they were like this from the beginning they come together not joined in matrimony but in seduction. If both are not like this, I dare to say that either the wife is in a fashion the harlot of her husband or he is an adulterer with his own wife . . . .

Two points bear noting: (1) Augustine moves easily from a condemnation of attempts to obstruct procreation to a condemnation of abortion and infanticide. Each violates the requirement of a procreative intent in intercourse stated at the beginning of the passage.[5] (2) Augustine shows a willingness to add to the moral force of his condemnation by using terms which, properly speaking, are inapplicable. For a man to be an adulterer with his own wife is, strictly speaking, an impossibility. Other early churchmen, in a similar inflation of moral rhetoric, branded persons using contraceptive potions, men who had castrated themselves, and even homosexuals as "parricides" and "murderers" . . . . That the latter terms were so loosely used should be kept in mind when assessing the Roman Catholic claim that the Church has always opposed abortion as a sin of killing.

Beginning with the words "Sometimes this lustful cruelty," the passage was incorporated into the *Decretum* compiled by Gratian in 1140. The *Decretum* was treated as part of the basic law of the Roman Catholic Church until the enactment of the new *Code of Canon Law* in 1917. It was also incorporated into Peter Lombard's *Sentences,* a theological text of signal influence. Thus, in what Noonan . . . calls the most important teaching on contraception in the Middle Ages, abortion is discussed together with contraception as *sexual* sin.

Another classical text linking abortion and contraception was contributed by a bishop committed to the Augustinian doctrine that a procreative intent is morally required for intercourse. A letter written by Caesarius, a 6th-century bishop of Arles, contains a condemnation of abortion as homicide, followed by these words:

> Who is he who cannot warn that no woman may take a potion so that she is unable to conceive or condemns in herself the nature which God willed to be fecund. As often as she could have conceived or given birth, *of that many homicides she will be held guilty,* and, unless she undergoes suitable penance, she will be damned by eternal death in hell. If a woman does not wish to have children, let her enter into a religious agreement with her husband; for chastity is the sole sterility of a Christian woman. (. . . , italics added)

The force of the condemnation of abortion as a sin of killing is completely undercut by Caesarius's subsequent treatment of the use of contraceptive potions as homicide.[6] The last sentence in this passage suggests that the sin which is uppermost in the author's mind is not that of killing an innocent human being, but that of having sexual intercourse without the desire of procreating. Again, a term applicable to killing is wrenched from its proper context to impress upon the reader the true gravity of nonprocreative sex.

The following text, repeating the teaching of Caesarius, appears in the 11th-century *Decretum* of Buchard.

> If someone to satisfy his lust or in deliberate hatred does something to a man or woman so that no children be born of him or her, or gives them to drink, so that he cannot generate or she conceive, let it be held as homicide. . . .

This text became canon law in the 13th century, and was also preserved in the law of the Catholic Church until 1917. Although it treats both abortion and the use of contraceptive potions as homicide, it is again clear that the sin which links the two is really lust.

By the 12th century, Augustine's doctrine of procreative intent was well established. There were, however, mild dissents.

A minority of theologians maintained that intercourse might also be initiated for the purpose of avoiding extramarital sex. Although this view conflicted with Augustine's, it did not displace procreation as the sole positive value of sexual activity.

Another dispute developed over whether the seeking of pleasure in intercourse was venial sin, as Augustine had taught, or mortal sin. Some theologians holding the more severe view that the seeking of pleasure was mortal sin also believed that the mere *experiencing* of sexual pleasure during intercourse was a venial sin.

Two popes held this belief: Pope Gregory the Great (in office at the turn of the 7th century), and the 13th-century Pope Innocent III. Innocent III queried, "Who does not know that conjugal intercourse is never committed without itching of the flesh, and heat and foul concupiscence, whence the conceived seeds are befouled and corrupted?" . . . To Gregory, it was a miracle if, even with a procreative intent, one could manage to have intercourse without sin. Responding to this problem, William of Auxerre, writing at the beginning of the 16th century, was driven to propose a highly refined distinction between enjoying and suffering sexual pleasure, only the latter being free from sin.

In the 13th century, St. Thomas Aquinas accepted Augustine's requirement of procreative intent, his synthesis of original sin and sex, and his low opinion of women. In Aquinas's teaching, however, the objective rather than subjective aspect of sexual acts is prominent.

The basic Thomist assumption is that sexual acts are "by nature" ordained toward procreation. Acts which violate this natural order are injuries against God, and as such occupy the supreme position in Thomas's hierarchy of sexual sin. As a criterion of "natural," Thomas adopted the depositing of semen in the "fit vessel." . . . Thomas . . . does not shrink from drawing the conclusion that rape (in which semen is properly deposited) is a lesser sin than "unnatural" sex with one's spouse.

On Thomas's view, neither intercourse with a sterile partner nor the use of contraceptive potions was unnatural. Although both were wrong on the Augustinian view adopted by Thomas, neither impeded the depositing of semen in the vagina. Thus, one could engage in a particular sexual act which precluded procreation without sinning against nature. This, of course, does not mean that Thomas's notion of what was natural was unrelated to what was procreative. Intercourse was the only sexual act from which procreation can result.

Thomas . . . argued that the preservation of the species requires that sexual acts be directed to generation. So rational a man as he, however, must have been aware that species survival does not require that no unnatural sexual activity occur, but only that some natural activity occur. Furthermore, that Thomas was not unduly worried about the preservation of the species is evident from his preference for virginity, and for complete sexual abstinence even among the married.

During the period 1450–1750 the Augustinian doctrine was somewhat weakened. The nonprocreative purpose of avoiding fornication was accepted as a lawful one for initiating intercourse. In addition, several major theologians defended the view that to seek pleasure in marital intercourse was licit. This view, however, failed to gain majority support. Furthermore, its promoters made no mention of a connection between sexual pleasure and the expression of love.

Sanchez, a 17th-century Jesuit moralist who specialized in marriage, came closest to acknowledging the possibility of such a connection. He proposed that a marital couple might engage in "embraces, kisses, and other touching" for the purpose of showing and fostering mutual love, even though there was a foreseen "risk of pollution" (ejaculation). The very phrasing of Sanchez's thesis makes clear that he was not so temerous as to apply his analysis to *genital* touching . . . .

As the influence of Augustinian doctrine lessened, the criterion of a licit sexual act came to be the Thomist criterion of naturalness. It will be recalled that Thomas had regarded a sexual act as natural so long as it involves depositing semen in the vagina. Some theologians expanded this doctrine to condemn as unnatural any attempt to frustrate the procreative end of intercourse, even though semen be properly deposited . . . . On this analysis, abortion is again illicit for the same reason that the use of contraceptive methods in intercourse is illicit. Both impede the procreative aspect of intercourse.

It is essentially this doctrine which is held today by the Roman Catholic Church, even though recent developments have deprived it of its ancient rationale and introduced a fatal inconsistency.

One important development is the recognition of a relationship between love and sexual pleasure. Beginning in the latter part of the 19th century, Catholic theologians recognized the expression and fostering of marital love as a legitimate purpose of intercourse . . . . Since the expression of love in sexual activity is related to the mutual ability to produce expressive modulations of physical sensations which are deeply gratifying, this development in doctrine implies that it is not intrinsically evil to seek sexual pleasure.

I have suggested here that it was a hostility toward sexual pleasure which led to the Church's initial insistence that sex be linked to procreation. Procreation was the value selected to control and, so to speak, to legitimate the experience of sensuous delight in sexual experience. Consequently, if the seeking of sexual pleasure is no longer regarded as sinful, then the initial rationale for maintaining a link between sex and procreation is eliminated.

Notes

1. In what follows, I rely heavily on Noonan's . . . monumental study of the history of the Roman Catholic treatment of contraception. Noonan obviously is not responsible for my speculative interpretation of that history. John T. Noonan, Jr., *Contraception: A History of Its Treatment by the Catholic Theologians and Canonists* (Cambridge, Mass.: Harvard University Press, 1966).
2. *Meditations* contains numerous admiring references to Socrates's conduct.
3. One particularly dramatic passage in the *Phaedo* (83d) compares bodily pleasures to rivets which nail the soul to the body, thereby rendering the soul unfit for the contemplation of truth. This language is easily adaptable to Christian use by a substitution of God for truth.
4. An exception to the requirement of procreative intent was made in circumstances where inter-

course was requested, for whatever reasons, by one's spouse. In such circumstances, a response was permitted and moreover required. This exception in doctrine appears to be aimed at keeping within marital bounds the sexual activity of a spouse who was too "weak" to obey the strict procreative rule. The exception is curious in that it makes it a duty to respond to what it is a sin to initiate. . . .

5. There is, of course, the possibility that a woman who aborts engaged in intercourse with a procreative intent, but has since changed her mind. Augustine does not consider this possibility.

6. Noonan[, *op. cit.*], pp. 88–90, concludes from a survey of the biological theories of that time that no one believed that the male seed was ensouled, or was itself a human being.

Gay Basics: Some Questions, Facts, and Values

RICHARD D. MOHR

for Robert W. Switzer

Who Are Gays Anyway?

A recent Gallup poll found that only one in five Americans reports having a gay or lesbian acquaintance.[1] This finding is extraordinary given the number of practicing homosexuals in America. Alfred Kinsey's 1948 study of the sex lives of 5,000 white males shocked the nation: 37 percent had at least one homosexual experience to orgasm in their adult lives; an additional 13 percent had homosexual fantasies to orgasm; 4 percent were exclusively homosexual in their practices; another 5 percent had virtually no heterosexual experience; and nearly one-fifth had at least as many homosexual as heterosexual experiences.[2]

Two out of five men one passes on the street have had orgasmic sex with men. Every second family in the country has a member who is essentially homosexual, and many more people regularly have homosexual experiences. Who are homosexuals? They are your friends, your minister, your teacher, your bank teller, your doctor, your mail carrier, your secretary, your congressional representative, your sibling, parent, and spouse. They are everywhere, virtually all ordinary, virtually all unknown.

Several important consequences follow. First, the country is profoundly ignorant of the actual experience of gay people. Second, social attitudes and practices that are harmful to gays have a much greater overall harmful impact on society than is usually realized. Third, most gay people live in hiding—in the closet—making the "coming out" experience the central fixture of gay consciousness and invisibility the chief characteristic of the gay community.

Ignorance, Stereotype, and Morality

Ignorance about gays, however, has not stopped people from having strong opinions about them. The void which ignorance leaves has been filled with stereotypes. Society holds chiefly two groups of antigay stereotypes; the two are an oddly contradictory lot. One set of stereotypes revolves around alleged mistakes in an individual's gender identity: Lesbians are women that want to be, or at least look and act like, men—bulldykes, diesel dykes; while gay men are those who want to be, or at least look and act like, women—queens, fairies, limp-wrists, nellies. These stereotypes of mismatched genders provide the materials through which gays and lesbians become the butts of ethnic-like jokes. These stereotypes and jokes, though derisive, basically view gays and lesbians as ridiculous.

Another set of stereotypes revolves around gays as a pervasive sinister conspiratorial threat. The core stereotype here is the gay person as child molester and, more generally, as sex-crazed maniac. These stereotypes carry with them fears of the very destruction of family and civilization itself. Now, that which is essentially ridiculous can hardly have such a staggering effect. Something must be afoot in this incoherent amalgam.

Sense can be made of this incoherence if the nature of stereotypes is clarified. Stereotypes are not *simply* false generalizations from a skewed sample of cases examined. Admittedly, false generalizing plays some part in the stereotypes a society holds. If, for instance, one takes as one's sample homosexuals who are in psychiatric hospitals or prisons, as was done in nearly all early investigations, not surprisingly one will probably find homosexuals to be of a crazed and criminal cast. Such false generalizations, though, simply confirm beliefs already held on independent grounds, ones that likely led the investigator to the prison and psychiatric ward to begin with. Evelyn Hooker, who in the late '50s carried out the first rigorous studies to use non-clinical gays, found that psychiatrists, when presented with case files including all the standard diagnostic psychological profiles—but omitting indications of sexual orientation—were unable to distinguish gay files from straight ones, even though they believed gays to be crazy and supposed themselves to be experts in detecting craziness.[3] These studies proved a profound embarrassment to the psychiatric establishment, the financial well-being of which has been substantially enhanced by "curing" allegedly insane gays. The studies led the way to the American Psychiatric Association finally dropping homosexuality from its registry of mental illnesses in 1973.[4] Nevertheless, the stereotype of gays as sick continues apace in the mind of America.

False generalizations *help maintain* stereotypes, they do not *form* them. As the history of Hooker's discoveries shows, stereotypes have a life beyond facts; their origin lies in a culture's ideology—the general system of beliefs by which it lives—and they are sustained across generations by diverse cultural transmissions, hardly any of which, including slang and jokes, even purport to have a scientific basis. Stereotypes, then, are not the products of bad science but are social constructions that perform central functions in maintaining society's conception of itself.

On this understanding, it is easy to see that the antigay stereotypes surrounding gender identification are chiefly means of reinforcing still powerful gender roles in society. If, as this stereotype presumes and condemns, one is free to choose one's social roles independently of gender, many guiding social divisions, both domestic and commercial, might be threatened. The socially gender-linked distinctions between breadwinner and homemaker, boss and secretary, doctor and nurse, protector and protected would blur. The accusations "fag" and "dyke" exist in significant part to keep women in their place and to prevent men from breaking ranks and ceding away theirs.

The stereotypes of gays as child molesters, sex-crazed maniacs, and civilization destroyers function to displace (socially irresolvable) problems from their actual source to a foreign (and so, it is thought, manageable) one. Thus, the stereotype of child molester functions to give the family unit a false sheen of absolute innocence. It keeps the unit from being examined too closely for incest, child abuse, wife battering, and the terrorism of constant threats. The stereotype teaches that the problems of the family are not internal to it, but external.[5]

One can see these cultural forces at work in society's and the media's treatment of current reports of violence, especially domestic violence. When a mother kills her child or a father rapes his daughter—regular Section B fare even in major urbane papers—this is never taken by reporters, columnists, or pundits as evidence that there is something wrong with heterosexuality or with traditional families. These issues are not even raised. But when a homosexual child molestation is reported, it is taken as confirming evidence of the way homosexuals are. One never hears of heterosexual murders, but one regularly hears of "homosexual" ones. Compare the social treatment of Richard Speck's sexually motivated mass murder of Chicago nurses with that of John Wayne Gacy's murders of Chicago youths. Gacy was in the culture's mind taken as symbolic of gay men in general. To prevent the possibility that "The Family" was viewed as anything but an innocent victim in this affair, the mainstream press knowingly failed to mention that most of Gacy's adolescent victims were homeless hustlers. That knowledge would be too much for the six o'clock news and for cherished beliefs.

Because "the facts" largely don't matter when it comes to the generation and maintenance of stereotypes, the effects of scientific and academic research and of enlightenment generally will be, at best, slight and gradual in the changing fortunes of lesbians and gay men. If this account of stereotypes holds, society has been profoundly immoral. For its treatment of gays is a grand scale rationalization, a moral sleight-of-hand. The problem is not that society's usual standards of evidence and procedure in coming to judgments of social policy have been misapplied to gays; rather, when it comes to gays, the standards themselves have simply been ruled out of court and disregarded in favor of mechanisms that encourage unexamined fear and hatred.

Are Gays Discriminated Against? Does It Matter?

Partly because lots of people suppose they don't know any gay people and partly through willful ignorance of its own workings, society at large is unaware of the many ways in which gays are subject to discrimination in consequence of widespread fear and hatred. Contributing to this social ignorance of discrimination is the difficulty for gay people, as an invisible minority, even to complain of discrimination. For if one is gay, to register a complaint would suddenly target one as a stigmatized person, and so in the absence of any protections against discrimination, would simply invite additional discrimination. Further, many people, especially those who are persistently downtrodden and so lack a firm sense of self to begin with, tend either to blame themselves for their troubles or to view injustice as a matter of bad luck rather than as indicating something wrong with society. The latter recognition would require doing something to rectify wrong, and most people, especially the already beleaguered, simply aren't up to that. So for a number of reasons discrimination against gays, like rape, goes seriously underreported.

First, gays are subject to violence and harassment based simply on their perceived status rather than because of any actions they have performed. A recent extensive study by the National Gay Task Force found that over 90 percent of gays and lesbians had been victimized in some form on the basis of their sexual orientation.[6] Greater than one in five gay men and nearly one in ten lesbians had been punched, hit, or kicked, a quarter of all gays had had objects thrown at them, a third had been chased, a third had been sexually harassed, and 14 percent had been spit on—all just for being perceived as gay.

The most extreme form of antigay violence is queerbashing—where groups of young men target a person who they suppose is a gay man and beat and kick him unconscious and sometimes to death amid a torrent of taunts and slurs. Such seemingly random but in reality socially encouraged violence has the same social origin and function as lynchings of blacks—to keep a whole stigmatized group in line. As with lynchings of the recent past, the police and courts have routinely averted their eyes, giving their implicit approval to the practice.

Few such cases with gay victims reach the courts. Those that do are marked by inequitable procedures and results. Frequently judges will describe queerbashers as "just all-American boys." Recently a District of Columbia judge handed suspended sentences to queerbashers whose victim had been stalked, beaten, stripped at knifepoint, slashed, kicked, threatened with castration, and pissed on, because the judge thought the bashers were good boys at heart—after all, they went to a religious prep school.[7]

Police and juries will simply discount testimony from gays; they typically construe assaults on and murders of gays as "justified" self-defense—the killer need only claim his act was a panicked response to a sexual overture. Alternatively, when guilt seems patent, juries will accept highly implausible "diminished capacity" defenses, as in the case of Dan White's 1978 assassination of openly gay San Francisco city [supervisor] Harvey Milk—Hostess Twinkies made him do it.[8]

These inequitable procedures and results collectively show that the life and liberty of gays, like those of blacks, simply count for less than the life and liberty of members of the dominant culture.

The equitable rule of law is the heart of an orderly society. The collapse of the rule of law for gays shows that society is willing to perpetrate the worst possible injustices against them. Conceptually there is only a difference in degree between the collapse of the rule of law and systematic extermination of members of a population simply for having some group status independently of any act an individual has performed. In the Nazi concentration camps, gays were forced to wear pink triangles as identifying badges, just as Jews were forced to wear yellow stars. In remembrance of that collapse of the rule of law, the pink triangle has become the chief symbol of the gay rights movement.[9]

Gays are subject to widespread discrimination in employment—the very means by which one puts bread on one's table and one of the chief means by which individuals identify themselves to themselves and achieve personal dignity. Governments are leading offenders here. They do a lot of discriminating themselves, require that others do it ([such as] government contractors), and set precedents favoring discrimination in the private sector. The federal government explicitly discriminates against gays in the armed forces, the CIA, FBI, National Security Agency, and the State Department. The federal government refuses to give security clearances to gays and so forces the country's considerable private-sector military and aerospace contractors to fire known gay employees. State and local governments regularly fire gay teachers, policemen, firemen, social workers, and anyone who has contact with the public. Further, states through licensing laws officially bar gays from a vast array of occupations and professions—everything from doctors, lawyers, accountants, and nurses to hairdressers, morticians, and used car dealers. The American Civil Liberties Union's handbook *The Rights of Gay People* lists 307 such prohibited occupations.[10]

Gays are subject to discrimination in a wide variety of other ways, including private-sector employment, public accommodations, housing, immigration and naturalization, insurance of all types, custody and adoption, and zoning regulations that bar "singles" or "nonrelated" couples. All of these discriminations affect central components of a meaningful life; some even reach to the means by which life itself is sustained. In half the states, where gay sex is illegal, the central role of sex to meaningful life is officially denied to gays.

All these sorts of discriminations also affect the ability of people to have significant intimate relations. It is difficult for people to live together as couples without having their sexual orientation perceived in the public realm and so becoming targets for discrimination. Illegality, discrimination, and the absorption by gays of society's hatred of them all interact to impede or block altogether the ability of gays and lesbians to create and maintain significant personal relations with loved ones. So every facet of life is affected by discrimination. Only the most compelling reasons could justify it.

But Aren't They Immoral?

Many people think society's treatment of gays is justified because they think gays are extremely immoral. To evaluate this claim, different sense of *moral* must be distinguished. Sometimes by *morality* is meant the overall beliefs affecting behavior in a society—its mores, norms, and customs. On this understanding, gays certainly are not moral: Lots of people hate them and social customs are designed to register widespread disapproval of gays. The problem here is that this sense of morality is merely a *descriptive* one. On this understanding *every* society has a morality—even Nazi society, which had racism and mob rule as central features of its "morality" understood in this sense. What is needed in order to use the notion of morality to praise or condemn behavior is a sense of morality that is *prescriptive* or *normative*— a sense of morality whereby, for instance, the descriptive morality of the Nazis is found wanting.

As the Nazi example makes clear, that something is descriptively moral is nowhere near enough to make it normatively moral. [The fact that] a lot of people in a society say something is good, even over eons, does not make it so. Our rejection of the long history of socially approved and state-enforced slavery is another good example of this principle at work. Slavery would be wrong even if nearly everyone liked it. So consistency and fairness require that we abandon the belief that gays are immoral simply because most people dislike or disapprove of gays or gay acts, or even because gay sex acts are illegal.

Furthermore, recent historical and anthropological research has shown that opinion about gays has been by no means universally negative. Historically, it has varied widely even within the larger part of the Christian era and even within the church itself.[11] There are even societies—current ones—where homosexuality is not only tolerated but a universal compulsory part of social maturation.[12] Within the last thirty years, American society has undergone a grand turnabout from deeply ingrained, near total condemnation to near total acceptance on two emotionally charged "moral" or "family" issues: contraception and divorce. Society holds its current descriptive morality of gays not because it has to, but because it chooses to.

If popular opinion and custom are not enough to ground moral condemnation of homosexuality, perhaps religion can. Such argument[s] proceed along two lines. One claims that the condemnation is a direct revelation of God, usually through the Bible; the other claims to be able to detect condemnation in God's plan as manifested in nature.

One of the more remarkable discoveries of recent gay research is that the Bible may not be as univocal in its condemnation of homosexuality as has been usually believed.[13] Christ never mention[ed] homosexuality. Recent interpreters of the Old Testament have pointed out that the story of Lot at Sodom is probably intended to condemn inhospitality rather than homosexuality. Further, some of the Old Testament condemnations of homosexuality seem simply to be ways of tarring those of the Israelites' opponents who happen to accept homosexual practices when the Israelites themselves did not. If so, the condemnation is merely a quirk of history and rhetoric rather than a moral precept.

What does seem clear is that those who regularly cite the Bible to condemn an activity like homosexuality do so by reading it selectively. Do ministers who cite what they take to be condemnations of homosexuality in Leviticus maintain in their lives all the hygienic and dietary laws of Leviticus? If they cite the story of Lot at Sodom to condemn homosexuality, do they also cite the story of Lot in the cave to praise incestuous rape? It seems then not that the Bible is being used to ground condemnations of homosexuality as much as society's dislike of homosexuality is being used to interpret the Bible.[14]

Even if a consistent portrait of condemnation could be gleaned from the Bible, what social significance should it be given? One of the guiding principles of society, enshrined in the [U.S.] Constitution as a check against the government, is that decisions affecting social policy are not made on religious grounds. If the real ground of the alleged immorality invoked by governments to discriminate against gays is religious (as it has explicitly been even in some recent court cases involving teachers and guardians), then one of the major commitments of our nation is violated.

But Aren't They Unnatural?

The most noteworthy feature of the accusation of something being unnatural (where a moral rather than an advertising point is being made) is that the plaint is so infrequently made. One used to hear the charge leveled against abortion, but that has pretty much faded as antiabortionists have come to lay all their chips on the hope that people will come to view abortion as murder. Incest used to be considered unnatural but discourse now usually assimilates it to the moral machinery of rape and violated trust. The charge comes up now in ordinary discourse only against homosexuality. This suggests that the charge is highly idiosyncratic and has little, if any, explanatory force. It fails to put homosexuality in a class with anything else so that one can learn by comparison with clear cases of the class just exactly what it is that is allegedly wrong with it.

Though the accusation of unnaturalness looks whimsical, in actual ordinary discourse when applied to homosexuality, it is usually delivered with venom of forethought. It carries a high emotional charge, usually expressing disgust and evincing queasiness. Probably it is nothing but an emotional charge. For people get equally disgusted and queasy at all sorts of things that are perfectly natural—to be expected in nature apart from artifice—and that could hardly be fit subjects for moral condemnation. Two typical examples in current American culture are some people's responses to mothers' suckling in public and to women who do not shave body hair. When people have strong emotional reactions, as they do in these cases, without being able to give good reasons for them, we think of them not as operating morally, but rather as being obsessed and manic. So the feelings of disgust that some people have to gays will hardly ground a charge of immorality. People fling the term *unnatural* against gays in the same breath and with the same force as when they call gays "sick" and "gross." When they do this, they give every appearance of being neurotically fearful and incapable of reasoned discourse.

When *nature* is taken in *technical* rather than ordinary usage, it looks like the notion also will not ground a charge of homosexual immorality. When *unnatural* means "by artifice" or "made by humans," it need only be pointed out that virtually everything that is good about life is unnatural in this sense, that the chief feature that distinguishes people from other animals is their very ability to make over the world to meet their needs and desires, and that their well-being depends upon these departures from nature. On this understanding of human nature and the natural, homosexuality is perfectly unobjectionable.

Another technical sense of *natural* is that something is natural, and so, good, if it fulfills some function in nature. Homosexuality on this view is unnatural because it allegedly violates the function of genitals, which is to produce babies. One problem with this view is that lots of bodily parts have lots of functions and just because some one activity can be fulfilled by only one organ (say, the mouth for eating) this activity does not condemn other functions of the organ to immorality (say, the mouth for talking, licking stamps, blowing bubbles, or having sex). So the possible use of the genitals to produce children does not, without more, condemn the use of the genitals for other purposes, say, achieving ecstasy and intimacy.

The functional view of nature will only provide a morally condemnatory sense to the unnatural if a thing which might have many uses has but one proper function to the exclusion of other possible functions. But whether this is so cannot be established simply by looking at the thing. For what is seen is all its possible functions. The notion of function seemed like it might ground moral authority, but instead it turns out that moral authority is needed to define proper function. Some people try to fill in this moral authority by appeal to the "design" or "order" of an organ, saying, for instance, that the genitals are designed for the purpose of procreation. But these people cheat intellectually if they do not make explicit *who* the designer and orderer is. If it is God, we are back to square one—holding others accountable for religious beliefs.

Further, ordinary moral attitudes about childrearing will not provide the needed supplement, which, in conjunction with the natural function view of bodily parts, would produce a positive obligation to use the genitals for procreation. Society's attitude toward a childless couple is that of pity not censure—even if the couple could have children. The pity may be an unsympathetic one, that is, not registering a course one would choose *for oneself,* but this does not make it a course one would *require* of others. The couple who discovers it cannot have children is viewed not as having thereby had a debt canceled, but rather as having to forgo some of the richness of life, just as a quadriplegic is not viewed as absolved from some moral obligation to hop, skip, and jump, but is viewed as missing some of the richness of life. Consistency requires then that, at most, gays who do not or cannot have children are to be pitied rather than condemned. What *is* immoral is the willful preventing of people from achieving the richness of life. Immorality in this regard lies with those social customs, regulations, and statutes that prevent lesbians and gay men from establishing blood or adoptive families, not with gays themselves.

Sometimes people attempt to establish authority for a moral obligation to use bodily parts in a certain fashion simply by claiming that moral laws are natural laws and vice versa. On this account, inanimate objects and plants are good in that they follow natural laws by necessity, animals by instinct, and persons by a rational will. People are special in that they must first discover the laws that govern them. Now, even if one believes the view—dubious in the post-Newtonian, post-Darwinian world—that natural laws in the usual sense ($e = mc^2$, for instance) have some moral content, it is not at all clear how one is to discover the laws in nature that apply to people.

If, on the one hand, one looks to people themselves for a model—and looks hard enough—one finds amazing variety, including homosexuality as a social ideal (upper-class 5th-century Athenians) and even as socially mandatory (Melanesia today). When one looks to people, one is simply unable to strip away the layers of social custom, history, and taboo in order to see what's really there to any degree more specific than that people are the creatures that make over their world and are capable of abstract thought. That this is so should raise doubts that neutral principles are to be found in human nature that will condemn homosexuality.

On the other hand, if one looks to nature apart from people for models, the possibilities are staggering. There are fish that change gender over their lifetimes: Should we "follow nature" and be operative transsexuals? Orangutans, genetically our next of kin, live completely solitary lives without social organization of any kind: Ought we to "follow nature" and be hermits? There are many species where only two members per generation reproduce: Shall we be bees? The search in nature for people's purpose—far from finding sure models for action—is likely to leave one morally rudderless.

But Aren't Gays Willfully the Way They Are?

It is generally conceded that if sexual orientation is something over which an individual—for whatever reason—has virtually no control, then discrimination against gays is especially deplorable, as it is against racial and ethnic classes, because it holds people accountable without regard for anything they themselves have done. And to hold a person accountable for that over which the person has no control is a central form of prejudice.

Attempts to answer the question whether or not sexual orientation is something that is reasonably thought to be within one's own control usually appeal simply to various claims of the biological or "mental" sciences. But the ensuing debate over genes, hormones, twins, early childhood development, and the like is as unnecessary as it is currently inconclusive.[15] All that is needed to answer the question is to look at the actual experience of gays in current society, and it becomes fairly clear that sexual orientation is not likely a matter of choice. For coming to have a homosexual identity simply does not have the same sort of structure that decision-making has.

On the one hand, the "choice" of the gender of a sexual partner does not seem to express a trivial desire which might be as easily well fulfilled by a simple substitution of the desired object. Picking the gender of a sex partner is decidedly dissimilar, that is, to such activities as picking a flavor of ice cream. If an ice-cream parlor is out of one's flavor, one simply picks another. And if people were persecuted, threatened with jail terms, shattered careers, loss of family and housing and the like for eating, say, rocky road ice cream, no one would ever eat it; everyone would pick another easily available flavor. That gay people abide in being gay even in the face of persecution shows that being gay is not a matter of easy choice.

On the other hand, even if establishing a sexual orientation is not like making a relatively trivial choice, perhaps it is nevertheless relevantly like making the central and serious life choices by which individuals try to establish themselves as being of some type. Again, if one examines gay experience, this seems not to be the case. For one never sees anyone setting out to become a homosexual, in the way one does see people setting out to become doctors, lawyers, and bricklayers. One does not find gays-to-be picking some end—"At some point in the future, I want to become a homosexual"—and then set[ting] about planning and acquiring the ways and means to that end, in the way one does see people deciding that they want to become lawyers, and then sees them plan[ning] what courses to take and what sort of temperaments, habits, and skills to develop in order to become lawyers. Typically gays-to-be simply find themselves having homosexual encounters and yet at least initially resisting quite strongly the identification of being homosexual. Such a person even very likely resists having such encounters but ends up having them anyway. Only with time, luck, and great personal effort, but sometimes never, does the person gradually come to accept her or his orientation, to view it as a given material condition of life, coming as materials do with certain capacities and limitations. The person begins to act in accordance with his or her orientation and its capacities, seeing its actualization as a requisite for an integrated personality and as a central component of personal well-being. As a result, the experience of coming out to oneself has for gays the basic structure of a discovery, not the structure of a choice. And far from signaling immorality, coming out to others affords one of the few remaining opportunities in ever more bureaucratic, mechanistic, and socialistic societies to manifest courage.

How Would Society at Large Be Changed If Gays Were Socially Accepted?

Suggestions to change social policy with regard to gays are invariably met with claims that to do so would invite the destruction of civilization itself: After all, isn't that what did Rome in? Actually Rome's decay paralleled not the flourishing of homosexuality, but its repression under the later Christianized emperors.[16] Predictions of

American civilization's imminent demise have been as premature as they have been frequent. Civilization has shown itself rather resilient here, in large part because of the country's traditional commitments to a respect for privacy, to individual liberties, and especially to people minding their own business. These all give society an open texture and the flexibility to try out things to see what works. And because of this one now need not speculate about what changes reforms in gay social policy might bring to society at large. For many reforms have already been tried.

Half the states have decriminalized homosexual acts. Can you guess which of the following states still have sodomy laws? Wisconsin, Minnesota; New Mexico, Arizona; Vermont, New Hampshire; Nebraska, Kansas. One from each pair does and one does not have sodomy laws. And yet one would be hard pressed to point out any substantial difference between the members of each pair. (If you're interested: It is the second of each pair with them.) Empirical studies have shown that there is no increase in other crimes in states that have decriminalized [homosexual acts].[17] Further, sodomy laws are virtually never enforced. They remain on the books not to "protect society" but to insult gays and, for that reason, need to be removed.

Neither has the passage of legislation barring discrimination against gays ushered in the end of civilization. Some 50 counties and municipalities, including some of the country's largest cities (like Los Angeles and Boston) have passed such statutes and among the states and [counties] Wisconsin and the District of Columbia have model protective codes. Again, no more brimstone has fallen in these places than elsewhere. Staunchly antigay cities, like Miami and Houston, have not been spared the AIDS crisis.

Berkeley, California, has even passed domestic partner legislation giving gay couples the same rights to city benefits as married couples, and yet Berkeley has not become more weird than it already was.

Seemingly hysterical predictions that the American family would collapse if such reforms would pass proved false, just as the same dire predictions that the availability of divorce would lessen the ideal and desirability of marriage proved completely unfounded. Indeed, if current discriminations, which drive gays into hiding and into anonymous relations, were lifted, far from seeing gays raze American families, one would see gays forming them.

Virtually all gays express a desire to have a permanent lover. Many would like to raise or foster children—perhaps [from among the] alarming number of gay kids who have been beaten up and thrown out of their "families" for being gay. But currently society makes gay coupling very difficult. A life of hiding is a pressure-cooker existence not easily shared with another. Members of nongay couples are here asked to imagine what it would take to erase every trace of their own sexual orientation for even just a week.

Even against oppressive odds, gays have shown an amazing tendency to nest. And those gay couples who have survived the odds show that the structure of more usual couplings is not a matter of destiny but of personal responsibility. The so-called basic unit of society turns out not to be a unique immutable atom but can adopt different parts, be adapted to different needs, and even be improved. Gays might even have a thing or two to teach others about divisions of labor, the relation of sensuality and intimacy, and stages of development in such relations.

If discrimination ceased, gay men and lesbians would enter the mainstream of the human community openly and with self-respect. The energies that the typical gay person wastes in the anxiety of leading a day-to-day existence of systematic disguise would be released for use in personal flourishing. From this release would be generated the many spin-off benefits that accrue to a society when its individual members thrive.

Society would be richer for acknowledging another aspect of human richness and diversity. Families with gay members would develop relations based on truth and trust rather than lies and fear. And the heterosexual majority would be better off for knowing that they are no longer trampling their gay friends and neighbors.

Finally and perhaps paradoxically, in extending to gays the rights and benefits it has reserved for its dominant culture, America would confirm its deeply held vision of itself as a morally progressing nation, a nation itself advancing and serving as a beacon for others—especially with regard to human rights. The words with which our national pledge ends—"with liberty and justice for all"—are not a description of the present but a call for the future. Ours is a nation given to a prophetic political rhetoric which acknowledges that morality is not arbitrary and that justice is not merely the expression of the current collective will. It is this vision that led the black civil rights movement to its successes. Those congressmen who opposed that movement and its centerpiece, the 1964 Civil Rights Act, on obscurantist grounds, but who lived long enough and were noble enough came in time to express their heartfelt regret and shame at what they had done. It is to be hoped and someday to be expected that those who now grasp at anything to oppose the extension of that which is best about America to gays will one day feel the same.

Notes

1. "Public Fears—and Sympathies," *Newsweek* (August 12, 1985), p. 23.
2. Alfred C. Kinsey, *Sexual Behavior in the Human Male* (Philadelphia: Saunders, 1948), pp. 650–51. On the somewhat lower incidences of lesbianism, see Alfred C. Kinsey, *Sexual Behavior in the Human Female* (Philadelphia: Saunders, 1953), pp. 472–75.
3. Evelyn Hooker, "The Adjustment of the Male Overt Homosexual," *Journal of Projective Techniques* 21 (1957), pp. 18–31, reprinted in Hendrik M. Ruitenbeek, ed., *The Problem of Homosexuality* (New York: Dutton, 1963), pp. 141–61.
4. See Ronald Bayer, *Homosexuality and American Psychiatry* (New York: Basic Books, 1981).
5. For studies showing that gay men are no more likely—indeed, are less likely—than heterosexuals to be child molesters and that the largest classes and most persistent sexual abusers of children are the children's fathers, stepfathers, or mother's boyfriends, see Vincent De Francis, *Protecting the Child Victim of Sex Crimes Committed by Adults* (Denver: The American Humane Association, 1969), pp. *vii*, 38, 69–70; A. Nicholas Groth, "Adult Sexual Orientation and Attraction to Underage Persons," *Archives of Sexual Behavior* 7 (1978), pp. 175–81; Mary J. Spencer, "Sexual Abuse of Boys," *Pediatrics* 78:1 (July 1986), pp. 133–38.
6. See National Gay Task Force, *Antigay/Lesbian Victimization* (New York: NGTF,1984).
7. "2 St. John's Students Given Probation in Assault on Gay," *The Washington Post* (May 15, 1984), p. 1.

8. See Randy Shilts, *The Mayor of Castro Street: The Life and Times of Harvey Milk* (New York: St. Martin's, 1982), pp. 308–25.
9. See Richard Plant, *The Pink Triangle: The Nazi War Against Homosexuals* (New York: Holt, 1986).
10. E. Carrington Boggan, *The Rights of Gay People: The Basic ACLU Guide to a Gay Person's Rights,* 1st ed. (New York: Avon, 1975), pp. 211–35.
11. John Boswell, *Christianity, Social Tolerance, and Homosexuality: Gay People in Western Europe from the Beginning of the Christian Era to the Fourteenth Century* (Chicago: The University of Chicago Press, 1980).
12. See Gilbert Herdt, *Guardians of the Flute: Idioms of Masculinity* (New York: McGraw-Hill, 1981), pp. 232–39, 284–88, and see generally Gilbert Herdt, ed., *Ritualized Homosexuality in Melanesia* (Berkeley: University of California Press, 1984). For another eye-opener, see Walter J. Williams, *The Spirit and the Flesh: Sexual Diversity in American Indian Culture* (Boston: Beacon, 1986).
13. See especially Boswell, *op. cit.,* Chapter 4.
14. For Old Testament condemnations of homosexual acts, see Leviticus 18:22, 21:3. For hygienic and dietary codes, see, for example, Leviticus 15:19–27 (on the uncleanliness of women) and Leviticus 11:1–47 (on not eating rabbits, pigs, bats, finless water creatures, legless creeping creatures, and so on). For Lot at Sodom, see Genesis 19:1–25. For Lot in the cave, see Genesis 19:30–38.
15. The preponderance of the scientific evidence supports the view that homosexuality is either genetically determined or a permanent result of early childhood development. See the Kinsey Institute's study by Alan Bell, Martin Weinberg, and Sue Hammersmith, *Sexual Preference: Its Development in Men and Women* (Bloomington: Indiana University Press, 1981); Frederick Whitam and Robin Mathy, *Male Homosexuality in Four Societies* (New York: Praeger, 1986), Chapter 7.
16. See Boswell, *op. cit.,* Chapter 3.
17. See Gilbert Geis, "Reported Consequences of Decriminalization of Consensual Adult Homosexuality in Seven American States," *Journal of Homosexuality* 1:4 (1976), pp. 419–26; Ken Sinclair and Michael Ross, "Consequences of Decriminalization of Homosexuality: A Study of Two Australian States," *Journal of Homosexuality* 12:1 (1985), pp. 119–27.

Consensual Homosexuality and the Constitutional Right to Privacy

DAVID A. J. RICHARDS

From its recognition in *Griswold* v. *Connecticut,* . . . the constitutional right to privacy commonly has been attacked as expressing subjective judicial ideology, as lacking a constitutionally neutral principle, and as being, in substance, a form of legislative policy not properly pursued by the courts. . . . In particular, critics, both on . . . and off the Supreme Court, . . . have questioned the methodology of the Court in inferring an independent constitutional right to privacy that is not within the contours of the rights expressly guaranteed by the Constitution; in brief, how can the Court legitimately appeal to an unwritten constitution when the *point* of the constitutional design was to limit governmental power by a written text?

The summary affirmance in *Doe* v. *Commonwealth's Attorney for Richmond,*[1] which could be read as excluding homosexual acts between consenting adults from the scope of the constitutional right to privacy, may give compelling force to these kinds of objections. The Court may have summarily limited the right to privacy in a way that suggests fiat, not articulated principle, for how can the Court in a principled way sustain the constitutional right to privacy of married and unmarried people to use contraceptives, . . . or to have abortions, . . . or to use pornography in the privacy of one's home, . . . and not sustain the rights of consenting adult homosexuals to engage in the form of sex they find natural?

I believe that the constitutional right to privacy is a sound and defensible development in our constitutional jurisprudence that *Doe* betrays. . . .

From David A.J. Richards, *Sex, Drugs, Death, and the Law: An Essay on Human Rights and Overcriminalization* (Totowa, N.J.: Rowman and Littlefield, 1982), pp. 29–43 and 63. Reprinted by permission of the publisher.

The Concept of Human Rights as an Unwritten Constitution

The constitutional power of judicial review is marked by two salient structural features. First, such review is intrinsically countermajoritarian. The Constitution clearly was intended to put legal constraints on majority power, whether exercised by the legislature or by the executive. Second, the basis of this countermajoritarian appeal appears to be ideas of human rights that, by definition, government has no moral title to transgress. Under the constitutional order, certain human rights are elevated into legally enforceable rights, so that if a law infringes on these moral rights, the law is not valid. . . .

Ronald Dworkin has recently described these structural features in terms of his rights thesis, . . . which rests on an analytical claim regarding the force of rights as trump cards that, by definition, outweigh utilitarian or quasi-utilitarian considerations and can legitimately be weighed only against other rights. Moreover, the weighing of *rights* cannot be a sham appeal to vague and speculative consequences. Finally, the force of the rights thesis in American constitutional law is shown by the fact that violation of constitutional rights establishes not merely a permission but an affirmative right and even a duty to disobey the challenged law. This principle derives from the force of the case or controversy requirement for federal litigation, . . . which typically requires that people have standing to make constitutional arguments about violations of human rights only when they have disobeyed the law in question and are about to be prosecuted for violations thereof. . . . Accordingly, the vindication and elaboration of constitutional rights require willingness to disobey the law on a suitable occasion.

Dworkin's description of the institutionalization of the rights thesis in American constitutional law directly challenges current constitutional theories that do not take seriously the rights thesis and the consequent proper scope of the countermajoritarian judicial review that enforces constitutional rights. These theories rest either on utilitarianism, . . . which became the dominant American moral jurisprudence in the late nineteenth century with [Justice Oliver Wendell] Holmes's *The Common Law*, . . . or on twentieth-century value skepticism. . . . Neither moral view can be squared with the rights thesis as it underlies American constitutional law. Accordingly, the constitutional theories that assume or presuppose these viewpoints either skeptically question the very legitimacy of judicial review . . . or urge that the scope of judicial review be sharply circumscribed. . . . The American practice of constitutional law, as Dworkin's descriptive thesis shows, does not conform to this theory; American judges, like Holmes and [Learned] Hand, did not decide constitutional cases in the way their theory of law would require. . . . This dissonance of American theory and practice indicates, I believe, not a defect in the practice of American constitutional law, which rests on sound moral foundations, but a focal inadequacy in American legal theory that has not, in a memorable phrase of Dworkin's, taken rights seriously.

In order to understand and interpret the constitutional design, we must take seriously the radical vision of human rights that the Constitution was intended to express and in terms of which the written text of the Constitution was intended to be interpreted; I call this vision the unwritten constitution. . . .

[T]he idea of human rights was a major departure in human thought, and . . . the philosophers who best articulated its radical implications for the significance of respect for moral personality (Locke, Rousseau, and Kant) called for corresponding practical reforms. The political implications of this way of thinking are a matter of history. The idea of human rights was among the central moral concepts in terms of which a number of great political revolutions conceived and justified their demands. . . . Once introduced, the idea of human rights could not be confined. In this country it provided the foundation for the distinctly American innovation of judicial review—the idea that an enforceable charter of human rights requires a special set of governing institutions that, in principle, protect these rights from incursions of the governing majority. . . . Thus, there is little question that the Bill of Rights was part of and gave expression to a developing moral theory regarding the rights of individuals that had been theoretically stated by Milton . . . and Locke . . . and that was given expression by Rousseau . . . and Kant. . . . The founding fathers believed some such theory . . . and regarded the Bill of Rights, inter alia, as a way of institutionalizing it. . . . Nevertheless, attempts to define the specific content of constitutionally protected moral rights are frustrated by the fact that articulation of such rights typically rests on constitutional provisions strikingly general in form ([for example], "freedom of speech or of the press"; "due process of law"; "equal protection of the law") and often lacking any convincing legal history regarding the intended application of the provision. A consensus, to the extent one existed when these clauses were drafted, was reached on the ambiguous generalities of political compromise. . . . Even when circumstances at the time strongly suggest a certain interpretation, such legal history has not conventionally been regarded as dispositive. . . . In order to understand how constitutional provisions of these kinds are interpreted, we must advert to the underlying concepts of human rights that they express.

Often, in order to articulate a hermeneutics of the meanings that language properly bears, we invoke an underlying theory of the kind of communication that a specific form of discourse exemplifies. . . . When a critic of the arts, for example, interprets the meaning of a complex work of art, he or she invokes, inter alia, conventions of communication of the genre in question, because such conventions are part of the assumed and well-understood background of shared communicative understandings that the artist invoked in creating the work. . . . In the law, the canons of statutory interpretation importantly attempt to specify an underlying theory of the proper communicative purposes that may reasonably be imputed to the choice of legislative language in the context of constitutional values and the institutional separation of powers. . . . Correspondingly, the meaning of constitutional provisions necessarily rests on the background theory of human values that the Constitution assumes as its communicative context.

When referring, then, to the concept of human rights as the unwritten constitution, I do not mean to suggest that these underlying understandings are in some sense a secret and impalpable mist. . . . On the contrary, the idea of human rights is the necessary hermeneutical principle that alone enables us to understand how it is that constitutional provisions have any meaning at all. Indeed, alternative, legal-realist constitutional theories are notoriously inadequate in that they fail to take seriously the kinds of normative meaning that constitutional provisions conventionally and often unambiguously express. That the interpretation of constitutional meaning should invoke background communicative understandings is *in principle* no more mysterious than the fact of human linguistic communication. . . .

Since the central task of a constitutional theory is to explicate the background understandings that constitutional language invokes, we must take as our central analytical focus the unwritten constitution, the idea of human rights. Accordingly, the philosophical explication of the concept of human rights . . . necessarily must clarify the proper structure of constitutional argument relevant to many issues. Let us consider how the . . . autonomy-based interpretation of treating persons as equals—in particular, the contractarian interpretation of equal concern and respect for autonomy—clarifies the moral basis of the constitutional right to privacy in general and the application of this right to consensual homosexuality in particular.

A Moral Theory of the Constitutional Right to Privacy

All discussions of the right of privacy must begin with the famous law review article by [Samuel D.] Warren and [Louis D.] Brandeis in which they recommended the recognition of privacy as an independent legal right.[2] Warren and Brandeis were immediately concerned with the failure of existing tort law to provide a clear remedy for the public disclosure of private facts. Nevertheless, basing their argument on the rights "of an inviolate personality," . . . they spoke more broadly of the human need for "some retreat from the world," . . . of the effect of unwarranted intrusion on a person's "estimate of himself and upon his feelings," . . . and of the "general right of the individual to be let alone." . . . The latter suggestion that the right of privacy is broader than the tort remedies under immediate examination was confirmed by the famous dissent in *Olmstead* v. *United States* . . . in which Brandeis invoked "the right to be let alone," not in support of a private tort remedy but in support of an expanded interpretation of fourth amendment constitutional rights of private parties against the state. . . .

Of course, we now perceive the interests of privacy torts and fourth amendment guarantees as analytically similar—rights of information control protected in the one case against individuals, in the other against the state. . . . But the spirit of Brandeis's argument cuts deeper than this analytical point on which he places no great weight. Brandeis, rather, is appealing to an underlying moral argument about the place of human rights in the American contractarian conception of the relation of individuals among themselves and to the state. In his *Olmstead* dissent, for example, he notes:

The makers of our Constitution undertook to secure conditions favorable to the pursuit of happiness. They recognized the significance of man's spiritual nature, of his feelings and of his intellect. They knew that only a part of the pain, pleasure, and satisfactions of life are to be found in material things. They sought to protect Americans in their beliefs, their thoughts, their emotions, and their sensations.[3]

When Brandeis summarized this foundational right as "the most comprehensive of rights and the right most valued by civilized men," . . . he was, I believe, invoking the general conception of human rights, founded on autonomy and equal concern and respect. Certain of the principles of constitutional justice upon which Brandeis relied are concerned with issues having deep connection with personal dignity and the right to control highly personal information about oneself. Such information control is one of the primary ways in which persons autonomously establish their self-conception and their varying relations to other persons through selective information disclosure. . . . Without some legally guaranteed right to control such information, personal autonomy is degraded at its core. From *personal* self-definition and self-mastery it is debased into the impersonal and fungible conventionalism that uncontrolled publicity inevitably facilitates. . . . Accordingly, arguments, premised on the foundational values of equal concern and respect for autonomy, justify the protection of conventional privacy interests under tort law, as well as under various constitutional guarantees.

Actions protected by principles enunciated in *Griswold* and subsequent cases are denominated "private," not because they rest on information control, but because substantive constitutional principles define conclusive reasons why they may not properly be the subject of encroachment by the state or by private individuals. Such rights are sensibly called "rights to privacy" in the sense that constitutional principles debar forms of state and private regulatory or prohibitory intrusion into the relevant areas of people's lives; on the basis of these principles, interference in these areas is unwarranted.

What is at stake here is nothing less than the basic moral vision of persons as having human rights: that is, as autonomous and entitled to equal concern and respect. This vision, correctly invoked by Warren and Brandeis in developing rights to information control, similarly underlies the constitutional right to privacy. In order to explain with care how this is so, we now turn to a deeper examination of the content of the moral principles involved in this latter right, and how they express the underlying values of autonomy and equal concern and respect to which Brandeis appeals. This examination will show why the constitutional right to privacy is a natural and defensible development rooted in the unwritten constitution, which gives sense to the constitutional design.

The Concept of Morality and the Transvaluation of Values.   The constitutional right of privacy cases typically arise in areas where there is a strong conventional wisdom that certain conduct is morally wrong and where the justice of that wisdom is under fundamental attack. It is no accident that the right of privacy is conceived by its proponents not merely as an advisable or charitable or even wise thing to concede, but as a *right*. . . . Proponents conceive matters involving rights, not as human weaknesses or excusable defects that others should benevolently overlook, but as positive moral goods that one may demand and enforce as one's due. Accordingly, the constitutional right to privacy is, in part, to be understood in terms of a transvaluation of values: Certain areas of conduct, traditionally conceived as morally wrong and thus the proper object of public regulation and prohibition, are now perceived as affirmative goods the pursuit of which does not raise serious moral questions and which thus is no longer a proper object of public critical concern. . . .

How, philosophically, are we to interpret and understand such changes? First, as used here to explain the constitutional right to privacy, transvaluation of values refers to changes in the lower-order rules and conventions—namely, in the light of contemporary evidence and conditions, certain lower-order conventions are no longer justified by ultimate moral considerations. For example, according to one influential model, sex is proper only for the purpose of procreation. Many would argue, however, that the distinctive force of human, as opposed to animal, sexuality is that it is *not* rigidly procreational. To the extent that the traditional model of sexuality is discarded in favor of a nonprocreational model, rigid moral rules prohibiting forms of nonprocreational sex are no longer perceived as justified by ultimate moral considerations.

In order to provide reasonable criteria to assess the justifiability of such shifts, we must return to our discussion of the foundations of constitutional morality. As we saw, autonomy and equal concern and respect justify the constitutional immunity of human rights from political bargaining. Since one crucial ground for political bargaining is public morality, constitutional values require that the content of the public morality must be squared with the underlying values of constitutional morality. The primacy of the free exercise and establishment of religion clauses shows that at the core of constitutional values is religious toleration, understood as neutrality between those visions of the good life that are fundamental to autonomous capacities. Conceptually, contractarians give expression to this moral value by the ignorance assumption that deprives the contractors of any basis for keying the choice of ultimate principles to their possibly parochial vision of the good life. These values of constitutional morality ineluctably put determinate constraints on the content of the public morality, which is the foundation of the criminal law and the enforcement of which pervades the entire legal system. . . .

What is the constitutionally permissible content of the legal enforcement of morals? Regarding this question, recent moral philosophy has been increasingly occupied with the clarification of the conceptual structure of ordinary moral reasoning. . . . The concept of morality or ethics is not an openly flexible one; there are certain determinate constraints on the kind of beliefs that can be counted as ethical in nature. . . . Some examples of these constraints are the principles of mutual respect—treating others as you would like to be treated in comparable circumstances; . . . universalization—judging the morality of principles by the consequences of their universal application; . . . and minimization of fortuitous human differences (like clan, caste, ethnicity, gender, and color) as a basis for differential treatment. . . . It follows from this conception that a view is not a moral one merely because it is passionately and sincerely held, or because it has a certain emotional depth, . . . or because it is the view of one's father or mother or clan, or because it is conventional. On the contrary, the moral point of view affords an impartial way of assessing whether any of these beliefs, which may often press one to action, is in fact worthy of ethical commitment. . . .

In similar ways and for similar reasons, not everything invoked by democratic majorities as justified by "public morality" is, in fact, morally justified. From the moral point of view, we must always assess such claims by whether they can be sustained by the underlying structure of normal reasoning—by principles of mutual respect, universalization, and minimization of fortuity. In this regard, constitutional morality is at one with the moral point of view. The values of equal concern and respect for personal autonomy, which we have unearthed at the foundations of American constitutionalism, are the same values that recent moral theory, following Kant, . . . has identified as the fundamental values of the moral point of view. This kind of moral analysis affords definite constraints on what may permissibly or justifiably be regarded as an ethical belief. . . . In an area where public attitudes about public morality are, in fact, demonstrably not justified by underlying moral constitutional principles, laws resting on such attitudes are constitutionally dubious. There being no defensible moral principle to sustain state interference, the matter is not a proper object of state concern. In this soil, the constitutional right to privacy took root in *Griswold*.

The understanding of *Griswold* and its progeny begins with repudiation of the procreational model of sexual love, which was given its classic formulation by St. Augustine. . . . For Augustine, sexuality was a natural object of continuing shame because it involved loss of control. . . . Accordingly, the only proper form of sex was that which was done with the controlled intention to procreate; sexuality without procreation or independent of such intentions was, for Augustine, intrinsically degrading. It follows from this view that certain rigidly defined kinds of intercourse in conventional marriage, always with the intention to procreate, are alone moral; contraception, whether within or outside marriage, extramarital and, of course, homosexual intercourse are forbidden since these do not involve the intent to procreate. . . .

Augustine's argument rests on a rather remarkable fallacy. Augustine starts with two anthropological points about human sexual experience: First, humans universally insist on having sex alone and unobserved by others, . . . and second, humans universally cover their genitals in public. . . . Augustine argues that the only plausible explanation for these two empirical facts about human sexuality is that humans experience sex as intrinsically degrading because it involves the loss of control; . . . this perception of shame, in turn, must rest on the fact that the only proper form of sex is having it with the controlled intention to procreate; . . . sexuality is intrinsically degrading because we tend to experience it without or independent of the one intention that alone can validate it. . . . Assuming, *arguendo,* the truth of Augustine's anthropological assumptions, . . . it does not follow that humans must find sex intrinsically shameful. These facts are equally well explained by the fact that people experience embarrassment in certain forms of publicity of their sexuality, not shame in the experience of sex itself. Shame is conceptually distinguishable from embarrassment in that its natural object is a failure of personally esteemed competent self-control, whether the failure is public or private; embarrassment, in contrast, is experienced when a matter is made public that properly is regarded as private. . . . The twin facts adduced by Augustine are, indeed, better explained by the hypothesis of embarrassment, not shame. Surely many people experience no negative self-evaluations when they engage in sex in private, which is what the hypothesis of embarrassment, not shame, would lead us to expect. For example, people may experience pride in knowing that other people know or believe that they are having sex (the recently married young couple). There is no shame here, but there would be severe embarrassment if the sex act were actually observed. That people would experience such embarrassment reveals something important about human sexual experience, but it is not Augustine's contempt for the loss of control of sexual passion. Sexual experience is, for human beings, a profoundly personal, spontaneous, and absorbing experience in which they express intimate fantasies and vulnerabilities which typically cannot brook the sense of an external, critical observer. That humans require privacy for sex relates to the nature of the experience; there is no suggestion that the experience is, *pace* Augustine, intrinsically degrading.

The consequence of Augustine's fallacy is to misdescribe and misidentify natural features of healthy sexual experience, namely, the privacy required to express intimate sexual vulnerabilities, in terms of putatively degraded properties of sexual experience per se. In fact, this latter conception of sexuality relies on and expresses an overdeveloped willfulness that fears passion itself as a form of loss of control, . . . as though humans cannot with self-esteem indulge emotional spontaneity outside the rule of the iron procreational will. Such a conception both underestimates the distinctly human capacity for self-control and overestimates the force of sexuality as a dark, unreasoning, Bacchie possession whose demands inexorably undermine the rational will. It also fails to fit the empirical facts, indeed contradicts them. Human, as opposed to animal, sexuality is crucially marked by its control by higher cortical functions and thus its involvement with the human symbolic imagination, so that sexual propensities and experience are largely independent of the reproductive cycle. Consequently, humans use sexuality for diverse purposes—to express love, for recreation, or for procreation. No one purpose necessarily dominates; rather, human self-control chooses among the purposes depending on context and person.

The constitutional right to privacy was developed in *Griswold* and its progeny because the procreational model of sexuality could no longer be sustained by sound empirical or conceptual argument. Lacking such support, the procreational model could no longer be legally enforced on the grounds of the "public morality," for it failed to satisfy the postulate of constitutional morality that legally enforceable moral ideas be grounded on equal concern and respect for autonomy and demonstrated by facts capable of empirical validation. Accordingly, since anticontraceptive laws are based on the concept that nonprocreational sex is unnatural, the *Griswold* Court properly invoked the right of privacy to invalidate the Connecticut statute. For similar reasons, laws prohibiting the use of pornography in the home were invalidated. . . . Subsequently, abortion laws were also struck down because the traditional objection to them rested, in large part, on the procreational model and the residuum of moral condemnation that was not clearly sustained by sound argument. . . .

If the right to privacy extends to sex among unmarried couples . . . or even to autoeroticism in the home, . . . it is difficult to understand how in a principled way the Court could decline to consider fully the application of this right to private, consensual, deviant sex acts. The Court might distinguish between heterosexual and homosexual forms of sexual activity, but could this distinction be defended rationally? At bottom, such a view must rest on the belief that homosexual or deviant sex is unnatural. . . .

The use of so imprecise a notion as "unnatural" to distinguish between those acts not protected by the constitutional right to privacy and those which are so protected is clearly unacceptable. The case where the constitutional right to privacy had its origin was one involving contraception—a practice which the Augustinian view would deem unnatural. Yet the Court has apparently concluded that the "unnaturalness" of contraception or abortion is constitutionally inadmissible and cannot limit the scope of the right to privacy. In considering the constitutional permissibility of allowing majoritarian notions of the unnatural to justify limitations on the right to privacy, the Court must take into account two crucial factors: (1) the absence of empirical evidence or sound philosophical argument that these practices are unnatural; and (2) the lack of any sound moral argument, premised on equal concern and respect, that these practices are in any sense immoral. In particular, as we saw in the contraception and abortion decisions, the Court impliedly rejected the legitimacy of both the classic Augustinian view of human sexuality and the associated judgments about the exclusive morality of marital procreational sex. The enforcement of majoritarian prejudices, without any plausible empirical basis, could be independently unconstitutional as a violation of due process rationality in legislation. . . . To enforce such personal tastes in matters touching basic autonomous life choices violates basic human rights. The moral theory of the Constitution, built as a bulwark against "serious oppressions of the minor party in the community,"[4] . . . requires that such human rights be upheld and protected against majoritarian prejudices.

For the same reasons that notions of the unnatural are constitutionally impermissible in decisions involving contraception, abortion, and the use of pornography in the home, these ideas are also impermissible in the constitutional assessment of laws prohibiting private forms of sexual deviance between consenting adults. No empirical evidence compels a finding that homosexuality is unnatural. . . . Indeed, there have been cultures that possessed normative assumptions of what is natural that nevertheless did not regard homosexuality as unnatural. . . . Some societies (including ancient Greece) have included or include homosexuality among legitimate sexual conduct, and some prescribe it in the form of institutional pederasty. . . . Individuals within our own culture have assailed the view that homosexuality is unnatural by adducing various facts which traditionalists either did not know or did not understand. . . . For example, it is now known that homosexual behavior takes place in the animal world, suggesting that homosexuality is part of our mammalian heritage of sexual responsiveness. . . .

Some have attempted to distinguish between individuals who are exclusively homosexual and the general population based on symptoms of mental illness[5] or measures of self-esteem and self-acceptance. . . . In general, however, apart from their sexual preference, exclusive homosexuals are psychologically indistinguishable from the general population. . . .

The view sometimes expressed that male homosexuality necessarily involves the loss of desirable character traits probably rests on the idea that sexual relations between males involve the degradation of one or both parties to the status of a woman. . . . This view, however, rests on intellectual confusion and unacceptable moral premises since it confuses sexual preference with gender identity, whereas, in fact, no such correlation exists. Male homosexuals or lesbians may be quite insistent about their respective gender identities and have quite typical "masculine" or "feminine" personalities. Their homosexuality is defined only by their erotic preference for members of the same gender. . . . The notion that the status of woman is a degradation is morally repugnant to contemporary jurisprudence . . . and morality. . . . If such crude and unjust sexual stereotypes lie at the bottom of antihomosexuality laws, they should be uprooted, as is being done elsewhere in modern life.

Finally, homosexual preference appears to be an adaptation of natural human propensities to very early social circumstances of certain kinds, . . . so that the preference is settled, largely irreversibly, at a quite early age. . . .

The cumulative impact of such facts is clear. The notion of "unnatural acts," interpreted in terms of a fixed procreational model of sexual functioning, deviations from which result in inexorable damage or degradation, is not properly applied to homosexual acts performed in private between consenting adults. Such activity is clearly a natural expression of human sexual competences and sensitivities, and does not reflect any form of damage, decline, or injury.[6] To deny the acceptability of such acts is itself a human evil, a denial of the distinctive human capacities for loving and sensual experience without ulterior procreative motives—in a plausible sense, itself unnatural.

There is consequently no logically consistent explanation for the Court's refusal to enforce concepts of the "unnatural" in the case of contraception while permitting statutes based on similar concepts to prohibit sexual deviance. Indeed, the moral arguments in the latter case are more compelling. For one thing, at the time *Griswold* was decided, statutes condemning and prohibiting forms of contraception probably no longer reflected a majoritarian understanding of the unnaturalness of this form of birth control. . . . Accordingly, the need for constitutional protection, while proper, was not exigent. . . . In the case of homosexuality, however, there is good reason to believe that, as a group, homosexuals are subject to exactly the kind of unjust social hatred that constitutional guarantees were designed to combat. . . .

A second way by which the Court might justify its restricted application of the right of privacy would be to focus on the morality of the acts in question. Presumably, the naturalness of homosexual experience would not in itself legitimize such experience, if homosexuality were shown to be immoral. There is, however, no sound moral argument any longer to sustain the idea that homosexuality is intrinsically immoral.

The concept of morality, proposed herein, puts certain constraints—mutual respect, universalization, minimization of fortuity—on the kinds of beliefs and arguments that can properly be regarded as ethical in nature. Certainly, such constraints would dictate certain prohibitions and regulations of sexual conduct. For example, respect for the development of capacities of autonomous rational choice would require that various liberties, guaranteed to mature adults, might not extend to persons presumably lacking rational capacities, such as children. Nor is there any objection to the reasonable regulation of obtrusive sexual solicitations or, of course, to forcible forms of intercourse of any kind. Such regulations or prohibitions would secure a more equal expression of autonomy compatible with a like liberty for all, thus advancing underlying values of equal concern and respect. In addition, forms of sexual expression would be limited by other moral principles that would be universalized compatibly with equal concern and respect, for example: principles of not killing, harming, or inflicting gratuitous cruelty; principles of paternalism in narrowly defined circumstances; and principles of fidelity. . . . Thus, as formulated, the relevant limiting moral and constitutional principles permit some reasonable, legitimate restrictions on complete individual freedom.

Statutes that absolutely prohibit deviant sexual acts such as that considered in *Doe* . . . cannot be justified consistently with the principles just discussed. Such statutes are not limited to forcible or public forms of sexual intercourse, or to sexual intercourse by or with children, but extend to private, consensual acts between adults as well. To say that such laws are justified by their indirect effect of stopping homosexual intercourse by or with the underaged would be as absurd as to claim that absolute prohibitions on heterosexual intercourse could be similarly justified. There is no reason to believe that homosexuals as a class are any more involved in offenses with the young than heterosexuals. . . . Nor is there any reliable evidence that such laws inhibit children from being naturally homosexual who would otherwise be naturally heterosexual. Sexual preference is settled, largely irreversibly, in very early childhood, well before laws of this kind could have any effect. . . . If the state has any legitimate interest in determining the sexual preference of its citizens, which is doubtful, . . . that interest cannot constitutionally be secured by overbroad statutes that tread upon the rights of exclusive homosexuals of all ages[7] and that, in any event, irrationally pursue the claimed interest.

Other moral principles also fail to justify absolute prohibitions on consensual sexual deviance. Homosexual relations, for example, are not generally violent. Thus, prohibitory statutes could not be justified by moral principles of nonmaleficence. . . . There is no convincing evidence that homosexuality is either harmful to the homosexual or correlated with any form of mental or physical disease or defect. . . . To the contrary, there is evidence that antihomosexuality laws, which either force homosexuals into heterosexual marriage unnatural for them or otherwise distort and disfigure the reasonable pursuit of natural emotional fulfillment, harm homosexuals and others in deep and permanent ways. . . . Accordingly, principles of legitimate state paternalism do not here come into play.

One relevant set of facts that would justify prohibitions of homosexuality would be empirical support for the view that homosexuality is a kind of degenerative social poison that leads directly to disease, social disorder, and disintegration. . . . Principles of constitutional justice must be compatible with the stability of institutions of social cooperation. Thus, if the above allegation were true, prohibition of homosexuality might be justified on the ground that such prohibition would preserve the constitutional order, so that justice on balance would be secured. These beliefs are quite untenable today, however. Many nations, including several in western Europe, . . . have long allowed homosexual acts between adults, with no consequent social disorder or disease. . . .

The critics of the constitutional right to privacy are wrong. . . . It is they, not the Court, who have lost touch with the moral vision underlying the constitutional design. The institutional protection of moral personality requires that this right be recognized. A case like *Doe* . . . shows not that the constitutional right to privacy is incoherent, but that the Court has failed consistently to apply or articulately to understand its underlying principle. *Doe* is deeply, morally wrong. Sexual autonomy is a human right in terms of which people define the meaning of their lives. In particular, the persecution of homosexuals, for that is the name we may now properly give it, deserves not constitutional validation, but systematic and unremitting attack. To appeal to popular attitudes, in the way in which *Doe* implicitly does, is precisely to withhold human rights when, as a shield against majoritarian oppression, they are most exigently needed. Homosexuals have the right to reclaim the aspects of the self that society has traditionally compelled them to deny; they, like other persons, have the right to center work and love in a life they can authentically call their own.

Notes

1. 425 U.S. 901 (1976), . . . affirmed without opinion, 403 F.Supp. 1199 (E.D. Va. 1975) (three-judge court). In *Doe*, two homosexuals challenged the constitutionality of Virginia's criminal sodomy statute as applied to private acts between consenting adults. The challenge was based on the due process clauses of the fifth and fourteenth amendments, the first amendment guarantee of freedom of expression, the first and ninth amendment guarantee of the right to privacy, and the eighth amendment proscription against cruel and unusual punishment. Nevertheless, the district court found no constitutional bar to the criminalization of homosexual conduct.

2. Samuel D. Warren and Louis D. Brandeis, "The Right to Privacy," 4 *Harv. L. Rev.* 193 (1890).

3. *Olmstead* v. *United States,* 277 U.S. 438, 478 (1928).

4. Alexander Hamilton, *The Federalist* No. 78 (Hallowell ed. 1857), p. 359.

5. In the recent Kinsey Institute study of homosexuality, the authors divide homosexuals into five functional categories (close-coupleds, open-coupleds, functionals, dysfunctionals, and asexuals) and observe that failure to make such distinctions distorts one's realistic picture of the complex and diverse reality of homosexual relations. The close-coupleds, essentially monogamous and stable unions, evince considerable psychological health, which may exceed that of comparable heterosexual unions. In contrast, the asexuals appear to be quite psychologically ill-adjusted. The conflation of these distinct categories presents, the Kinsey study proposes, an unrealistic picture of homosexuality that fails to capture fundamental distinctions among forms of adaptation to homosexual preference in a hostile society. See A. Bell & M. Weinberg, *Homosexualities: A Study of Diversity among Men and Women* (1978), pp. 195–231.

6. Venereal disease is one health problem that might be adduced in this connection on the ground that it is common among homosexuals. In fact, however, there is no necessary connection between homosexuality and the incidence of venereal disease; in any event, there is reason to believe that the incidence of venereal disease among homosexuals has been fostered, not prohibited, by sodomy statutes. As regards the incidence of venereal disease among homosexuals,

two significant classes of homosexuals do not involve the venereal disease problem: (1) Lesbians do not in general suffer from venereal disease in that they "practically never become infected except through contact with men," G. Henry, *All the Sexes* (1955), p. 366. (2) Stable homosexual relations, male and female, do not implicate the disease. In general, the root of the venereal disease problem among homosexuals arises from isolated, promiscuous relations among male homosexuals, not from the form of intercourse itself. This promiscuity among homosexuals is fostered by absolute prohibitions on all forms of homosexual relations and concomitant forms of economic and social discrimination. Indeed, medical attempts to treat the problem are made more difficult by lack of candor by homosexuals about their sexual life and preference, arising from fears of criminal penalties and related forms of discrimination. See generally Note, "The Constitutionality of Laws Forbidding Private Homosexual Conduct," 72 *Mich.L.Rev.* 1613, 1631–33 (1974).

7. Consider, for example, the claims that prohibiting all homosexual conduct and homosexual teachers protects the young. . . . Adult homosexuals are often gifted teachers. . . . These prohibitions either penalize their being teachers or allow them to do so only on hypocritical terms which violate their rights of self-respect based on personal integrity. Society is thus deprived of a social asset or secures it only on immoral terms.

In addition, there is a fundamental unfairness in allowing teachers to be publicly heterosexual, which affords the heterosexual young role models of how to build a life around their sexuality, and not to allow teachers to be publicly homosexual, thus depriving the homosexual young of the education that is any person's right in how to build a life of sexual self-respect. The effect of such public knowledge on the heterosexual young is to discourage in them immoral stereotypes and to develop desirable ethical attitudes of tolerance and respect for the diversities of human fulfillment. Present prohibitions, on the contrary, teach and support immoral and inhumane attitudes that are destructive to the young and to society at large.

Consider, as a useful analogy, the first attacks on racial segregation in the area of elementary education, attacks that have since been enlarged to encompass all forms of state-supported racial discrimination. Such constitutional attacks understandably began in the area of elementary education because undoing racial segregation at this point cuts racist isolation and misunderstanding at its roots. A comparable argument of equivalent force could be made regarding the sexist stereotypes that underlie much antihomosexual prejudice. These sexist stereotypes retain their force because of compelled ignorance about the nature of homosexuality and homosexuals and the failure of people publicly to acknowledge the irrelevance of sexual preference to any fair measure of moral decency, humanity, or good citizenship. In order to cut at the roots of these unjust and immoral attitudes in ignorance and isolation, public acknowledgment and toleration of sexual diversity in teachers and students in early education appears as necessary and useful here as it was and is in the case of racism. Finally, of course, no teacher or guardian of the young, heterosexual or homosexual, has the right to seduce the underaged young.

Bowers v. Hardwick

White, J., delivered the opinion of the Court, in which Burger, C.J., and Powell, Rehn-quist, and O'Connor, JJ., joined. Burger, C.J., and Powell, J., filed concurring opinions. Blackmun, J., filed a dissenting opinion, in which Brennan, Marshall, and Stevens, JJ., joined. Stevens, J., filed a dissenting opinion, in which Brennan and Marshall, JJ., joined.

JUSTICE WHITE DELIVERED the opinion of the Court.

In August 1982, respondent was charged with violating the Georgia statute crimi-nalizing sodomy[1] by committing that act with another adult male in the bedroom of respondent's home. After a preliminary hearing, the District Attorney decided not to present the matter to the grand jury unless further evidence developed.

Respondent then brought suit in the Federal District Court, challenging the con-stitutionality of the statute insofar as it criminalized consensual sodomy.[2] He asserted that he was a practicing homosexual, that the Georgia sodomy statute, as admin-istered by the defendants, placed him in imminent danger of arrest, and that the stat-ute for several reasons violates the Federal Constitution. The District Court granted the defendants' motion to dismiss for failure to state a claim. . . .

A divided panel of the Court of Appeals for the Eleventh Court reversed. . . . [T]he court [held] that the Georgia statute violated respondent's fundamental rights be-cause his homosexual activity is a private and intimate association that is beyond the reach of state regulation by reason of the Ninth Amendment and the Due Process Clause of the Fourteenth Amendment. The case was remanded for trial, at which, to prevail, the State would have to prove that the statute is supported by a compelling interest and is the most narrowly drawn means of achieving that end.

[1] Because other Courts of Appeals have arrived at judgments contrary to that of the Eleventh Circuit in this case, . . . we granted the State's petition for certiorari questioning the holding that its sodomy statute violates the fundamental rights of homosexuals. We agree with the State that the Court of Appeals erred, and hence reverse its judgment. . . .

From an opinion delivered by the U.S. Supreme Court, 106 S.Ct. 2841[, 2842–56] (1986).

[2] This case does not require a judgment on whether laws against sodomy between consenting adults in general, or between homosexuals in particular, are wise or desirable. It raises no question about the right or propriety of state legislative decisions to repeal their laws that criminalize homosexual sodomy, or of state court decisions invalidating those laws on state constitutional grounds. The issue presented is whether the Federal Constitution confers a fundamental right upon homosexuals to engage in sodomy and hence invalidates the laws of the many States that still make such conduct illegal and have done so for a very long time. The case also calls for some judgment about the limits of the Court's role in carrying out its constitutional mandate.

We first register our disagreement with the Court of Appeals and with respondent that the Court's prior cases have construed the Constitution to confer a right of privacy that extends to homosexual sodomy and for all intents and purposes have decided this case. . . .

[T]hree cases were interpreted as construing the Due Process Clause of the Fourteenth Amendment to confer a fundamental individual right to decide whether or not to beget or bear a child. . . .

Accepting the decisions in these cases and the above description of them, we think it evident that none of the rights announced in those cases bears any resemblance to the claimed constitutional right of homosexuals to engage in acts of sodomy that is asserted in this case. No connection between family, marriage, or procreation on the one hand and homosexual activity on the other has been demonstrated, either by the Court of Appeals or by respondent. Moreover, any claim that these cases nevertheless stand for the proposition that any kind of private sexual conduct between consenting adults is constitutionally insulated from state proscription is unsupportable. . . .

Precedent aside, however, respondent would have us announce, as the Court of Appeals did, a fundamental right to engage in homosexual sodomy. This we are quite unwilling to do. It is true that despite the language of the Due Process Clauses of the Fifth and Fourteenth Amendments, which appears to focus only on the processes by which life, liberty, or property is taken, the cases are legion in which those Clauses have been interpreted to have substantive content, subsuming rights that to a great extent are immune from federal or state regulation or proscription. Among such cases are those recognizing rights that have little or no textual support in the constitutional language. . . .

Striving to assure itself and the public that announcing rights not readily identifiable in the Constitution's text involves much more than the imposition of the Justices' own choice of values on the States and the Federal Government, the Court has sought to identify the nature of the rights qualifying for heightened judicial protection. In *Palko* v. *Connecticut,* 302 U.S. 319, 325, 326 . . . (1937), it was said that this category includes those fundamental liberties that are "implicit in the concept of ordered liberty," such that "neither liberty nor justice would exist if [they] were sacrificed." A different description of fundamental liberties appeared in *Moore* v. *East Cleveland,* 431 U.S. 494, 503 . . . (1977) (opinion of Powell, J.), where they are characterized as those liberties that are "deeply rooted in this Nation's history and tradition." *Id.,* at 503 . . . .

It is obvious to us that neither of these formulations would extend a fundamental right to homosexuals to engage in acts of consensual sodomy. Proscriptions against that conduct have ancient roots. . . . Sodomy was a criminal offense at common law and was forbidden by the laws of the original thirteen States when they ratified the Bill of Rights. . . . In 1868, when the Fourteenth Amendment was ratified, all but 5 of the 37 States in the Union had criminal sodomy laws. . . . In fact, until 1961, . . . all 50 States outlawed sodomy, and today, 24 States and the District of Columbia continue to provide criminal penalties for sodomy performed in private and between consenting adults. . . . Against this background, to claim that a right to engage in such conduct is "deeply rooted in this Nation's history and tradition" or "implicit in the concept of ordered liberty" is, at best, facetious.

[3] Nor are we inclined to take a more expansive view of our authority to discover new fundamental rights imbedded in the Due Process Clause. The Court is most vulnerable and comes nearest to illegitimacy when it deals with judge-made constitutional law having little or no cognizable roots in the language or design of the Constitution. . . . There should be, therefore, great resistance to expand the substantive reach of those Clauses, particularly if it requires redefining the category of rights deemed to be fundamental. Otherwise, the Judiciary necessarily takes to itself further authority to govern the country without express constitutional authority. The claimed right pressed on us today falls far short of overcoming this resistance.

Respondent, however, asserts that the result should be different where the homosexual conduct occurs in the privacy of the home. He relies on *Stanley* v. *Georgia,* 394 U.S. 557 . . . (1969), where the Court held that the First Amendment prevents conviction for possessing and reading obscene material in the privacy of his home: "If the First Amendment means anything, it means that a State has no business telling a man, sitting alone in his house, what books he may read or what films he may watch." *Id.,* at 565 . . . .

Stanley did protect conduct that would not have been protected outside the home, and it partially prevented the enforcement of state obscenity laws; but the decision was firmly grounded in the First Amendment. The right pressed upon us here has no similar support in the text of the Constitution, and it does not qualify for recognition under the prevailing principles for construing the Fourteenth Amendment. Its limits are also difficult to discern. Plainly enough, otherwise illegal conduct is not always immunized whenever it occurs in the home. Victimless crimes, such as the possession and use of illegal drugs, do not escape the law where they are committed at home. *Stanley* itself recognized that its holding offered no protection for the possession in the home of drugs, firearms, or stolen goods. . . . And if respondent's submission is limited to the voluntary sexual conduct between consenting adults, it would be difficult, except by fiat, to limit the claimed right to homosexual conduct while leaving exposed to prosecution adultery, incest, and other sexual crimes even though they are committed in the home. We are unwilling to start down that road.

[4] Even if the conduct at issue here is not a fundamental right, respondent asserts that there must be a rational basis for the law and that there is none in this case other than the presumed belief of a majority of the electorate in Georgia that homosexual sodomy is immoral and unacceptable. This is said to be an inadequate rationale to

support the law. The law, however, is constantly based on notions of morality, and if all laws representing essentially moral choices are to be invalidated under the Due Process Clause, the courts will be very busy indeed. Even respondent makes no such claim, but insists that majority sentiments about the morality of homosexuality should be declared inadequate. We do not agree, and are unpersuaded that the sodomy laws of some 25 States should be invalidated on this basis. . . .

Accordingly, the judgment of the Court of Appeals is

Reversed.

Chief Justice Burger, concurring.

I join the Court's opinion, but I write separately to underscore my view that in constitutional terms there is no such thing as a fundamental right to commit homosexual sodomy.

As the Court notes, . . . the proscriptions against sodomy have very "ancient roots." Decisions of individuals relating to homosexual conduct have been subject to state intervention throughout the history of Western Civilization. Condemnation of those practices is firmly rooted in Judaeo-Christian moral and ethical standards. Homosexual sodomy was a capital crime under Roman law. See Code Theod. 9.7.6; Code Just. 9.9.31. See also D. Bailey, *Homosexuality in the Western Christian Tradition* 70–81 (1975). During the English Reformation when powers of the ecclesiastical courts were transferred to the King's Courts, the first English statute criminalizing sodomy was passed. 25 Hen. VIII, c. 6. Blackstone described "the infamous crime against nature" as an offense of "deeper malignity" than rape, an heinous act "the very mention of which is a disgrace to human nature," and "a crime not fit to be named." Blackstone's Commentaries *215. The common law of England, including its prohibition of sodomy, became the received law of Georgia and the other Colonies. In 1816 the Georgia Legislature passed the statute at issue here, and that statute has been continuously in force in one form or another since that time. To hold that the act of homosexual sodomy is somehow protected as a fundamental right would be to cast aside millennia of moral teaching.

This is essentially not a question of personal "preferences" but rather of the legislative authority of the State. I find nothing in the Constitution depriving a State of the power to enact the statute challenged here. . . .

Justice Blackmun, with whom Justice Brennan, Justice Marshall, and Justice Stevens join, dissenting.

This case is no more about "a fundamental right to engage in homosexual sodomy," as the Court purports to declare, . . . than *Stanley* v. *Georgia,* 394 U.S. 557 . . . (1969), was about a fundamental right to watch obscene movies, or *Katz* v. *United States,* 389 U.S. 347 . . . (1967), was about a fundamental right to place interstate bets from a telephone booth. Rather, this case is about "the most comprehensive of rights and the right most valued by civilized men," namely, "the right to be let alone." *Olmstead* v. *United States,* 277 U.S. 438 . . . (1928) (Brandeis, J., dissenting).

The statute at issue, Ga.Code Ann. § 16-6-2, denies individuals the right to decide for themselves whether to engage in particular forms of private, consensual sexual activity. The Court concludes that § 16-6-2 is valid essentially because "the laws of . . . many States . . . still make such conduct illegal and have done so for a very long time." . . . But the fact that the moral judgments expressed by statutes like § 16-6-2 may be "natural and familiar . . . ought not to conclude our judgment upon the question whether statutes embodying them conflict with the Constitution of the United States." *Roe* v. *Wade,* 410 U.S. 113 . . . (1973). . . . Like Justice Holmes, I believe that "[i]t is revolting to have no better reason for a rule of law than that so it was laid down in the time of Henry IV. It is still more revolting if the grounds upon which it was laid down have vanished long since, and the rule simply persists from blind imitation of the past." Holmes, "The Path of the Law," 10 *Harv.L.Rev.* 457, 469 (1897). I believe we must analyze respondent's claim in the light of the values that underlie the constitutional right to privacy. If that right means anything, it means that, before Georgia can prosecute its citizens for making choices about the most intimate aspects of their lives, it must do more than assert that the choice they have made is an "'abominable crime not fit to be named among Christians.'" *Herring* v. *State,* 119 Ga. 709, 721 . . . (1904).

I

In its haste to reverse the Court of Appeals and hold that the Constitution does not "confe[r] a fundamental right upon homosexuals to engage in sodomy," . . . the Court relegates the actual statute being challenged to a footnote and ignores the procedural posture of the case before it. A fair reading of the statute and of the complaint clearly reveals that the majority has distorted the question this case presents.

First, the Court's almost obsessive focus on homosexual activity is particularly hard to justify in light of the broad language Georgia has used. Unlike the Court, the Georgia Legislature has not proceeded on the assumption that homosexuals are so different from other citizens that their lives may be controlled in a way that would not be tolerated if it limited the choices of those other citizens. . . . Rather, Georgia has provided that "[a] person commits the offense of sodomy when he performs or submits to any sexual act involving the sex organs of one person and the mouth or anus of another." Ga. Code Ann. § 16-6-2(a). The sex or status of the persons who engage in the act is irrelevant as a matter of state law. In fact, to the extent I can discern a legislative purpose for Georgia's 1968 enactment of § 16-6-2, that purpose seems to have been to broaden the coverage of the law to reach heterosexual as well as homosexual activity. . . . I therefore see no basis for the Court's decision to treat this case as an "as applied" challenge to § 16-6-2, see *ante,* at 2842, n. 2, or for Georgia's attempt, both in its brief and at oral argument, to defend § 16-6-2 solely on the grounds that it prohibits homosexual activity. Michael Hardwick's standing may rest in significant part on Georgia's apparent willingness to enforce against homosexuals a law it seems not to have any desire to enforce against heterosexuals. . . . But his claim that § 16-6-2 involves an unconstitutional intrusion into his privacy and his right of intimate association does not depend in any way on his sexual orientation.

Second, I disagree with the Court's refusal to consider whether § 16-6-2 runs afoul of the Eighth or Ninth Amendments or the Equal Protection Clause of the Fourteenth Amendment . . . . I need not reach either the Eighth Amendment or the Equal Protection Clause issues because I believe that Hardwick has stated a cognizable claim that § 16-6-2 interferes with constitutionally protected interests in privacy and freedom of intimate association. But neither the Eighth Amendment nor the Equal Protection Clause is so clearly irrelevant that a claim resting on either provision should be peremptorily dismissed. . . . The Court's cramped reading of the issue before it makes for a short opinion, but it does little to make for a persuasive one.

II

"Our cases long have recognized that the Constitution embodies a promise that a certain private sphere of individual liberty will be kept largely beyond the reach of government." *Thornburgh* v. *American Coll. of Obst. & Gyn.,* . . . 106 S.Ct. 2169, 2184 . . . (1986). In construing the right to privacy, the Court has proceeded along two somewhat distinct, albeit complementary, lines. First, it has recognized a privacy interest with reference to certain *decisions* that are properly for the individual to make. . . . Second, it has recognized a privacy interest with reference to certain *places* without regard for the particular activities in which the individuals who occupy them are engaged. . . . The case before us implicates both the decisional and the spatial aspects of the right to privacy.

A.   The Court concludes today that none of our prior cases dealing with various decisions that individuals are entitled to make free of governmental interference "bears any resemblance to the claimed constitutional right of homosexuals to engage in acts of sodomy that is asserted in this case." . . . While it is true that these cases may be characterized by their connection to protection of the family, . . . the Court's conclusion that they extend no further than this boundary ignores the warning in *Moore* v. *East Cleveland,* 431 U.S. 494, 501 . . . (1977) (plurality opinion), against "clos[ing] our eyes to the basic reasons why certain rights associated with the family have been accorded shelter under the Fourteenth Amendment's Due Process Clause." We protect those rights not because they contribute, in some direct and material way, to the general public welfare, but because they form so central a part of an individual's life. "[T]he concept of privacy embodies the 'moral fact that a person belongs to himself and not others nor to society as a whole.'" *Thornburgh* v. *American Coll. of Obst. & Gyn.,* . . . 106 S.Ct., at 2187, n. 5 (Stevens, J., concurring), quoting Fried, Correspondence, 6 Phil. & Pub. Affairs 288–289 (1977). And so we protect the decision whether to marry precisely because marriage "is an association that promotes a way of life, not causes; a harmony in living, not political faiths; a bilateral loyalty, not commercial or social projects." *Griswold* v. *Connecticut,* 381 U.S., at 486 . . . . We protect the decision whether to have a child because parenthood alters so dramatically an individual's self-definition, not because of demographic considerations or the Bible's command to be fruitful and multiply. . . . And we protect the family because it contributes so powerfully to the happiness of individuals, not because of a preference for stereotypical households. . . . The Court recognized in *Roberts,* 468 U.S., at 619 . . . , that the "ability independently to define one's identity that is central to any concept of liberty" cannot truly be exercised in a vacuum; we all depend on the "emotional enrichment of close ties with others." *Ibid.*

Only the most willful blindness could obscure the fact that sexual intimacy is "a sensitive, key relationship of human existence, central to family life, community welfare, and the development of human personality," *Paris Adult Theatre I* v. *Slaton,* 413 U.S. 49, 63 . . . (1973). . . . The fact that individuals define themselves in a significant way through their intimate sexual relationships with others suggests, in a Nation as diverse as ours, that there may be many "right" ways of conducting those relationships, and that much of the richness of a relationship will come from the freedom an individual has to *choose* the form and nature of these intensely personal bonds. . . .

In a variety of circumstances we have recognized that a necessary corollary of giving individuals freedom to choose how to conduct their lives is acceptance of the fact that different individuals will make different choices. . . . "A way of life that is odd or even erratic but interferes with no rights or interests of others is not to be condemned because it is different." *Wisconsin* v. *Yoder,* 406 U.S. 205, 223–24 . . . (1972). The Court claims that its decision today merely refuses to recognize a fundamental right to engage in homosexual sodomy; what the Court really has refused to recognize is the fundamental interest all individuals have in controlling the nature of their intimate associations with others.

B. The behavior for which Hardwick faces prosecution occurred in his own home, a place to which the Fourth Amendment attaches special significance. The Court's treatment of this aspect of the case is symptomatic of its overall refusal to consider the broad principles that have informed our treatment of privacy in specific cases. Just as the right to privacy is more than the mere aggregation of a number of entitlements to engage in specific behavior, so too, protecting the physical integrity of the home is more than merely a means of protecting specific activities that often take place there. . . .

The Court's interpretation of the pivotal case of *Stanley* v. *Georgia,* 394 U.S. 557 . . . (1969), is entirely unconvincing. *Stanley* held that Georgia's undoubted power to punish the public distribution of constitutionally unprotected, obscene material did not permit the State to punish the private possession of such material. According to the majority here, *Stanley* relied entirely on the First Amendment, and thus, it is claimed, sheds no light on cases not involving printed materials. . . . But that is not what *Stanley* said. Rather, the *Stanley* Court anchored its holding in the Fourth Amendment's special protection for the individual in his home:

"'The makers of our Constitution undertook to secure conditions favorable to the pursuit of happiness. They recognized the significance of man's spiritual nature, of his feelings and of his intellect. They knew that only a part of the pain, pleasure, and satisfactions of life are to be found in material things. They sought to protect Americans in their beliefs, their thoughts, their emotions, and their sensations.' . . .

"These are the rights that appellant is asserting in the case before us. He is asserting the right to read or observe what he pleases—the right to satisfy his intellectual and emotional needs in the privacy of his own home." *Id.,* at 564–565, . . . quoting *Olmstead* v. *United States,* 277 U.S., at 478 . . . (Brandeis, J., dissenting).

The central place that *Stanley* gives Justice Brandeis's dissent in *Olmstead,* a case raising *no* First Amendment claim, shows that *Stanley* rested as much on the Court's understanding of the Fourth Amendment as it did on the First. Indeed, in *Paris Adult Theatre I* v. *Slaton,* 413 U.S. 49 . . . (1973), the Court suggested that reliance on the Fourth Amendment not only supported the Court's outcome in *Stanley* but actually was *necessary* to it: "If obscene material unprotected by the First Amendment in itself carried with it a 'penumbra' of constitutionally protected privacy, this Court would not have found it necessary to decide *Stanley* on the narrow basis of the 'privacy of the home,' which was hardly more than a reaffirmation that 'a man's home is his castle.'" *Id.,* 413 U.S., at 66 . . . . "The right of the people to be secure in their . . . houses," expressly guaranteed by the Fourth Amendment, is perhaps the most "textual" of the various constitutional provisions that inform our understanding of the right to privacy, and thus I cannot agree with the Court's statement that "[t]he right pressed upon us here has no . . . support in the text of the Constitution" . . . . Indeed, the right of an individual to conduct intimate relationships in the intimacy of his or her own home seems to me to be the heart of the Constitution's protection of privacy.

III

. . . First, petitioner asserts that the acts made criminal by the statute may have serious adverse consequences for "the general public health and welfare," such as spreading communicable diseases or fostering other criminal activity. . . . Inasmuch as this case was dismissed by the District Court on the pleadings, it is not surprising that the record before us is barren of any evidence to support petitioner's claim.[3] . . . Nothing in the record before the Court provides any justification for finding the activity forbidden by § 16-6-2 to be physically dangerous, either to the persons engaged in it or to others.[4]

The core of petitioner's defense of § 16-6-2, however, is that respondent and others who engage in the conduct prohibited by § 16-6-2 interfere with Georgia's exercise of the "'right of the Nation and of the States to maintain a decent society,'" *Paris Adult Theatre I* v. *Slaton,* 413 U.S., at 59–60 . . . . Essentially, petitioner argues, and the Court agrees, that the fact that the acts described in § 16-6-2 "for hundreds of years, if not thousands, have been uniformly condemned as immoral" is a sufficient reason to permit a State to ban them today. . . .

I cannot agree that either the length of time a majority has held its convictions or the passions with which it defends them can withdraw legislation from this Court's scrutiny. . . . As Justice Jackson wrote so eloquently for the Court in *West Virginia Board of Education* v. *Barnette*, 319 U.S. 624, 641–42 . . . (1943), "we apply the limitations of the Constitution with no fear that freedom to be intellectually and spiritually diverse or even contrary will disintegrate the social organization. . . . [F]reedom to differ is not limited to things that do not matter much. That would be a mere shadow of freedom. The test of its substance is the right to differ as to things that touch the heart of the existing order." . . . It is precisely because the issue raised by this case touches the heart of what makes individuals what they are that we should be especially sensitive to the rights of those whose choices upset the majority.

The assertion that "traditional Judeo-Christian values proscribe" the conduct involved . . . cannot provide an adequate justification for § 16-6-2. That certain, but by no means all, religious groups condemn the behavior at issue gives the State no license to impose their judgments on the entire citizenry. The legitimacy of secular legislation depends instead on whether the State can advance some justification for its law beyond its conformity to religious doctrine. . . . Thus, far from buttressing his case, petitioner's invocation of Leviticus, Romans, St. Thomas Aquinas, and sodomy's heretical status during the Middle Ages undermines his suggestion that § 16-6-2 represents a legitimate use of secular coercive power. . . . A State can no more punish private behavior because of religious intolerance than it can punish such behavior because of racial animus. "The Constitution cannot control such prejudices, but neither can it tolerate them. Private biases may be outside the reach of the law, but the law cannot, directly or indirectly, give them effect." *Palmore* v. *Sidoti*, 466 U.S. 429, 433 . . . (1984). No matter how uncomfortable a certain group may make the majority of this Court, we have held that "[m]ere public intolerance or animosity cannot constitutionally justify the deprivation of a person's physical liberty." *O'Connor* v. *Donaldson*, 422 U.S. 563, 575 . . . (1975). . . .

Nor can § 16-6-2 be justified as a "morally neutral" exercise of Georgia's power to "protect the public environment," *Paris Adult Theatre I*, 413 U.S., at 68–69 . . . . Certainly, some private behavior can affect the fabric of society as a whole. Reasonable people may differ about whether particular sexual acts are moral or immoral, but "we have ample evidence for believing that people will not abandon morality, will not think any better of murder, cruelty, and dishonesty, merely because some private sexual practice which they abominate is not punished by the law." H.L.A. Hart, "Immorality and Treason," reprinted in *The Law as Literature* 220, 225 (L. Blom-Cooper, ed., 1961). Petitioner and the Court fail to see the difference between laws that protect public sensibilities and those that enforce private morality. Statutes banning public sexual activity are entirely consistent with protecting the individual's liberty interest in decisions concerning sexual relations: The same recognition that those decisions are intensely private, which justifies protecting them from governmental interference, can justify protecting individuals from unwilling exposure to the sexual activities of others. But the mere fact that intimate behavior may be punished when it takes place in public cannot dictate how States can regulate intimate behavior that occurs in intimate places. . . .

This case involves no real interference with the rights of others, for the mere knowledge that other individuals do not adhere to one's value system cannot be a legally cognizable interest, . . . let alone an interest that can justify invading the houses, hearts, and minds of citizens who choose to live their lives differently.

IV

It took but three years for the Court to see the error in its analysis in *Minersville School District* v. *Gobitis,* 310 U.S. 586 . . . (1940), and to recognize that the threat to national cohesion posed by a refusal to salute the flag was vastly outweighed by the threat to those same values posed by compelling such a salute. . . . I can only hope that here, too, the Court soon will reconsider its analysis and conclude that depriving individuals of the right to choose for themselves how to conduct their intimate relationships poses a far greater threat to the values most deeply rooted in our Nation's history than tolerance of nonconformity could ever do. Because I think the Court today betrays those values, I dissent.

Notes

1. Ga.Code Ann. § 16-6-2 (1984) provides, in pertinent part, as follows: "(a) A person commits the offense of sodomy when he performs or submits to any sexual act involving the sex organs of one person and the mouth or anus of another. . . . (b) A person convicted of the offense of sodomy shall be punished by imprisonment for not less than one nor more than 20 years . . . ."
2. John and Mary Doe were also plaintiffs in the action. They alleged that they wished to engage in sexual activity proscribed by § 16-6-2 in the privacy of their home, App. 3, and that they had been "chilled and deterred" from engaging in such activity by both the existence of the statute and Hardwick's arrest. . . . The District Court held, however, that because they had neither sustained, nor were in immediate danger of sustaining, any direct injury from the enforcement of the statute, they did not have proper standing to maintain the action. . . . The Court of Appeals affirmed the District Court's judgment dismissing the Does' claim for lack of standing, . . . and the Does do not challenge that holding in this Court. . . .
3. Even if a court faced with a challenge to § 16-6-2 were to apply simple rational-basis scrutiny to the statute, Georgia would be required to show an actual connection between the forbidden acts and the ill effects it seeks to prevent. The connection between the acts prohibited by § 16-6-2 and the harms identified by petitioner in his brief before this Court is a subject of hot dispute, hardly amenable to dismissal under Federal Rule of Civil Procedure 12(b)(6). Compare . . . Brief for Petitioner 36–37 and Brief for David Robinson, Jr., as *Amicus Curiae* 23–28, on the one hand, with *People* v. *Onofre,* 51 N.Y.2d 476, 489, . . . (1980); Brief for the Attorney General of the State of New York, joined by the Attorney General of the State of California, as *Amici Curiae* 11–14; and Brief for the American Psychological Association and American Public Health Association as *Amici Curiae* 19–27, on the other.
4. Although I do not think it necessary to decide today issues that are not even remotely before us, it does seem to me that a court could find simple, analytically sound distinctions between certain private, consensual sexual conduct, on the one hand, and adultery and incest (the only two vaguely specific "sexual crimes" to which the majority points . . . , on the other. For example, marriage, in addition to its spiritual aspects, is a civil contract that entitles the contracting parties to a variety of governmentally provided benefits. A State might define the contractual commitment

necessary to become eligible for these benefits to include a commitment of fidelity and then punish individuals for breaching that contract. Moreover, a State might conclude that adultery is likely to injure third persons, in particular, spouses and children of persons who engage in extramarital affairs. With respect to incest, a court might well agree with respondent that the nature of familial relationships renders true consent to incestuous activity sufficiently problematical that a blanket prohibition of such activity is warranted. . . . Notably, the Court makes no effort to explain why it has chosen to group private, consensual homosexual activity with adultery and incest rather than with private, consensual heterosexual activity by unmarried persons or, indeed, with oral or anal sex within marriage.

Brief of *Amici Curiae* American Psychological Association and American Public Health Association in Support of Respondents

Filed in conjunction with *Bowers* v. *Hardwick*

The Georgia statute disserves the legitimate objectives of improving the public health and individual mental health.

The question whether and to what extent the statute serves any legitimate state objectives is not properly before this Court. These issues remain to be determined on remand. Nevertheless, one *amicus* brief supporting the State asserts erroneously that O.C.G.A. § 16-6-2 is justified as a health measure. Brief of David Robinson, Jr. *Amici* APHA and APA submit that this is simply not true.[1]

A. THE STATUTE IS NOT A PUBLIC HEALTH MEASURE AND IS COUNTERPRODUCTIVE TO PUBLIC HEALTH GOALS.

1. The statute does not significantly contribute to combating the spread of acquired immunodeficiency syndrome (AIDS) or to any other public health goal.

The state cannot seriously contend that the statute is justified generally as advancing the public health or specifically as combating acquired immunodeficiency syndrome ("AIDS") or any other sexually transmitted disease. The statute was enacted in 1816, long before AIDS was known. . . . Its purpose, as the State concedes, was to perpetuate in Georgia the English common law's harsh moral condemnation of the specified sexual conduct, including male homosexuality. Any claim that the statute is justified as protecting the public or individual health is a transparent and unfounded *post-hoc* attempt to capitalize on the current climate of fear about AIDS.

The statute's lack of public health rationale can be seen first by the very loose relationship between its prohibitions and the health problems that Georgia and *amicus* Robinson assert it addresses. The viral agent associated with AIDS appears to be transmitted through exchange of semen or blood, as can occur during anal intercourse and fellatio. . . . But the statute prohibits *all* oral-genital sexuality, and there is no evidence that AIDS is communicated through heterosexual or lesbian cunnilingus. Moreover, those heterosexuals who have been exposed to AIDS can transmit the virus through vaginal intercourse as well as through some types of conduct forbidden by Georgia. . . . Thus, even to the extent heterosexuals are at risk, deterring the prohibited conduct has minimal impact on heterosexual transmission of AIDS.

As applied to homosexual behavior, the Georgia statute is also overly broad. Lesbians as a group are not at risk for AIDS. Among gay men, oral and anal sex are not inevitably associated with transmission of the virus, even when one gay male partner has been exposed. Use of a condom during oral or anal intercourse greatly reduces the risk of transmission of the AIDS virus. . . .

Most important, given what we know about the fundamental nature and strength of the sex drive in humans, it is unrealistic to think that fear of criminal sanction will effectively deter forbidden sexual conduct in private between consenting adults. If the risk of contracting AIDS, a fatal and thus far incurable disease, to say nothing of the threat of social ostracism, humiliation, and loss of job and friends, does not deter variant sexual conduct, then surely the very slim possibility of arrest and prosecution for private conduct does not do so.[2] The experience of the many jurisdictions in which consensual sexual conduct is not criminal seems to be that the prevalence of homosexuality is about the same as in jurisdictions in which it is illegal. . . . Thus, consensual sodomy laws deter at most a negligible amount of overt homosexual behavior. . . . As a result, even with respect to that subset of sexual conduct prohibited by the statute that does pose a risk of spreading AIDS, the statute has no beneficial public health effect.

2. The statute disserves the public health.

The statute does not deter conduct that spreads AIDS, but it may deter conduct essential to combating it. The achievement of the public health goals of health maintenance, disease prevention, and disease detection and treatment depends upon the cooperation of many individuals, including patients, physicians, hospital personnel, researchers, and government officials. To make sound decisions about individual treatment and public health, both individual physicians and public health personnel must be able to obtain accurate information. Criminal statutes such as Georgia's can seriously undermine these essential public health strategies by causing individuals to conceal or distort relevant information and by inhibiting effective public education efforts. In the case of sexually transmitted diseases such as AIDS, substantial harm to individuals and the public may result. Indeed, researchers have discovered that societies with harsh penalties for homosexual conduct suffer from poorer reporting and treatment of sexually transmitted diseases among homosexuals than more lenient societies.[3]

a. The statute may adversely affect the health and treatment of individuals.

Fearing both social disapproval and legal penalties, many homosexual men and women do not tell their personal physicians about their sexual orientation.[4] A patient runs the risk that members of a physician's or hospital's staff may make accidental or unauthorized disclosure of his or her sexual orientation. Such disclosure presents a risk of prosecution, as well as of intensified discrimination.[5] This concealment may adversely affect the medical care an individual receives,[6] with potentially serious consequences for the individual whose illness is misdiagnosed for some period of time. Fear of punitive government actions also can lead to failure to seek treatment at all. Thus, some people who have been exposed to AIDS may avoid reporting their own exposure, fearing that their report may lead to criminal prosecution.[7]

b. The statute may adversely affect scientific investigation directed toward containing disease and finding a cure.

The process of understanding and controlling newly identified diseases such as AIDS urgently requires prompt gathering of accurate information. Diagnosis of individual cases, identification of relevant attributes of the population, finding individuals who may be unknowing or unreported sources of infection, and testing of hypotheses about the origin and spread of a disease, all depend on careful collection of data. . . . A statutory scheme that creates a realistic fear of punishment if certain behavior is disclosed runs the risk of obscuring important data, as individuals simply refuse to volunteer for studies or provide needed information, and of creating false data, as individuals try to conform what they reveal to what they believe is legal. Thus, people who, due to incomplete disclosure, are wrongly diagnosed may continue to be sources of infection without knowing it. Others, who fail to report early symptoms or their own exposure to the disease, also may spread it. Moreover, the public health technique of treating people with whom the patient has had sexual contact requires "the patient's cooperation . . . by assuring that each [contact] is promptly referred, evaluated, and given any indicated therapeutic or preventive treatment."[8] The prospect of criminal penalties against themselves and their partner may well deter individuals from making such referrals. A punitive scheme like Georgia's may also inhibit health care professionals from fulfilling the important public health role of passing on relevant information about the incidence of a disease to researchers and public health officials. Historically, such forces have interfered substantially with efforts to control other forms of venereal disease.[9]

The short history of AIDS shows that fear of punishment has already hindered the current investigation. With respect to at least two important issues—the existence of potentially high risk to recent immigrants from Haiti,[10] and the transmissibility of the

AIDS virus from women to men[11]—there is reason to believe that falsifications of information, caused by fear of punishment, have distorted the epidemiological picture. Finding these and other crucial pieces of the AIDS puzzle should not have to depend on the ability of epidemiologists to guess whether patients are not telling the truth because they fear being punished.

c. The statute interferes with health education efforts designed to encourage safer sexual practices.

The statute also may harm the public health by interfering with efforts intended to advise the public how to minimize or avoid contracting the disease. Public health officials and private groups have been actively encouraging people to change to "safe sex" behavior. . . . "[T]he best chance of controlling the AIDS epidemic at present is through education and counseling to enhance behavioral change and personal responsibility."[12] Researchers report dramatic changes in sexual behavior to reduce the risk of AIDS in areas where major educational efforts are underway, demonstrating the urgent importance of such efforts.[13]

Such community effort and support are made more difficult in an environment in which a concomitant of participating in educational efforts is self-incrimination. Attending an educational presentation on "safe sex," for example, could be seen as an admission of engaging in sexual practices prohibited by the statute. Criminalization is likely to compromise the efficacy of informal educational networks by making people more cautious about what they reveal about themselves to acquaintances. It also presents state public health officials with the awkward choice of appearing to suppress information about safe sex techniques or appearing to condone felonious conduct.

In short, the statute is likely to deter *only* conduct necessary to *improve* the public health. From a public health standpoint, the statute is simply counterproductive.

B. The Georgia Statute Does Not Further Any Mental Health Objectives and Injures the Mental Health of Many Members of Society, with Harmful Repercussions for Individual Physical Health.

The statute is also counterproductive with respect to mental health goals. Because freedom to choose whether to engage in the prohibited conduct *benefits,* rather than harms, individual mental health, deterring individuals from engaging in the types of sexual conduct specified—even if criminal laws could do so—cannot be defended as a mental health objective. Similarly, because homosexuality is not pathological, individual mental health is not served by official attempts to "deter" people from becoming homosexuals.

Even assuming, *arguendo,* that lowering the incidence of homosexual orientation in society were in some other way a legitimate governmental objective, criminalization of homosexual conduct does not have this effect. Although it is clear that same-sex orientation and activity do not indicate mental disorder and illness, it is less clear why some people have a same-sex orientation. Few of the theories advanced to explain the formation of sexual orientation are supported by reliable data.[14] Certainly, homosexual orientation is not a matter of simple choice. It is a set of emotions and proclivities often established early in life. Research indicates that sexual orientation develops independently of isolated sexual experiences, and the data do not support the idea that early childhood homosexual activity has any direct relationship to later sexual orientation.[15] Indeed, there are no empirical data to support the popular myth that homosexual orientation or behavior results from "contagion" by other homosexuals. The only consistent findings are that homosexuals have many more and much stronger sexual fantasies about members of their own sex, and that these fantasies usually appear during childhood and early adolescence. . . .

Once established, homosexual orientation is not easily modified. Researchers agree that the sexual orientation of only a small fraction of homosexual people who are highly motivated to change has been or can be modified through therapy.[16] Consensual sodomy laws thus have little or no effect on the incidence of homosexual orientation. . . .

Furthermore, statutes outlawing variant sexual behavior do cause substantial psychological harm, which, in turn, may have serious consequences for physical health. In part because their behavior is punishable by criminal law,[17] homosexuals become stigmatized as "deviants"[18] and are viewed in terms of undesirable stereotypes. This process results in prejudice—called *homophobia*—against homosexuals by many heterosexual people. Homosexuals develop coping mechanisms, which are common traits in most persecuted groups. These traits can include excessive concern with minority group membership, feelings of insecurity, withdrawal, militancy, and neuroticism. They can also include denial of membership in the group, self-derision, self-hatred, hatred of others in the group, and acting out self-fulfilling prophecies about one's own inferiority. . . . The great majority of gay people come to terms with their sexual orientation and integrate it into their lives. Studies demonstrate that these homosexuals are the most psychologically well-adjusted. But the small group of homosexuals who do not overcome this are more troubled and dysfunctional, and may act in self-destructive ways and destructively toward other gay people.[19] This clinically observed psychological condition is known as "internalized homophobia." . . . This psychological harm is a significant health cost of the Georgia statute.

By contributing to imposing internalized homophobia, criminal sodomy statutes also harm the effort to combat AIDS. Despite major shifts in the at-risk population to "safe sex" practices, a small minority of gay men continue to engage in dangerous conduct. To a significant extent, internalized homophobia may cause this destructive and self-destructive behavior. Although this group is very small as a percentage of all gay men, . . . for a disease with the etiology of AIDS the consequences are tragic.

In terms of both physical and mental health, the statute is counterproductive.

Conclusion

For the foregoing reasons, *amici* respectfully urge this Court to affirm the decision of the United States Court of Appeals for the Eleventh Circuit.

Notes

1. The application of heightened scrutiny to protect individual privacy will not interfere with the operation of legitimate public health laws, which, unlike the law at issue, are narrowly drawn to meet specific problems of compelling importance. See . . . *Jacobson* v. *Massachusetts,* 197 U.S. 11 (1905).

2. See *State* v. *Saunders,* 75 N.J. 200, 381 A.2d 333, 341–42 (1977) (criminal penalties add no deterrent force to fear of contracting serious illness).

3. Ostrow and Altman, "Sexually Transmitted Diseases and Homosexuality," 10 *Sexually Transmitted Diseases* 208, 212 (1983).

4. See . . . Dardick and Grady, "Openness between Gay Persons and Health Professionals," 93 *Annals of Internal Medicine* 115, Part 1 (1980).

5. See *State* v. *Saunders,* 381 A.2d at 342 (a criminal statute "operates as a deterrent to . . . voluntary participation" in treatment programs).

6. For example, physicians may not include in their list of possible diagnoses certain conditions that appear in homosexual men.

7. A clear analogy is provided by the effects of the U.S. Army's venereal disease policy during World War I. American soldiers in Europe were subject to court martial if they were diagnosed as having contracted a venereal disease. A. Brandt, *No Magic Bullet* (1985), p. 102. Many military physicians believed that the threat of court martial induced soldiers to conceal their illness for as long as possible. *Ibid.,* pp. 102, n. 20, 103–05. But the threat of court martial certainly did not prevent the contraction of venereal diseases: More than 380,000 soldiers were diagnosed as having a venereal disease during the period from April 1917 to December 1919. *Ibid.,* p. 115.

8. "1985 STD Treatment Guidelines," 34 *Morbidity and Mortality Weekly Rep.* 1085 (Oct. 18, 1985).

9. Early in the century, for example, many private physicians believed that they would be violating their duty to their patients if they reported syphilis cases. A. Brandt, *op. cit.,* pp. 43, 183–84. Nonreporting by physicians has persisted, frustrating public health efforts to control syphilis and gonorrhea. *Ibid.,* p. 46.

10. One explanation for epidemiologists' failure to identify an overlap between the Haitians and other identified high-risk groups, such as homosexual men and intravenous drug users, is that many Haitian patients were afraid to tell investigators the truth. Admitting to illegal behavior in one's new country—and thereby risking deportation—may have seemed too great a risk to take simply to provide information to doctors.

11. A study of military personnel done at Walter Reed Army Medical Center shows a much higher incidence of female-to-male transmission of HTLV-III/LAV virus than most other United States reports. . . . The question of the incidence of female-to-male transmission is an important area of current inquiry. It is possible that the other reports show an artifically low incidence of such transmission. But another explanation for the disparity is that the military personnel in the Walter Reed study were reluctant to admit to homosexual activity or intravenous drug use, either of which could lead to discharge. See . . . *Rich* v. *Secretary of the Army,* 735 F.2d 1220 (10th Cir. 1984) (Army discharge of homosexual man).

12. Dr. James O. Mason, acting assistant secretary for health, Department of Health and Human Services, testimony before the Republican Study Committee, House of Representatives (Nov. 7, 1985).

13. See . . . "Self-Reported Behavioral Changes among Gay and Bisexual Men—San Francisco," 34 *Morbidity and Mortality Weekly Rep.* 613 (Oct. 11, 1985); . . . "Declining Rates of Rectal and Pharyngeal Gonorrhea among Males—New York City," 33 *Morbidity and Mortality Weekly Rep.* 295 (June 1, 1984), reprinted in MMWR Reports, p. 59.

14. Several popular theories have been disproved. See A. Bell, M. Weinberg, and S. Hammersmith, *Sexual Preference: Its Development in Men and Women* (1981).

15. See A. Bell, et al., *op. cit.,* pp. 97–113 (62 percent of heterosexual men reported that their first sexual encounter was with another male; 39 percent of homosexual men reported such experience).

16. Moreover, for many homosexuals, seeking to change sexual orientation would be an inappropriate goal of psychotherapy.

17. Although sodomy statutes apply to heterosexual conduct as well as homosexual conduct, in practice they are enforced almost exclusively against homosexuals. . . . It is well known, in both law, see *Brown* v. *Board of Education,* 347 U.S. 483, 494–95 (1954), and psychology, see . . . J. Jones, *Prejudice and Racism,* pp. 138–40 (1972), that social or moral pronouncements as expressed through the law and imposed by a majority on a minority can through the process of stigmatization significantly injure the mental health of members of the minority.

18. The term *deviant* as used in the social sciences refers to the social *reaction* to behavior, not to the intrinsic characteristics of the behavior itself.

19. Homosexuals who have been able to express their homosexuality are psychologically healthier than those who have repressed it.

Glossary[*]

AIDS (acquired immune deficiency syndrome): A disease believed to be caused by the retrovirus HTLV-III (human T-lymphotropic virus, type III) and characterized by a deficiency of the immune system. The primary defect in AIDS is an acquired, persistent, quantitative functional depression within the T4 subset of lymphocytes. This depression often leads to infections caused by microorganisms that usually do not produce infections in individuals with normal immunity or to the development of a rare type of cancer (Kaposi's sarcoma) usually seen only in elderly people or in individuals who are severely immunocompromised from other causes. Other associated diseases are currently under investigation and will probably be included in the final definition of AIDS.

ARC (AIDS-related complex): A variety of chronic but nonspecific symptoms and physical findings that appear to be related to AIDS, such as chronic generalized lymphadenopathy, recurrent fevers, weight loss, minor alterations in the immune system, and minor infections. Some people with AIDS-related complex may develop full-blown AIDS, while in others, the condition may represent the height of clinical illness in reaction to infection with HTLV-III. AIDS-related complex is sometimes known as "pre-AIDS." (Compare "lymphadenopathy syndrome.")

Antibody: A blood protein produced by mammals in response to exposure to a specific antigen. Antibodies are a critical component of the mammalian immune system.

Antigen: A large molecule—usually a protein or carbohydrate—that, when introduced into the body, stimulates the production of an antibody that will react specifically with that antigen.

DNA (deoxyribonucleic acid): A linear polymer, made up of deoxyribonucleotide repeating units, that is, the carrier of genetic information in living organisms.

Immune: Being highly resistant to a disease because of the formation of humoral antibodies or the development of cellular immunity (or both), or as a result of some other mechanism (such as interferon activity in viral infections).

Kaposi's sarcoma: A multifocal, spreading cancer of connective tissue, principally involving the skin; it usually begins on the toes or the feet as soft, reddish-blue or brownish nodules and tumors.

LAV (lymphadenopathy-associated virus): A retrovirus recovered from a person with lymphadenopathy (enlarged lymph nodes) who is also in a group at high risk for AIDS; it is now believed to be the same virus as HTLV-III.

Lymphadenopathy syndrome (LAS): A condition, characterized by persistent, generalized, enlarged lymph nodes (sometimes accompanied by signs of minor illness, such as

*Drawn from "Technical Memorandum of the Office of Technology Assessment." *Review of the Public Health Service's Response to AIDS* (February 1985), pp. 145–148.

fever and weight loss), that apparently represents a milder reaction to infection with HTLV-III than full-blown AIDS. Some patients with LAS have gone on to develop full-blown AIDS, while in others, LAS may represent the height of clinical illness in reaction to infection with HTLV-III. LAS is also known as "generalized lymphadenopathy syndrome."

Lymphocytes: Specialized white blood cells involved in the immune response.

Opportunistic infection: A disease or infection caused by a microorganism that does not ordinarily cause disease but may, under certain conditions (such as impaired immune response), become pathologic.

Pneumocystis carinii pneumonia: A type of pneumonia primarily found in infants and now commonly occurring in patients with AIDS.

Retroviruses: Viruses that contain RNA, not DNA, and that produce a DNA analog of their RNA through the production of an enzyme known as "reverse transcriptase." The resulting DNA is incorporated in the genetic structure of the invaded cell.

RNA (ribonucleic acid):   Any of various nucleic acids that contain ribose and uracil as structural components and that are associated with the control of cellular chemical activities.

T-lymphocytes (or T-cells):   Lymphocytes that mature in the thymus and that mediate cellular immune reactions. T-lymphocytes also release factors that induce proliferation of T-lymphocytes and B-lymphocytes.

Vaccine: A preparation—consisting of nonliving organisms, living attenuated organisms, living fully virulent organisms, or parts of microorganisms—that is administered to produce or artificially increase immunity to a particular disease.

Viruses: Any of a large group of submicroscopic agents, capable of infecting plants, animals, and bacteria, and characterized by a total dependence on living cells for reproduction and by a lack of independent metabolism.

Selected Readings

Books

Altman, Dennis, *AIDS in the Mind of America* (Garden City, N.Y.: Doubleday, 1986).

Baumgartner, Gail H., *AIDS: Psychological Factors in the Acquired Immune Deficiency Syndrome* (Springfield, Ill.: Charles C. Thomas Publishing, 1985).

Black, David, *The Plague Years: A Chronicle of AIDS, the Epidemic of Our Times* (New York: Simon & Schuster, 1986).

Brandt, Allan M., *No Magic Bullet: A Social History of Venereal Disease in the United States since 1880,* 2nd ed. (New York: Oxford University Press, 1987).

Cahill, Kevin M., ed., *The AIDS Epidemic* (New York: St. Martin's Press, 1983).

Cantwell, Alan, *AIDS: The Mystery and the Solution* (Los Angeles: Aries Rising Press, 1983).

DeVita, Vincent T., Samuel Hellman, and Steven Rosenberg, eds., *AIDS: Etiology, Diagnosis, Treatment, and Prevention* (New York: J. B. Lippincott, 1985).

Fettner, Ann Giudici, and William A. Check, *The Truth about AIDS* (New York: Holt, Rinehart & Winston, 1984).

Gong, Victor, ed., *Understanding AIDS: A Comprehensive Guide* (New Brunswick: Rutgers University Press, 1985).

Gupta, Sudhir, ed., *AIDS: Associated Syndromes* (New York: Plenum Press, 1985).

Institute of Medicine of the National Academy of Science, *Mobilizing Against AIDS* (Cambridge, Mass.: Harvard University Press, 1986).

Kulstad, Ruth, ed., *AIDS: Papers from* Science *1982–1985* (Washington, D.C.: American Association for the Advancement of Science, 1986).

Leibowitch, Jacques, *A Strange Virus of Unknown Origin* (New York: Ballantine Books, 1985).

Liebmann-Smith, Richard, *The Question of AIDS* (New York: The New York Academy of Sciences, 1985).

Mcleod, Donald W., and Alan V. Miller, eds., *Medical and Social Aspects of the Acquired Immune Deficiency Syndrome: A Bibliography* (Toronto: Canadian Gay Archives, 1985).

Nungesser, Lon G., *Epidemic of Carnage: Facing AIDS in America* (New York: St. Martin's Press, 1986).

Patton, Cindy, *Sex and Germs: The Politics of AIDS* (Boston: South End Press, 1985).

Peabody, Barbara, *The Screaming Room: A Mother's Journal of Her Son's Struggle with AIDS* (San Diego: Oak Tree Publishers, 1986).

Siegal, Frederick P., and Marta Siegal, *AIDS: The Medical Mystery* (New York: Grove Press, 1983).

Slaff, James I., and John Brubacker, *The AIDS Epidemic* (New York: Warner Books, 1985).

Sontag, Susan, *Illness As Metaphor* (New York: Farrar, Straus & Giroux, 1978).

Supplementary volume on AIDS, *The Milbank Quarterly* 64 (1986).

Articles

"AIDS: Deadly but Hard to Catch," *Consumer Reports* (November 1986), pp. 724–728.

Bayer, Ronald, "AIDS and the Gay Community: Between the Specter and the Promise of Medicine," *Social Research* 52 (Autumn 1985), pp. 581–606.

"The Constitutional Rights of AIDS Carriers," *Harvard Law Review* 99 (1986), pp. 1274–1292.

"The Constitutional Status of Sexual Orientation: Homosexuality as a Suspect Classification," *Harvard Law Review* 98 (March 1985), pp. 1285–1309.

"The Constitutionality of Laws Forbidding Private Homosexual Conduct," *Michigan Law Review* 72 (August 1974), pp. 1613–1637.

Gallo, Robert C., "The First Human Retrovirus," Part I of a two-part article on the human retroviruses (Part II is on AIDS), *Scientific American* 255 (December 1986), pp. 88–98.

Gostin, Larry, and William J. Curran, "The First Line of Defense in Controlling AIDS: Compulsory Casefinding—Testing, Screening, and Reporting," *American Journal of Law and Medicine* 12 (1986), in press.

Grady, Denise, "'Look, Doctor, I'm Dying. Give Me the Drug,'" *Discover* (August 1986), pp. 78–86.

Huber, Peter, "AIDS and Lawyers," *The New Republic* (May 5, 1986), pp. 14–15.

Koop, C. Everett, "Surgeon General's Report on Acquired Immune Deficiency Syndrome" (Washington, D.C.: Government Printing Office, 1986), pp. 1–36.

Langone, John, "AIDS," *Discover* (December 1985), pp. 28–53.

———. "AIDS Update: Still No Reason for Hysteria," *Discover* (September 1986), pp. 28–47.

Levine, Carol, and Joyce Bermel, eds., "AIDS: The Emerging Ethical Dilemmas," *Hastings Center Report, A Special Supplement* (August 1985), pp. 1–31.

Lieberson, Jonathan, "The Reality of AIDS," *The New York Review of Books* XXXII (January 16, 1986), pp. 43–48.

Mohr, Richard D., "AIDS: What to Do—And What Not to Do," *Report from The Center for Philosophy and Public Policy* 5 (1985), pp. 6–9.

The New York Times, Series on AIDS (March 16–19, 1987).

Nichols, Chris D., "AIDS—A New Reason to Regulate Homosexuality?" *Journal of Contemporary Law* 11 (1984), pp. 315–343.

Osborn, June E., "The AIDS Epidemic: Multidisciplinary Trouble," *The New England Journal of Medicine* 314 (March 20, 1986), pp. 779–782.

TRB from Washington, "Moral Anemia," *The New Republic* (December 1, 1986), pp. 6 and 41.

Van Atta, Dale, "Faint Light, Dark Print: Roy Cohn, AIDS, and the Question of Privacy," *Harper's* (November 1986), pp. 54–57.

Plays

The AIDS Show: Artists Involved with Death & Survival in *West Coast Plays 17/18* (Los Angeles: California Theatre Council, 1985); *Unfinished Business: The AIDS Show* (revised and updated script) and videotape of same available from Theatre Rhinoceros, 2926 16th Street #9, San Francisco, CA 94103. (Videotape of the PBS documentary available from Direct Cinema Ltd., P. O. Box 69589, Los Angeles, CA 90069.)

Hoffman, William M., *As Is* (New York: Random House, 1985).

Holsclaw, Doug, *Life of the Party,* in *West Coast Plays* (Los Angeles: California Theatre Council, in press). (Also available from Theatre Rhinoceros, 2926 16th Street #9, San Francisco, CA 94103.)

Kramer, Larry, *The Normal Heart* (New York: New American Library, 1985).

Sources of Information

AIDS Action Council
729 Eighth Street, S.E.
Suite 200
Washington, D.C. 20003

American Association of Physicians for Human Rights
P.O. Box 14366
San Francisco, CA 94114

American Red Cross
AIDS Education Office
1730 D Street, N.W.
Washington, D.C. 20006

CDC AIDS Weekly
Dept. 1-A
1409 Fairview Road
Atlanta, GA 30306–4611

CDC Hotline
1-800-342-AIDS (Recorded information)
1-800-447-AIDS (Specific questions)

Gay Men's Health Crisis
P.O. Box 274
132 West 24th Street
New York, NY 10011

Hispanic AIDS Forum
c/o APRED
853 Broadway, Suite 2007
New York, NY 10003

U.S. Public Health Service
Public Affairs Office
Hubert H. Humphrey Building
Room 725-H
200 Independence Avenue, S.W.
Washington, D.C. 20201